The Juice Lady's

REMEDIES

FOR ASTHMA AND ALLERGIES

CHERIE CALBOM, MS, CN

SILOAM

Most Charisma House Book Group products are available at special quantity discounts for bulk purchase for sales promotions, premiums, fund-raising, and educational needs. For details, write Charisma House Book Group, 600 Rinehart Road, Lake Mary, Florida 32746, or telephone (407) 333-0600.

The Juice Lady's Remedies for Asthma and Allergies
by Cherie Calbom
Published by Siloam
Charisma Media/Charisma House Book Group
600 Rinehart Road
Lake Mary, Florida 32746
www.charismahouse.com

Cover design by Justin Evans
Design Director: Bill Johnson

Visit the author's website at www.juiceladycherie.com.

Library of Congress Cataloguing-in-Publication Data:
An application to register this book for cataloging has been submitted to the Library of Congress.
International Standard Book Number: 978-1-62136-601-0

14 15 16 17 18 — 9 8 7 6 5 4 3 2 1
Printed in the United States of America

CONTENTS

INTRODUCTION

ALLERGIC REACTIONS SERVE no purpose. They're simply misguided immune system reactions to a normally harmless substance that you eat, inhale, or touch. But allergies and asthma, a respiratory condition that can accompany allergies, are nothing to take lightly. The two are common and often annoying. Without proper treatment they can sometimes be fatal.

The job of your immune system is to protect your body from harmful invaders (antigens), such as germs, viruses, and other foreign substances. Your immune system is continuously searching for and destroying unwanted organisms.

Fortunately your immune system doesn't attack everything foreign that enters your body. Most of the foods, drinks, and pharmaceutical drugs that you ingest don't trigger an immune response. Occasionally though the immune system goes astray and reacts— or rather overreacts—to an innocent invader such as pollen or cat dander, causing allergies. Your immune system perceives the substance as harmful and launches an attack against it.

A Healthier Life Awaits You!

Juicing can help you achieve the abundant health you long for. If you suffer from allergies (as I did) or its companion affliction, asthma, this book is for you. The program I suggest goes far beyond salads and V8 juice. In fact, juices that are canned, commercially frozen (with the exception of wheat grass juice), or bottled have been pasteurized, which means that many of their life-giving nutrients, such as enzymes and vitamins, have been killed in the process. And while these processed options are certainly better than soda, they are a poor substitute when compared with freshly made juice. Raw juices offer an abundance of nutrients. They make your body feel alive!

I want you to discover how easy juicing can be. I hope you look forward to drinking the fresh juices you make each day so you can experience their life-giving benefits as I did. I'm thrilled to pass on to you the knowledge about juicing, delicious recipes, and dietary choices that I've discovered are effective, on my own journey toward health, through what my clients have taught me, and through the dedicated scientific research of others.

Juicing is an easy, delicious way to add the goodness of fruits and vegetables to your daily diet. A good juicer and fresh produce will allow you to enjoy a wealth of nutrients every day, which is important even if your health is good. If your health is not good, juicing is even more vital. You may never know how good you can feel until you make juicing fresh organic vegetables a way of life.

In this book you'll learn how juicing can help you naturally and safely eliminate toxins from your body so your organs can function more efficiently. You'll discover how your allergies and asthma symptoms will subside the more natural foods you consume in your daily diet. You will experience more energy and a higher level of wellness. Best of all you'll discover a way of life that will help you feel and look alive and vibrant each and every day of your life. A healthier life truly does await you!

1

MY OWN JOURNEY
to HEALTH

SITTING BY THE window one day in my father's home staring at the snow-topped mountains in the distance, I imagined that people were enjoying the hiking trails and perhaps someone was climbing the mountain that day. It was early June, and the weather was beautiful. I wished I had the strength to just walk around the block. But I was too sick and tired—I could barely walk around the house. I had been sick for a couple of years and just kept getting worse. "Will I ever be well again?" I wondered.

When I turned thirty, I had to quit my job. I had chronic fatigue syndrome and fibromyalgia that made me so sick I couldn't work. I felt as though I had a never-ending flu. Constantly feverish with swollen glands and perennially lethargic, I was also in constant pain. My body ached as though I'd been bounced around in a washing machine.

I had moved back to my father's home in Colorado to try and recover. But not one doctor had an answer as to what I should do to facilitate healing. So I went to some health food stores and browsed around, talked with employees, and read a few books. I decided that everything I'd been doing—such as eating fast food, granola for dinner, and not eating vegetables—was tearing down my health rather than healing my body. I read about juicing and whole foods, and it made sense. So I bought a juicer and designed a program I could follow.

I juiced and ate a nearly perfect diet of live and whole foods for three months. There were ups and downs throughout. I had days where I felt encouraged that I was making some progress but other days when I felt worse. Those were discouraging and made me wonder if health was the elusive dream. No one told me about detox reactions, which was what I was experiencing. I was obviously very toxic, and my body was cleansing away all that stuff that had made me sick. This caused some not-so-good days amid the promising ones.

But one morning I woke up early—early for me,

which was around 8:00 a.m.—without an alarm sounding off. I felt like someone had given me a new body in the night. I had so much energy I actually wanted to go jogging. What had happened? This new sensation of health had just appeared with the morning sun. But actually my body had been healing all along; it just had not manifested until that day. What a wonderful sense of being alive! I looked and felt completely renewed.

With my juicer in tow and a new lifestyle fully embraced, I returned to Southern California a couple weeks later to finish writing my first book. For nearly a year it was "ten steps forward" with great health and more energy and stamina than I'd ever remembered. Then, all of a sudden, I took a giant step back.

The Event That Took My Breath Away

July fourth was a beautiful day like so many others in Southern California. I celebrated the holiday with friends that evening at a backyard barbecue. We put on jackets to insulate against the cool evening air and watched fireworks light up the night sky. I returned just before midnight to the house I was sitting for vacationing friends who lived in a lovely neighborhood not far from some family members. I was in bed just a bit after midnight.

I woke up shivering some time later. "Why is it so cold?" I wondered as I rolled over to see the clock; it was 3:00 a.m. That's when I noticed that the door was open to the backyard. "Wonder how that happened?" I thought as I was about to get up to close and lock it. That's when I noticed him crouched in the shadows of the corner of the room—a shirtless young guy in shorts. I blinked twice, trying to deny what I was seeing. Instead of running, he leaped off the floor and ran toward me. He pulled a pipe from his shorts and began attacking me, beating me repeatedly over the head and yelling, "Now you are dead!" We fought, or I should say I tried to defend myself and grab the pipe. It finally flew out of his hands. That's when he choked me to unconsciousness. I felt life leaving my body.

In those last few seconds I knew I was dying. "This is it, the end of my life," I thought. I felt sad for the people who loved me and how they would feel about this tragic event. Then I felt my spirit leave in a sensation of popping out of my body and floating upward. Suddenly everything was peaceful and still. I sensed I was traveling, at what seemed like the speed of light, through black space. I saw what looked like lights twinkling in the distance. But all of a sudden I was back in my body, outside the house, clinging to a fence at the end of the dog run. I don't know how I got there. I screamed for help with all the breath I had. It was my third scream that took all my strength. I felt it would be my last. Each time I screamed, I passed out and landed on the cement. I then had to pull myself up again. But this time a neighbor heard me and sent her husband to help. Within a short time I was on my way to the hospital.

Lying on a cold gurney at 4:30 a.m. chilled to the bone, in and out of consciousness, I tried to assess my injuries, which was virtually impossible. When I finally looked at my right hand, I almost passed out again. My ring finger was barely hanging on by a small piece of skin. My hand was split open, and I could see deep inside. The next thing I knew, I was being wheeled off to surgery. Later I learned that I had suffered serious injuries to my head, neck, back, and right hand, with multiple head wounds and part of my scalp torn from my head. I also incurred numerous cracked teeth that resulted in several root canals and crowns months later.

My right hand sustained the most severe injuries,

with two knuckles crushed to mere bone fragments that had to be held together by three metal pins. Six months after the attack I still couldn't use it. The cast I wore—with bands holding up the ring finger, which had almost been torn from my hand, and various odd-shaped molded parts—looked like something from a science-fiction movie. I felt and looked worse than hopeless, with a shaved top of my head, totally red and swollen eyes, a gash on my face, a useless right hand, terrorizing fear, and barely enough energy to get dressed in the morning. I was an emotional wreck. I couldn't sleep at night—not even a minute. It was torturous. Never mind that I was staying with a cousin and his family. There was no need to worry about safety from a practical point of view, but that made no difference emotionally. I'd lie in bed all night and stare at the ceiling or the bedroom door. I had five lights that I kept on all night. I'd try to read, but my eyes would sting. I could sleep for only a little while during the day.

But the worst part was the pain in my soul that nearly took my breath away. All the emotional pain of the attack joined up with the pain and trauma of my past for an emotional tsunami. My past had been riddled with loss, trauma, and anxiety. My brother died when I was two. My mother had died of cancer when I was six. I couldn't remember much about her death—the memories seemed blocked. But my cousin said I fainted at her funeral. That told me the impact was huge.

I lived for the next three years with my maternal grandparents and father. But Grandpa John, the love of my life, died when I was nine—the loss was immeasurable. Four years later my father was involved in a very tragic situation that would take far too long to discuss here, but to sum it up—it was horrific. He was no longer in my daily life. I felt terrified about my future. My grandmother was eighty-six. I had no idea how many more years she would live. The next year I moved to Oregon to live with an aunt and uncle until I graduated from high school.

As you can probably imagine, wrapped in my soul was a huge amount of anguish and pain with all sorts of triggers for emotional and binge eating. I know firsthand about eating-disorder behavior—binge eating and then not eating anything for a few days. I know what it is to get triggered emotionally and be clueless as to what set off an eating binge. Food is immediate comfort. It's often the first thing we turn to. It was for me. But not wanting to gain a lot of weight, I would then avoid food for a day or two after binge eating.

After the attack it took every ounce of my will, faith, and trust in God, deep spiritual work, alternative medical help, extra vitamins and minerals, vegetable juicing, emotional release, healing prayer, and numerous detox programs to heal physically, mentally, and emotionally. I met a nutritionally minded physician who had healed his own slow mending broken bones with lots of vitamin-mineral IVs. He gave me similar IVs. Juicing, cleansing, nutritional supplements, a nearly perfect diet, prayer, and physical therapy helped my bones and other injuries heal.

After following this regimen for about nine months, what my hand surgeon said would be impossible became real—a fully restored, fully functional hand. He had told me I'd never use my right hand again and that it wasn't even possible to put in plastic knuckles because of its poor condition. But my knuckles did indeed re-form primarily through prayer, and function of my hand returned. A day came when he told me I was completely healed, and though he admitted he didn't believe in miracles, he said, "You're the closest thing I've seen to one."

The healing of my hand was indeed a miracle! I

had a useful hand again, and my career in writing was not over as I thought it would be. My inner wounds were what seemed severest in the end and the hardest to heal. Nevertheless, they mended too. I experienced healing from the painful memories and trauma of the attack and the wounds from the past through prayer, laying on of hands, and deep emotional healing work. I called them the *kitchen angels*—the ladies who prayed for me around their kitchen table week after week until my soul was healed. I cried endless buckets of tears that had been pent up in my soul. It all needed release. Forgiveness and letting go came in stages and was an integral part of my total healing. I had to be honest about what I really felt and willing to face the pain and toxic emotions confined inside, and then let them go. Finally, one day after a long journey—I felt free. A time came when I could celebrate the Fourth of July without fear.

Today I know more peace and health than I ever thought would be possible. I have experienced what it is to feel whole—complete; not damaged, broken, wounded, or impaired; but truly healed and restored in body, soul, and spirit. And I'm not plagued with emotional eating anymore.

When I look back to that first day in the hospital

after many hours of surgery, it's amazing to me that I made it. My hand was resting in a sling hanging above my head. It was wrapped with so much stuff it looked like George Foreman's boxing glove. My face was black and blue and my eyes were red—no whites—they were completely red. A maintenance man came into my room for a repair and did a double take. He asked if I'd been hit by a truck! I felt like I had. As I lay there alone with tears streaming down my face, I asked God if He could bring something good out of this horrific situation. I needed something to hang onto. My prayer was answered. Eventually I knew my purpose was to love people to life through my writing and nutritional information to help them find their way to health and healing. If I could recover from all that had happened to me, they could too. No matter what anyone faced, there was hope.

I want you to know that you are loved, and I send you my love between the lines of this book and with the juice and raw food recipes. There is hope for you. You do not have to continue suffering the results of stress and exhaustion. No matter what challenges you face, there are answers that will heal your body, mind, and spirit. There's a purpose for your life, just as there was for mine. You need to be strong and well to complete your purpose. You can be greatly served by a positive mind and an optimistic attitude. To that end I have specially designed *The Juice Lady's Remedies for Asthma and Allergies* just for you. With God's help and the latest nutritional data in this book, you can facilitate abundant health and learn the right way to live your life to the fullest and finish well.

2

ALLERGIES: WHEN GOOD IMMUNE SYSTEMS GO BAD

SNEEZING AND WHEEZING. Itchy, watery eyes. Hives and rash on the skin. Upset stomach and diarrhea. Even anaphylactic shock. When the immune system goes into overdrive, it can be anything from a nuisance to a life-and-death situation. Allergies run the gamut of symptoms, but all are caused by your immune system overreacting to typically "innocent," or harmless triggers—these can include dust mites, pollen, mold, animal dander, or, in the case of food allergies certain dietary items (for example, milk is a common culprit). These triggers are called *allergens*, and they can be found throughout the environment.

Do you or a loved one have an allergy to one or more of the following?

- Tree pollen or grasses
- Mold and/or mildew
- Pet dander
- Milk or dairy items
- House dust mites

If so your body is releasing histamine and other substances as an overreaction to these otherwise harmless allergens. Your immune system is causing an *allergic reaction* to take place, creating inflammation in various parts of the body and symptoms such as the following:

- Hay fever: includes itchy, watery eyes; sneezing; post-nasal drip; coughing; and sinus headaches
- Asthma: commonly related to allergies; causes coughing, wheezing, chest tightness, and shortness of breath
- Eczema: a skin rash that is frequently itchy and scaly
- Hives: a more severe rash of the skin
- Upset stomach and/or diarrhea: frequently caused by food allergens

- Anaphylactic shock: a life-threatening reaction in the entire body; the throat may swell and close off and blood pressure may drop, as a result of blood vessels' sudden and extreme dilation.

COMMON MYTHS

Myth: *Allergies are all in your head.*

Fact: For most people allergies are a real medical condition. However, allergy symptoms may be aggravated by stress or emotions. Although stress and emotions don't cause allergies, they can exaggerate your body's response to the allergens. Scientists don't fully understand the relationship yet between allergic responses and emotions.

Myth: *Moving to Arizona will cure allergies.*

Fact: For years people bothered by seasonal allergies to pollens and molds thought that if they moved to the desert Southwest, where the foliage and climate are different from other regions, their allergies would disappear. Although the desert is lacking in maple trees and ragweed, it does have other pollen-producing plants, such as sagebrush and cottonwood, ash, and olive trees. People who are sensitive to some pollens and molds often find that in a new environment they eventually develop sensitivities to new allergens. For example, people sensitive to ragweed may become sensitive to sagebrush pollen.

Myth: *Most people outgrow hay fever.*

Fact: Many people believe that hay fever is a childhood disorder that you outgrow by the time you reach adulthood. On the contrary, hay fever can develop at any life stage, and you can recover from it at any point in your life.

Myth: *No one ever dies from allergies.*

Fact: Although it's true that many allergies are more of an inconvenience than anything else, some allergic reactions can be serious. People who are highly sensitive to allergens can experience life-threatening shock (anaphylaxis) after being stung by a certain insect, being injected with a certain drug, or eating a certain food. Asthma attacks can also be fatal. Severe reactions must be taken seriously and treated promptly and properly.

How Your Immune System Works

To fully understand allergies and asthma, it's important to know how your body's immune system works.

The main players in the majority of allergic reactions are white blood cells known as lymphocytes.

Lymphocytes are manufactured in bone marrow. Some migrate to your thymus, where they develop into specialized types of immune cells. Some lymphocytes migrate from bone marrow and the thymus to your lymph nodes and other organs, including your spleen, tonsils, adenoids, appendix, and small intestine. Other lymphocytes circulate throughout your body in blood and lymphatic vessels.

The role of lymphocytes is to seek out and destroy harmful foreign invaders that enter the body. In allergy sufferers lymphocytes view innocent substances such as pollen, dust mites, and dander as harmful and launch an attack against them. These are known as allergens.

When allergens enter your body, certain lymphocytes combat them by releasing a variety of chemicals. One of these is called histamine, which acts as an irritating stimulant. Often other white blood cells respond to allergens by releasing powerful chemicals intended to destroy them.

These immune responses result in a host of signs and symptoms that vary in severity. When histamine and other chemicals are released in the lungs, lung tissue becomes inflamed, causing the secretion of mucus and the swelling and narrowing of air passages. This leads to wheezing, coughing, and sometimes, shortness of breath.

When these chemicals are released in nasal cavities, they cause a runny nose, teary eyes, and itching in the nose, throat, roof of the mouth, and eyes. Histamine in the skin produces hives and other rashes. When the chemicals are activated in the digestive system, abdominal cramps and diarrhea may result.

Occasionally your entire body is affected in a serious allergic response known as anaphylactic shock (anaphylaxis). Blood vessels dilate and air passageways narrow, causing a drop in blood pressure, difficulty breathing, and other signs and symptoms. Unconsciousness or death may result.

Each allergen stimulates its own specific set of antibodies. For this reason a person may be sensitive to ragweed, but not to mold allergens. It is, however, fairly common for a person who's allergic to one substance to be allergic to others.

A surprising number of substances found outdoors, indoors, or in foods can cause an allergic reaction.

You may be allergic to substances in certain medications, parts of plants (such as pollen), dust mites in household dust, animal dander, molds, fungi, or insect venom released during a sting, such as a bee sting. Some people are also sensitive to chemical changes that occur in the body in response to exercise or to exposure to heat or cold.

Treating the Root of the Problem

Because allergies have so many different symptoms, it may seem impossible to treat all of them. You may decide to choose which symptoms to treat—for example, you may attempt to treat hay fever with antihistamines, a runny nose with a nasal spray, or an upset stomach with antacids. But if your allergies are more pervasive or difficult to treat, you may need to do something more. Prescription medications are a common "next step" in the battle against allergies—drugs such as steroids can give at least temporary relief, but they can also suppress parts of your healthy immune system in addition to the part of the immune system that has gone awry. Boosting your natural immunity is frequently a better solution to the problem of allergies.

WHEN TO CALL 911

If you are experiencing swelling in the tongue or throat, a sudden drop in blood pressure, and/or trouble breathing, especially after encountering a known allergen, call 911 immediately. You may be experiencing the extreme allergic reaction called anaphylaxis.

Treating the root of the problem rather than the symptoms is always a better idea—and the same is true for allergies. Focusing on shoring up the entire immune system can bring true health rather than just the alleviation of symptoms.

First, a determination is needed to discover exactly what is causing your allergies—what allergens are triggering your system. There are a number of tests available to help you determine what your allergens are: skin tests, blood tests, or an elimination diet to pinpoint food allergies.

Once you understand what your body is overreacting to, you can then work to desensitize your immune system to its potential triggers. The standard medical procedure is through allergy shots, injections that contain a small amount of each allergen. You will receive increasing doses of the allergen in injections that you receive on a frequent to semi-frequent basis. As the amount of the allergen increases in your shots, your immune system is able to build up a tolerance to those allergens—and it will no longer respond with an allergic reaction each time you encounter it in the "real world." Be aware that some people have a worsening of symptoms with new and strange symptoms that accompany them after receiving allergy shots.

There are many other things you can do that are natural and don't have harmful effects. Read on and you'll discover natural remedies that work.

Various Types of Allergies

There are various types of allergies that people regularly experience. Hay fever, which is characterized by itchy eyes, nose, and skin; sneezing; and a runny nose, is usually caused by *airborne allergens*. These allergens typically float through the air and include materials such as pollen, dander, and dust mites. The inflammatory chemical called histamine causes the miserable symptoms; histamine is released by the immune system as an overreaction to something usually considered harmless. Up to one-third of people who experience airborne allergies—especially of the seasonal variety—may also suffer *oral allergy syndrome* (OAS), which results from sensitivity to and cross-reactions between seasonal airborne pollen proteins (found in weeds, grass, and trees) and proteins found in some fresh fruits, vegetables, nuts, seeds, and herbs.

Are you allergic to ragweed pollen? Then you might experience OAS symptoms if you eat bananas, cucumbers, melons, zucchini, sunflower seeds, chamomile tea, or take the herb Echinacea. If you are allergic to birch tree pollen, you might suffer from symptoms if you consume peaches, apples, pears, cherries, carrots, hazelnuts, kiwifruit, or almonds.

THAT PESKY POLLEN

Wherever plants grow, pollen is in the air at some time of the year. Trees, both deciduous and evergreen, produce pollen in spring. Grasses and most flowers produce their pollen during summer months. Late-blooming plants such as ragweed produce pollen in early fall. In warm climates with long growing seasons, pollen may be present in the air for ten months of the year. In climates with shorter growing seasons the pollen is present for less time.

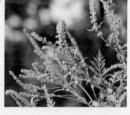

Ragweed, a roadside plant, heads the list of hay fever–causing plants east of the Rocky Mountains. Other plant pollens that produce allergy symptoms include sagebrush, tumbleweed, pigweed, spiny amaranth, burning bush, and English plantain.

Grasses that cause troublesome pollens include rye, timothy, redtop, Bermuda, orchard, sweet vernal, and bluegrass. Most trees, including maple, oak, ash, birch, poplar, elm, pecan, juniper, and cottonwood, produce pollens that can trigger hay fever.

Pollens that are carried by insects from one plant to another tend to be larger grains that are relatively harmless. Those carried by the wind are lighter and smaller and can cause hay fever. The amount of pollen in the air depends on the weather. Hot, dry breezes stir up pollen, whereas dampness washes the pollen to the ground.

Most pollen particles are so small that they can be carried by the air into a house through doors and screens. It doesn't take much pollen to produce an allergic reaction—as little as twenty particles per cubic yard. Many plants can produce up to a million such particles!

The most effective way to avoid pollen is to stay indoors, especially when pollen counts are high. Keep doors and windows closed. Air conditioning can also be helpful.

In addition to hay fever and OAS, *food allergies* are an unfortunate fact of life for many people. They occur when the body's immune system, again, over-reacts to something ordinarily considered harmless—usually a protein in a certain food or ingredient. Food allergies have risen alarmingly in the general population over the past several years. Food allergy symptoms vary widely among different people—and can even differ at various times in the same individual. People with food allergies commonly experience either skin reactions—rash, hives, psoriasis, or eczema—or gastrointestinal irritation, including nausea, vomiting, irritable bowel, inflammatory bowel disease, and/or diarrhea. Incidentally, hay fever–type symptoms can result from food allergies; in other words, some foods may cause some people to sneeze, wheeze, and cough. Also, consider the following list of symptoms, which can be the result of food allergies:

- Allergies
- Arthritis
- Ear infections
- Sinusitis
- Anxiety

- Depression
- Hyperactivity
- Postnasal drip
- Dizziness
- Fatigue
- Headaches
- Panic attacks
- Dark circles or puffiness under the eyes
- Chronic fluid retention
- Swollen glands

I would be remiss to discuss food allergies without mentioning the serious reaction called anaphylaxis, caused by some food allergens in certain individuals. There are approximately thirty thousand episodes of anaphylaxis yearly—and one hundred to two hundred deaths per year in the United States from this syndrome alone. The leading cause of deadly food allergies (leading to anaphylactic shock)? Nuts—especially peanuts, which are actually legumes.

Certain individuals may not be *allergic* to certain foods, but they may have a *sensitivity* to them, meaning they should avoid those foods to in turn avoid adverse symptoms. There is an endless number of foods that can cause an allergy or sensitivity, but the most common culprits include dairy, wheat (gluten), corn, eggs, fish, nuts, soy, chocolate, peanuts, shellfish, the night shades (tomato, potato, pepper, eggplant), citrus fruit, preservatives, and colorings. Food intolerances, or sensitivities, are mistaken for food allergies, but they are not exactly the same, as food allergies must always involve the immune system. Lactose intolerance is one of the most common types of food intolerance, occurring when an individual is missing an important enzyme necessary to digest milk sugars. It does *not* involve an overreaction of the immune system, and as such, it is not a food *allergy*, but it can make sufferers miserable through gas, bloating, and abdominal pain. In such individuals, milk and dairy products should be avoided.

There are a number of reasons for the drastic rise in the number of food allergies in this country over recent years. A primary underlying condition, which can promote the development of food allergies, including poor digestion, is "leaky gut." This condition allows too many intact food proteins to be absorbed into the bloodstream and chronic intestinal infections by yeast, bacteria, or parasites.

Another contributor seems to be genetically

modified (GM) foods. In 1960 we saw the introduction of "miracle seeds"—improved varieties of wheat, corn, and rice, which dramatically increased the crop yields of American farmers. Through the use of pesticides, irrigation, and genetic engineering, these miracle seeds doubled or tripled harvests on the same size plots as previous harvests. The seeds and growing practices quickly spread to farmers in other countries with the hope that they would help end world hunger.

This dramatic increase in crop production was called the "Green Revolution." It was a revolution without a doubt, but far from green—which has come to mean buying organic, purchasing foods locally, and promoting sustainable farming and animal husbandry (compassionate care for domestic animals). The hybrid seeds and genetically engineered crops gave us wheat with more gluten so manufacturers could make fluffier bread as I just mentioned, which caused allergies and gastrointestinal problems such as Crohn's disease, colitis, and irritable bowel syndrome.

Pesticides killed bugs, but they also killed songbirds; they are wiping out our bee population, and they are contributing to cancer, digestive problems, and other diseases in humans. In the end, they have killed many of us. (Studies show there is an increased incidence of cancer among farmers, indicating the impact that pesticides have on the human body.[1]) And we must ask ourselves why birds and fish are mysteriously dying by the thousands. Are they the "canaries in the coal mine"? Are we next?

Then along came "designer foods" concocted by food scientists, promising specific health benefits, belched out by big factories, and most often devoid of life-promoting ingredients. They led us astray with their "good health promises" that didn't deliver what they said. As a whole, people are sicker than ever before in history. As you can see, we can't trust the jingles, commercials, and marketing ads. They gave us slogans like "Reach for a Lucky instead of a sweet!" And, "More doctors smoke Camels." Here's the truth: we've been the human guinea pigs for decades.

We continue to learn, often too late, that many popular products have caused food allergies, made us sick, caused deaths, and took our money to boot! Do you want these people guiding your food choices? There's a little voice inside calling you home—away from the clamor and spin of the big companies with clever marketing slogans and foods designed to hook you to crave more unhealthy stuff—to the simple goodness of the earth, free of chemicals, genetic tampering, and the fluff that's killing you. The voice is calling you to compassionate eating, sustainability, and supporting local organic farmers. It's time to rethink your perception of food and to discover that you are not too busy to make the time to prepare whole, living foods. You're too busy not to. It's time for a revolution in the way you eat and the way you think about food. If you return to nature's living bounty, you can heal your body and mind along with the earth.

See the next chapter on food allergies for more information on this subject.

Food Choices to Help Our Bodies Heal

Though I recommend that you buy all organically grown produce, it is especially important for sufferers from allergies to avoid conventionally grown foods on the "dirty dozen" list.

The Dirty Dozen List[2]

- Apples
- Celery
- Cherry tomatoes
- Cucumbers
- Grapes

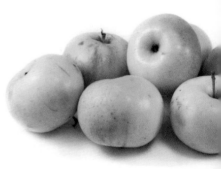

- Hot peppers
- Nectarines (imported)
- Peaches
- Potatoes
- Spinach
- Strawberries
- Bell peppers

The Cleanest Foods List[3]

- Asparagus
- Avocados
- Cabbage
- Cantaloupe
- Sweet corn (no GMO corn)
- Eggplant
- Grapefruit
- Kiwi
- Mangoes
- Mushrooms
- Onions
- Papayas

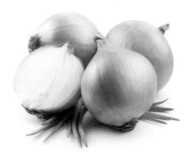

- Pineapples
- Sweet peas (frozen)
- Sweet potatoes

Lifestyle Recommendations for Allergy Sufferers

1. *Eliminate airborne allergies as much as possible.* Clean your environment as frequently as you can, paying careful attention to carpets, rugs, upholstered furniture, and other surfaces where dust and other particulate allergens can collect. Take special care to keep your bedroom allergy-proofed. Enclose your mattress, box spring, and pillows in allergen-resistant coverings, and frequently wash your bedding, towels, curtains, and clothing in hot water, using a fragrance-free detergent. Install an air purifier that has a HEPA filter (one that can trap tiny particles), and only vacuum using a machine with such a HEPA filter. Clean your furnace and air ducts annually. Clean any place where dust can collect—frequently and well.

2. *Get rid of the stress in your life.* Your immune system can be weakened by stress—and this weakened state can leave you vulnerable to allergic reactions.

Diet Recommendations for Allergy Sufferers

1. *For food allergies, keep track of any offending food(s) and avoid them as much as possible.* Use the Elimination Diet to determine which foods create the worst symptoms. And don't forget that a food allergy or intolerance may be caused by something you like and eat often—people often develop cravings for foods to which they are allergic. After you have determined which foods you are allergic to or intolerant of, be sure to rotate all of the food that you eat, both to control allergies you already are aware of and to prevent the development of new allergies or intolerances (the more you eat a certain food, the more likely you are to develop an allergy or intolerance). And finally, as much as possible, be sure to avoid all foods to which you are sensitive in any way.

THE ELIMINATION DIET

Many times, the best way to identify food allergies is with something called the "oral food challenge." Any potential food allergens are initially eliminated from the diet altogether, and then gradually reintroduced to see if symptoms then occur.

For the first seven days, eat only the foods listed in the diet—usually with many restrictions to help cleanse your system. (Read labels carefully to be sure you are eliminating all other foods, as some foods may "sneak in" without your being aware.) If your symptoms (such as rash or stomach upset) are related to food sensitivities or allergies, they will usually vanish by the end of the seven-day period. If they don't, a reaction to a food still remaining in your diet may be responsible. In that case, proceed to an even more restricted diet. When the period of time is complete (typically another seven days), you may then introduce one food every two days. Keep a detailed food diary as to when each food or ingredient was reintroduced and what symptoms appeared (or did not appear) after it was eaten. Some reactions may be delayed up to forty-eight hours, so keep that in mind as you analyze your diary.

2. *Consume more raw fruits, vegetables, and fresh vegetable juices.* Eating more raw foods in your diet can actually cause allergy symptoms to lessen over time.

3. *Avoid sugar and alcohol.* Sugar and alcohol both contribute to an acidic condition in the body that aggravates allergic reactions.

Nutrient Recommendations for Allergy Sufferers

1. *Bioflavonoids*, especially quercetin, molybdenum, and selenium, can reduce histamine levels and greatly relieve allergy symptoms. Yellow onions and shallots are good sources of quercetin and can help with allergies right away.

2. *Gamma-linolenic acid (GLA)* is produced by the body to reduce inflammation. You can ingest GLA through supplements of evening primrose oil.

3. *Vitamin C* supports the immune system, and thus provides many natural defenses against allergies.

4. *Amylase* is a digestive enzyme that breaks down complex carbohydrates into simple sugars. It's also present in saliva. So while we chew our food, it goes to work on carbs. That's why it's recommended that you chew each mouthful of food about thirty times. The pancreas also makes amylase. And amylase is plentiful in seeds that contain starch. (You can juice most seeds of fruits and vegetables.) Its therapeutic use is in the regulation of histamine, which is produced in response to recognized invaders to the body. Histamine is a responder in allergic reactions such as hay fever and is what causes hives, itchy, watery eyes, sneezing, and runny noses. Amylase breaks down the histamine produced by the body in response to allergens such as pollen or dust mites. Some health professionals believe it may help the body identify the allergen as not being harmful so it doesn't produce the histamine in the first place. This is one reason that people on a high raw plant diet often experience improvement in their allergies. For

the most effective approach to increasing enzymes such as amylase, you may want to take an enzyme supplement. I especially like an enzyme formula that is taken between meals—it cleans up any undigested particles of food floating around the system and greatly improves digestion. A popular side benefit is that your hair gets thicker and your nails grow stronger!

Help for Seasonal Airborne Allergies

Because seasonal airborne allergies typically cause problems from early spring to the time of the first frost, use these remedies during this time of year. Quercetin may be as helpful as over-the-counter medications in inhibiting histamine release, but without side effects such as drowsiness. By inhibiting histamine release at the outset, quercetin stands in direct contrast to many medications that attempt to nullify the *effects* of histamine—after an allergic reaction has already taken place. When combined with the herb nettle, quercetin is helpful to prevent or reduce sneezing, itching, and inflammation of the nasal passages. Use pantothenic acid, a B vitamin, to deal with the effects of nasal congestion.

Dosages:

- Quercetin: 500 mg two times daily. Take about twenty minutes before meals.

- Nettle: 250–300 mg on an empty stomach three times daily. Standardized to contain at least 1 percent of the herb silica.

- Vitamin C: 1,000 mg three times daily. If diarrhea develops, reduce the dose.

- Pantothenic acid: 500 mg three times daily. Take with food.

Herb Recommendations for Allergy Sufferers

To build up your immune system before allergy season starts, begin a daily dosage of *astragalus* at least one month before spring pollen begins to perpetuate. However, do not take astragalus if you have a fever or show any signs of an infection. Children with chronic allergies can be given a dose of astragalus two to three times each day for a week.

In addition, *licorice* is an inhibitor of phospholipase A, an enzyme that precipitates inflammatory reactions. Use a medicinal form of the herb. Do not use licorice candy. Use DGL (has no glycyrrhizin) if you have high blood pressure, kidney or liver disease, diabetes or heart disease, and do not use for more than six weeks.

Juice Therapy for Allergy Sufferers

Drink *alfalfa sprout* and *celery* juices to raise your blood alkalinity, which in turn helps prevent allergic reactions.

In addition, *parsley juice* can stop allergy attacks once they have started; drink it immediately upon experiencing allergic symptoms and it may soon help reduce them. (As always, however, if you are experiencing anaphylactic symptoms, call 911 right away.) Additionally, parsley juice contains more than three times the vitamin C of orange juice, so to help keep your immune system strong, add parsley juice as part of your juicing regimen. Parsley can be toxic if overused, and should be avoided by pregnant women, but a safe dose which will bring the most effectiveness is one-half cup of parsley per day.

Practical Remedies for Allergy Sufferers

- Neti pot. Also known as "nasal douche" or "nasal lavage," this irrigation uses salt water and a special little pot, which delivers a stream of salt water into the nasal cavities through one nostril and allows it to drain out through the other nostril. You may purchase a neti pot at many health stores and holistic pharmacies.

- Allergena. A homeopathic sublingual immunotherapy, Allergena reduces the body's negative reaction to allergens. These homeopathic allergy drops build immunity by giving microdoses of what a person is allergic to so the body becomes safely conditioned to tolerate those allergens and reduce allergic symptoms. Allergena is made for eight zones. Look online to determine your zone. Each zone is designed for the grasses, trees, and weeds of that zone. You will find these drops at health stores.

- Get an air purifier. Toxins can actually cause allergies in some people.

- Drink peppermint tea. Peppermint's essential oil acts as a decongestant. Also certain substances in peppermint contain anti-inflammatory and mild antibacterial constituents.

- Wasabi or horseradish makes sinuses and tear ducts open up because allyl isothiocyanate, a constituent in wasabi, promotes mucus flow. The tastiest way to get those allyl isothiocyanates is by putting horseradish on your meat or a bit of wasabi onto your favorite sushi. Another option is to purchase grated horseradish and take 1/4 teaspoon per day.

3

FOOD ALLERGIES: THE DANGERS in YOUR DINNER

F OOD ALLERGIES ARE not only common but also dangerous. Knowing which foods you are allergic to isn't always enough, as they can show up at any place and at any time. If you have a serious food allergy—one that would cause your throat to swell and threaten your life—it is important that you be vigilant at all times to avoid encountering the food allergen, and to be prepared with life-saving medication should it become necessary.

In one study of children who experienced life-threatening asthma, more than 50 percent of the children in the group were found to have food allergies, when compared to only 10 percent in the control group.[1] These results demonstrate that life-threatening asthma attacks can actually be triggered by food allergies.

Use of an elimination diet, in which you eliminate possible triggers one by one, can help you to learn which foods can trigger an asthma or allergy attack. Incidentally when you eat healthy, nourishing foods on a daily basis, your immune system will be healthier and more able to ward off toxins and allergens, without the severe inflammation of an asthma or allergy attack.

The following foods have been proven to boost your immune system, thus helping to prevent allergy attacks:

- Fresh fruits and vegetables; fresh vegetable juices
- Cold-water, wild-caught fish
- Extra-virgin olive oil
- Flaxseeds
- Herbal spices such as rosemary, ginger, and turmeric

Additionally you might consider changing to a vegetarian diet, if that is appropriate for your blood type. People who eat only fruits and vegetables rarely encounter any food allergy symptoms.

Children are most commonly affected by food

allergies. They are usually outgrown by adulthood, but some allergies, especially those involving peanuts and shellfish, can last a lifetime, says Talal M. Nsouli, MD, clinical associate professor of pediatrics and allergy/immunology at Georgetown University School of Medicine and director of the Watergate and Burke Allergy and Asthma Centers.[2]

There is a genetic component to food allergies. "Both my son and daughter have allergies," says Patricia Davis, MD, MSPH, president of Healthy U in Columbus, Ohio, who is also a preventive medicine specialist. If one of your parents has a food allergy, you have at least a 20 to 30 percent chance of having a food allergy, and if both of your parents are affected, your chance of having a food allergy yourself rises to 40 to 70 percent.[3]

Breastfeeding infants is one way to prevent food allergies in children later in life. Breastfed babies receive intestinal flora from their mothers' milk, which helps build their immune systems and prevents later allergies, says Jose Saavedra, MD, medical and scientific director of Nestlé Nutrition USA, and associate professor of pediatrics at Johns Hopkins University School of Medicine and Bloomberg School of Hygiene and Public Health in Baltimore.[4]

Little Bites Can Cause Big Problems

If you have only a mild food allergy, you might be able to eat a small bite or two of the allergen infrequently. But most people with food allergies experience severe symptoms when even a trace amount of the allergen is encountered. These symptoms can even bring about a life-threatening condition called anaphylaxis. Because of the extreme risk involved, most doctors would advise those with severe allergies to keep epinephrine syringes handy wherever they eat, all of the time. Epinephrine is known to stop an anaphylactic attack right away and prevent anaphylactic shock.

The best thing you can do to avoid food allergies is to avoid the offending foods altogether. Be sure to read the labels on any food you buy. If you are allergic to peanuts, for example, don't just look for the word *peanuts* but also watch out for any peanut powder or peanut oil that might have been used in the production of the food. And keep reading those labels! Food companies frequently change their "recipes," so a food that doesn't affect you today very well could tomorrow.

Even when you know what foods you are allergic to—and you can control the ingredients in your dinner at home—it is a bit more difficult to avoid offending foods when you eat out. If you are eating at a restaurant, ask the waiter or maître d' to check with the cook to be sure your offending food is not used in any way. Don't forget to inquire about oils and spices, as well.

Alkaline Diet

Eating alkalizing foods is also a great way to restore your health. Many diseases such as cancer thrive in an acidic state. Take away the acid, and they don't do as well. An alkaline diet also boosts your energy level, improves skin, reduces allergies, sustains the immune system, and enhances mental clarity.

To give your body a great start in rebalancing your pH, make sure 60 percent to 80 percent of your diet is made up of alkalizing foods such as green vegetables, raw juices, grasses such as wheatgrass, fresh fruit and vegetables, raw seeds and nuts, and sprouts. Greatly limit or avoid your consumption of acid-forming foods such as meat, dairy products, chocolate, sweets, bread (gluten) and all other yeast products, alcohol, carbonated drinks, sports drinks, coffee, and black tea.

Cleanse Your Liver

Optimizing liver function through seasonally cleansing and detoxifying your liver will reduce allergies and improve overall health. A liver cleanse focuses on cleansing, protecting, and nourishing the liver. The following foods and supplements can help you cleanse and support your liver. They are part of a liver cleanse program I describe in my book *Juicing, Fasting, and Detoxing for Life*, which contains recipes including a morning citrus-ginger-olive-oil shake, beet salad, carrot salad, and mineral broth, as well as a menu plan for a seven-day cleansing program. For quick reference and convenience I have also included some liver-supporting juices, smoothies, and food recipes in chapter 7.

- *Liver-friendly vegetables.* Juice and eat an abundance of these liver-friendly vegetables during your detoxification program: artichokes, beets, broccoli, brussels sprouts, cabbage, carrots, cauliflower, celery, chives, cucumber, eggplant, garlic, green beans, kale, kohlrabi, lettuce, mustard greens, okra, onion, parsley, parsnips, peas, pumpkin, spinach, squash, and sweet potatoes (yams).

- *Milk thistle (silymarin).* Milk thistle is an herb that protects the liver. Silymarin is the active ingredient in milk thistle, and because of its antioxidant properties, it helps prevent free-radical damage to the liver.

- *Artichoke powder.* A chemical found in artichoke that gives it a bitter taste actually aids your liver in the detoxification process. It helps increase bile production and strengthens the bile duct so that it's better able to contract. The phytochemicals in artichokes also strengthen liver cell walls, protecting them from damage. It also helps break up and mobilize fat stored in the liver, making it useful for lowering cholesterol as well.

- *Turmeric.* The key component in turmeric is curcumin. This golden spice helps cleanse the liver, purify the blood, improve digestion, and promote elimination. It stimulates

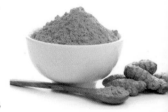

the gallbladder for bile production and scavenges free radicals.

- *N-acetyl-L-cysteine (NAC).* NAC protects the liver from free-radical damage caused by environmental pollution, radiation, cigarette smoke, and alcohol. Natural health practitioners often prescribe it for patients with mercury or heavy metal toxicity and environmental or dental amalgam mercury-filling toxicity because of its ability to bind to these toxins, allowing your body to excrete them.

- *L-methionine.* L-methionine is an amino acid used by the liver to create glutathione. It can help raise glutathione levels, thus improving the natural detoxification functions of the liver.

- *Beet leaf and black radish.* Beet leaf and black radish assist the liver's detoxification process and improve carbohydrate and fat metabolism. Beet leaf helps normalize the pH of the blood and stimulates bile flow, which can be helpful in lowering cholesterol. Black radish is rich in vitamins and bioflavonoids, which support heavy metal detoxification.

- *Dandelion.* Dandelion has been used for centuries for general detox. Herbalists and naturopathic doctors particularly like dandelion for cleansing the liver. It strengthens the liver by promoting bile secretion and provides a gentle cleansing action in the elimination of metabolic waste.

- *Garlic.* Love your liver with garlic. "Use garlic with equal abandon," says Dr. Oz. "In addition to adding oomph to almost any dish, it activates liver enzymes that support your filtration system, and it's good for another vital organ: your heart."[5] Just a small amount of this pungent white bulb has the ability to activate liver enzymes that help your body flush out toxins. Garlic is rich in allicin, the active ingredient, and selenium, two natural compounds that aid in liver cleansing.

- *Beet juice.* Beets have been used in naturopathic medicine to cleanse and support the liver. Beet juice, made with the root and the leaves, is an integral part of my seven-day liver-cleansing program. It's high in sugar, so always dilute with green veggies like cucumber and dark leafy greens. Also, beet salad is another key part of the program and can be made with the leftover beet pulp and a lemon juice–olive oil dressing. (The recipe is in *Juicing, Fasting, and Detoxing for Life*.)

- *Carrot juice.* Carrots help stimulate and improve overall liver function. They can be juiced as part of the liver-cleansing cocktails. The leftover pulp is made into a cleansing salad with a lemon juice–olive oil dressing. (The recipe is in *Juicing, Fasting, and Detoxing for Life*.)

- *Dark leafy green juice.* One of our most powerful allies in cleansing the liver, leafy greens can be juiced, eaten raw, and lightly cooked. Particularly high in plant chlorophyll, greens literally suck up toxins from the bloodstream. They also halt the progression of hyphae, the long, branching structures of yeast and fungus that cause it to spread systemically throughout the body. And with their distinct ability to neutralize heavy metals, chemicals, and pesticides, greens offer a powerhouse of cleansing for the liver.

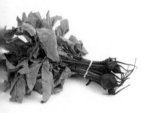

Excellent greens to juice include beet tops, arugula, dandelion greens, spinach, mustard greens, kale, chard, collards, kohlrabi leaves, and chicory. Green juice will help increase bile flow, which will help remove waste from the organs and blood.

- *The olive oil flush for liver and gallbladder cleansing.* The olive oil flush is used to purge out stones from the liver and gall-bladder. Follow the recipes and program in *Juicing, Fasting, and Detoxing for Life.*

NOTE: If you have a liver disease, consult your doctor first.

WILD FOODS AND LIVER DETOXIFICATION
(contributed by my dear friend Nina Walsh, ND)

Wild grown greens and herbs offer us some of the most cleansing, medicinal, and nutrient-dense foods we could find. And they are free! Here are some characteristics of wild foods:

- They are organic, clean, resilient, resistant to diseases, and nutrient and antioxidant rich.

- They are grown in rich soils and have greater access to and quality of nutrients.

- They come in a variety of species and offer a wide variety of nutrients.

- They have diversity of flavor—bitter, pungent, sour, bland, sweet, and salty.

- They are time-tested—wild plants have been used for thousands of years.

- They have enzyme systems and mechanisms for optimal digestion.

- Our human genome (inherited genetic information) is responsive to wild foods.

- They follow cycles and rhythms of nature, like our bodies.

- They cleanse and nourish our bodies and support optimal health.

- Specific plants cleanse and support specific organs.

Stinging Nettles

The stinging nettle is one of the first plants to come up in early spring. It is used traditionally for body cleansing. People who 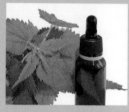 observe Lent in the Eastern Orthodox tradition abstain from heavy animal foods for about six weeks before Easter and eat spring herbs.

Nettle is a great tonic with unique healing and cleansing qualities. It flushes out toxins and cleanses the entire system. It's best known to detox the kidneys. It helps discharge metabolic wastes, such as uric acid crystals. And it's a good diuretic/aquaretic, meaning it will not waste electrolytes but will get rid of excess water. It gently tones the body, purifying the blood. It also helps cleanse the lymph and rid the body of the residues of months of sedentary winter lifestyle and heavy food. And it replenishes the body with nutrients—it's rich in iron, calcium, beta-carotene, and vitamin C.

In addition to all the cleansing it does, the tea of nettle tops also stimulates the formation of red blood cells. Further, it can lower blood sugar levels and is indicated for type 2 diabetics. This tea can be taken safely by anybody, though it may be particularly supportive for women during puberty, menopause, or pregnancy.

To make the best use of spring nettles, gather young leaves before the plants produce seeds. Use gloves to prevent stinging. You can add them to green smoothies and juice. They will not sting once they are juiced or blended. You can cook them; they are delicious in omelets, sautéed greens, nettle chips, soups, and teas. Also, you can add it to baths, body wash, and hair rinses.

Stinging Nettles Omelet

Start with a bunch of chopped young nettle leaves (use rubber gloves to prepare the nettles). Sauté with shallots or onions in 1 tablespoon of olive oil or coconut oil. Once the nettles are lightly cooked, they'll no longer sting. Add ½ cup sautéed sliced mushrooms and 2 eggs and finish cooking.

Dandelion

Dandelion is the quintessential digestive herb. Its bitter components stimulate production of stomach acid, enhance appetite, support action of the liver in breaking down nutrients, and cleanse the body of toxins. As a liver detox herb, it helps regulate hormones and alleviate hormonal ups and downs, such as those associated with the female menstrual cycle or menopause, and also low vitamin D levels.

One of the best herbs to use for a spring cleanse, dandelion acts as a cleansing agent on both the liver and the kidneys. It helps to purify the blood and flush out uric acid crystals that accumulate from eating a diet too rich in animal proteins and other acid-producing foods; it restores the alkalinity of the blood. Dandelion enhances bile flow. It also reduces and prevents inflammation in the liver and gallbladder. It contains choline, a substance that helps prevent fat from being deposited in the liver. Dandelion roots are particularly beneficial for the liver, while the leaves have a more pronounced effect on the kidneys as an aquaretic (it does not deplete potassium but actually adds potassium to the body). It is also rich in many other vitamins and minerals, including vitamin C, beta-carotene, calcium, iron, manganese, and phosphorus. Avoid picking dandelion leaves from lawns where chemical fertilizer was used. It is always best to collect wild foods in clean areas, away from traffic and pesticides. Every part of this plant can be used as food and medicine. Dandelion can be juiced and added to smoothies. (See Dr. Nina's Sweet Dandelion Smoothie in chapter 7.) For salads, it's best to mix with other milder-tasting spring greens. However, if you don't mind a slightly bitter tang, you can try a dandelion salad with 1 grated carrot and 1–2 cloves garlic. Add a fruity vinaigrette or a sweet and sour dressing made with yogurt, lemon juice, pepper, salt, garlic, and a little raw honey. (Or see Dr. Nina's Russian Cabbage Slaw in chapter 7.) Dandelion especially complements boiled eggs and cress type herbs. Like any greens, dandelion leaves and roots can be sautéed or stir-fried. Leaves can also be blended for soups. And you can make "coffee" from roasted roots.

Burdock

One of the best plants for cleansing, burdock is a wonderful digestive herb that supports liver function and detoxification, reduces liver inflammation, heals liver cells in fatty liver disease, and stimulates stomach acid production. It helps lymphatic flow and elimination of wastes from the tissues through the lymphatic system. It is a gentle diuretic and reduces water accumulation in extremities and around joints. It promotes healthy bowel flora and is healing for the intestinal lining. It's also a great source of fiber, protein, vitamins, and minerals.

It can be added to green smoothies and juices. You can use it as you would any root vegetable: sautéed, mixed with greens; added to puréed vegetables; or used in soups. It can be dehydrated as chips or made into a tea. You can also use the leaf and root for infusion for baths. To cook burdock with vegetables: Sauté 1/2 chopped medium onion in olive oil or coconut oil. Add 1 chopped burdock root, 1 chopped carrot, 1 chopped small beet, 2 chopped Jerusalem artichokes, 1 cup chopped broccoli or another green vegetable (like nettles), 2–3 cloves of chopped garlic, and 2–3 sprigs parsley. Sauté the onion until translucent and then add the rest of the vegetables with chopped garlic. When the vegetables are lightly cooked, add chopped parsley. Salt and pepper to taste. Sprinkle with lemon juice.[6]

Foods to avoid while cleansing your liver

Omit meat, dairy, sweets, alcohol, eggs, refined foods, sodas, all oils and spreads except olive oil and coconut oil, and all nonorganic foods.

FOOD ALLERGIES AND THYROID FUNCTION

When it comes to food-related allergies that impact the thyroid gland, it is not like eating a nut or a shrimp and getting an immediate reaction. The type of reaction that disrupts thyroid function is a delayed interaction with food antigens that can occur up to four days after eating the food. The two most prevalent food-related reactions come from dairy and wheat. These two foods are known in alternative medicine to be highly correlated with autoimmune thyroiditis. Dairy and wheat gluten are often removed from diets of thyroid patients with good success. The Journal of Clinical Gastroenterology demonstrated that those allergic to gluten had a much greater risk of thyroid abnormalities.[7]

4

ASTHMA: LEARNING to CATCH YOUR BREATH

ASTHMA SUFFERERS KNOW that living with this potentially deadly disease is challenging: all it takes is a change in the weather, a boost in tree pollen, even a simple run in the park—and sufferers can be breathing heavy and reaching for their rescue inhalers. Airways inside of the lungs can constrict at any time, in response to a huge number of triggers, leaving asthmatics feeling as though they are breathing through a straw. But it is possible to control asthma symptoms, even find a type of "remission" from the disease. A vital part of this healing strategy is what you eat. "Diet is the key," says Richard N. Firshein, DO, medical director of the Firshein Center for Comprehensive Medicine in New York City and author of *Reversing Asthma*.

Around 27 million Americans suffer from

asthma—bronchial inflammation and spasms that make it difficult for the body to breathe air in and out of the lungs. Each year, this disease causes more than five hundred thousand hospitalizations and four thousand deaths.[1]

Over the past twenty years, asthma has been on the increase in this country. In fact, the number of people with asthma has quadrupled, and the number of deaths from asthma attacks has doubled. Why is this dangerous disease on the rise? There is a genetic component to asthma: If one parent has the disease, chances are one in three that their children will also have it, and if both parents have asthma, the chances rise to seven in ten.[2]

On the other hand 50 percent of people with the disease have asthma attacks that are triggered by allergens (see the previous chapter), and the number of allergens (such as dust mites, tree pollen, molds, and animal dander) has been increasing steadily in today's environment. In addition, many of us consistently consume a high-sugar and high-fat inflammatory diet, and the nutritional deficiencies we experience alone can easily cause us to be more prone to any disease, including asthma. We also encounter immune-weakening toxins in our environment every day (including in our food); stress in our work and family lives; and air pollution in our cities—which, all together, bring about an increasing epidemic of asthma in our world.

What are the primary triggers for the wheezing, cough, shortness of breath, and chest tightness associated with asthma? Allergens are a primary cause: as such, asthma is essentially an "allergic reaction of the lungs."[3] Exercise may be a trigger, as can be tobacco smoke, burning wood, weather or climate changes, car exhaust fumes, stress in family life or at work, or even infections occurring in other parts of the body. Essentially asthma is a response of the immune system to any number of specific "triggers" and results in wheezing and being breathless. Of all of the triggers, an infection is one of the most common causes, and therefore, if you can maintain a strong and healthy immune system—and thus have fewer respiratory infections—you can have fewer asthma attacks as a result.

There are two basic forms of asthma: extrinsic and intrinsic. Extrinsic asthma is considered to be an allergic condition, which takes place when allergens to which a person is sensitive trigger the release of a chemical called histamine, which then causes an inflammatory response in the body. Intrinsic asthma, on the other hand, is triggered by such non-immune factors as physical exercise, emotional upset or stress, extreme heat or cold, chemical irritants or air pollutants, infections in the body (especially respiratory infections), aspirin, and food allergens, such as fish, seafood, eggs, nuts, milk, wheat, and soy.

As levels of air pollution increase, especially those immediately produced by cigarette smoke or perhaps a wood-burning stove, the frequency and severity of asthma attacks also increases. Tiny particles that can irritate lung tissue are present in wood smoke and in cigarette smoke, there are nitrogen oxides and toxic free radicals in the tar, which are then inhaled and become irritants. In addition to pollution and other toxins in the air asthma is closely linked to allergies. In fact, most, but not all, people with asthma also experience allergies.

Controlling Asthma

Your doctor can prescribe many helpful treatments and medications to help control your asthma. But if you do suffer from this life-altering disease, you can also find benefits in natural therapies that boost your immune system and level out its inflammatory responses to allergic stimuli. Such natural remedies, along with simple ways to alleviate allergens in your home, can make a world of difference for asthma sufferers. And when taken in conjunction with your doctor's medication prescription, these additional treatments can provide a "double whammy" against the disease and have you feeling much better for longer periods of time.

Fill up on nutrients.

There are many nutrients that have a beneficial effect on the disease of asthma, and which should

EXERCISE-INDUCED ASTHMA

Did you know that exercise can be a common trigger of asthma attacks? Exercise can even cause an asthma attack in people who have no other triggers and no other allergies and who do not experience asthma under any other circumstances.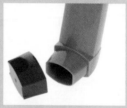

Interestingly it is thought that people with exercise-induced asthma are more sensitive to changes in the temperature and humidity of the air they are breathing. When you are at rest, you breathe through your nose, which warms, humidifies, and cleanses the air you inhale—thus making it more like the air in your lungs, and therefore easier to breathe.

However, when you are exercising, you usually breathe through your mouth, and as a result, the air that hits your lungs is colder and less humid. The contrast between the warmer air in the lungs and this colder, inhaled air (or even drier inhaled air and moist air in the lungs) can trigger an asthma attack.

Asthma cannot be cured, but it can be controlled through diet and medication. Fortunately in those with only exercise-induced asthma (EIA), maintenance therapy is often not required and medication can simply be taken before exercise. And happily, with appropriate treatment, almost everyone with EIA can enjoy the mental and physical benefits of exercise.

be taken daily to help improve asthmatic symptoms. These include magnesium, vitamins B_6 and B_{12}, vitamin C, vitamin D, vitamin E, selenium, molybdenum, beta-carotene, and quercetin. Here are some details about specific nutrients and natural treatments to help keep you breathing free and easy.

- *Vitamin D:* Vitamin D is a powerful tool in the fight against asthma. It balances the immune system, as well as prevents colds, flu, and pneumonia, which can exacerbate asthmatic symptoms. Vitamin D can even help asthmatics whose disease is not well managed with prednisone—a powerful and often dangerous drug that is not beneficial to remain on long-term.

- *Boswellia:* When taken at a dose of 300 milligrams, three times daily, this herb, which is also known as frankincense, acts as a powerful anti-inflammatory, reducing asthma symptoms within six weeks (and sometimes even within mere days of starting treatment).

- *Adrenal nutrients:* Prednisone is a common and powerful anti-inflammatory drug often used to treat asthma, but it is not a drug that should be maintained long-term. When the adrenal glands are strengthened through natural remedies, it can help control asthma to the point that prednisone may be lowered, even in severe cases. Nutrients that strengthen the adrenal glands include vitamin C, B_6, pantothenate, and licorice extract.

- *Lycopene:* At a dose of 30 to 45 milligrams daily, this antioxidant, which is found primarily in tomatoes, can be effective in preventing episodes of exercise-induced asthma (see earlier sidebar).

- *Omega-3 fatty acids:* These fatty acids, which are found primarily in fish, can be very helpful in controlling asthma in children, especially after environmental triggers have been removed as much as possible. Fish oil is especially prevalent in tuna, salmon, sardines, and other fatty fish, but it can also be taken in capsule or liquid form such as cod liver oil. Omega-3 fatty acids have also been shown to prevent asthma altogether. In one study children who ate fish more than once a week had one-third the risk of asthma compared with children eating lesser amounts of fish.

- *Thymus-supporting supplement:* There are many different types of supplements, including those with glandular tissue. The thymus gland regulates your immunity through the hormone thymulin, and it makes sense for asthma sufferers to boost their immunity as much as they can by using thymus extract for support. Any type of respiratory infection—including colds, the respiratory flu, or pneumonia—can trigger sensitive asthmatics to an episode. When you support your thymus gland, you support your asthma treatment! Therefore make sure you avoid all sucralose (Splenda), which has been shown to shrink the thymus gland.

Inhibit inflammation.

Inflammation is a primary enemy in the battle against asthma. Many asthmatics suffer from allergies to pollen and other airborne pollutants, and when these irritants are breathed into the lungs, the body's immune system reacts—defending you from "harm" by causing inflamed airways, thus causing labored breathing. A primary way to combat asthma is to combat the inflammatory process that is a result of the overreaction to allergens. Some evidence exists that antioxidants—especially vitamin C—help stop inflammation in the breathing passages of the lungs. "We know an asthma attack is inflammatory, and we know it produces a lot of oxygen radicals," says Gary E. Hatch, PhD, a research pharmacologist and branch chief of the pulmonary toxicology branch of the Environmental Protection Agency. "So antioxidants should help."[4] To help prevent asthma attacks, try adding vitamins C and E and the mineral selenium to your diet, along with fatty fish, which has been proven to reduce inflammation throughout the body.

Juice for good health.

There is a great deal of research that supports the idea that people who eat a great deal of fruits and vegetables have better lung function than those who do not. Vitamin C—as found in one glass of freshly made veggie juice per day—can increase lung capacity and diminish asthma symptoms significantly. Vitamin C is an antioxidant that helps to reduce inflammation, a common culprit in the disease of asthma. In one study conducted in Great Britain researchers compared the diets of 515 adults with asthma to 515 adults without the disease. Interestingly the more vitamin C the diet contained, the less risk there was that test subjects would contract symptomatic asthma.[5]

Super sources of vitamin C include citrus fruits and juices, red and green bell peppers, broccoli, brussels sprouts, parsley, dark leafy greens, and strawberries.

Ingest vitamin E.

Vitamin E is another vitamin that can drastically lower your risk of asthma. In one study conducted by

Harvard University, among 75,000 nurses, those getting the most vitamin E were 47 percent less likely to have asthma.[6]

Because vitamin E is primarily found in cooking oils, it can be difficult to get the necessary amounts in your diet. However, by adding wheat germ (one serving contains nearly 17 percent of the recommended daily dose) to other foods, such as smoothies and meat loaf, you can increase your intake of vitamin E and cut down on your asthma symptoms. Vitamin E is also found in almonds, sunflower seeds, whole grains, asparagus, salmon, brown rice, and the vegetables spinach and kale, so load up on these foods when you can![7]

Reduce your refined salt intake.

If you have asthma, it may be related to the sodium intake in your diet. Some research indicates that if you have the disease, a diet high in sodium chloride may actually worsen asthma symptoms. On the other hand, a lower-sodium diet may reduce the severity of exercise-induced asthma. A diet that contains more fruits and vegetables and less processed foods will naturally cause you to intake less salt, leading to a more healthy lifestyle overall.

You can use a little Celtic sea salt or pink

Himalayan salt, which has a full complement of minerals, unlike refined salt.

Fish your way to good health.

Lastly, the local fish market may be one place to go to help reduce your asthma symptoms. Omega-3 fatty acids, commonly found in oily fish such as salmon, tuna, or sardines, helps to reduce inflammation symptoms in the lungs. In one large study conducted in Australia, in families where people ate very little oily fish, almost 16 percent of the children had asthma. However, in families where fish was frequently consumed, only 9 percent of the children had asthma. And even more significant: In families where no fish was consumed, the rate of asthma in children increased to a whopping 23 percent.[8]

Nutrient Recommendations for Asthma Sufferers

If you suffer from asthma, in addition to the dietary changes suggested, you should consider taking the following nutrients and supplements to reduce the number of asthma attacks you suffer.

1. *Antioxidants* including vitamins C and E, beta-carotene, and selenium. Yellow, orange,

red, and dark green vegetables and fruit provide the most antioxidants.

2. *Essential fatty acids* (EFAs), especially eicosapentaenoic acid (EPA) and docosahexaenoic acid (DHA), two omega-3 fatty acids found in cold-water fish, are beneficial.

3. *Magnesium* as found in beetroot greens, spinach, parsley, dandelion greens, garlic, blackberries, beetroot, broccoli, cauliflower, carrots, and celery.

4. *Vitamin B_{12} (cobalamin)* successfully aids children with asthma. The best food sources of vitamin B^{12} are meat, poultry, and fish.

5. *Vitamin C* can cause an immediate decrease in airway constriction by reducing inflammation. Try eating more kale, parsley, broccoli, brussels sprouts, watercress, cauliflower, cabbage, strawberries, spinach, lemons, limes, turnips, and asparagus.

6. *Vitamin E* relaxes the smooth muscles of the lungs by reducing the inflammatory effects of histamine. Add more spinach,

watercress, asparagus, carrots, and tomatoes to your diet.

Juice Therapy for Asthma Sufferers

1. *Onion* juice reduces mucus in the respiratory tract.

2. *Parsley* juice can be toxic in overdose, so be sure to ingest only one-half cup juiced per day to treat asthma symptoms. Pregnant women should avoid parsley altogether.

3. *Radish* juice is another good remedy for asthma.

BEST TIPS for MAKING FRESH JUICES and SMOOTHIES

E VERY TIME YOU pour a glass of juice, picture a big vitamin-mineral cocktail with a wealth of nutrients that promote adrenal health and vitality. The veggies are broken down into an easily absorbable form that your body can use—right away. This food doesn't have to go through a big process of breaking everything down. So it goes to work in your body to give you energy and renew you right down to your cells. It also spares your organs all the work it takes to digest food, and that equates to more energy. It detoxifies your body as well because it's rich in antioxidants, so that lightens your toxic load, and the body doesn't have to work so hard to deal with all the toxic stuff coming from the environment.

The Nutritional Components of Fresh Juice

In addition to water and easily absorbed protein and carbohydrates, juice also provides essential fatty acids, vitamins, minerals, enzymes, biophotons, and phyto-nutrients. And researchers are continuing to explore how the nutrients found in juice help the body heal and shed unwanted pounds. The next time you make a glass of fresh juice, this is what you'll be drinking:

Protein

When you think of protein sources, does juice ever come to mind? Probably not, but surprisingly it does offer more than you might think. We use protein to form muscles, ligaments, tendons, hair, nails, and skin. Protein is needed to create enzymes, which direct chemical reactions, and hormones, which guide bodily functions. Fruits and vegetables contain lower quantities of protein than animal foods such as muscle meats and dairy products. Therefore they are thought of as poor protein sources. But juices are concentrated forms of vegetables and fruit and so provide easily absorbed amino acids, the building blocks that make up protein. For example, 16 ounces of carrot juice (2 to 3 pounds of carrots) provide about 5 grams of protein (the equivalent of about one chicken wing or 2 ounces of tofu). Vegetable protein is not complete protein, so it does not provide all the amino acids your body needs. In addition to lots of dark leafy greens, you'll want to eat other protein sources, such as sprouts, legumes (beans, lentils, and split peas), nuts, seeds, and whole grains. If you're not vegan, you can add eggs and free-range, grass-fed muscle meats such as chicken, turkey, lamb, and beef along with wild-caught fish.

Carbohydrates

Vegetable and fruit juices contain carbohydrates. Carbs provide fuel for the body, which uses it for movement, heat production, and chemical reactions. The chemical bonds of carbohydrates lock in the energy a plant takes up from the sun, and this energy is released when the body burns plant food as fuel. There are three categories of carbs: simple (sugars), complex (starches and fiber), and fiber. Choose more complex carbohydrates than simple carbs in your diet. There are more simple sugars in fruit juice than vegetable juice, which is why you should juice more vegetables and in most cases drink no more than 4 ounces of fruit juice a day. Both insoluble and soluble fibers are found in whole fruits and vegetables, and both types are needed for good health. Who said juice doesn't have fiber? Juice has the soluble form—pectin and gums, which are excellent for the digestive tract. Soluble fiber also helps to lower blood cholesterol levels, stabilize blood sugar, and improve good bowel bacteria.

Essential fatty acids

There is very little fat in fruit and vegetable juices, but the fats juice does contain are essential to your health. The essential fatty acids (EFAs)—linoleic and alpha-linolenic acids in particular—found in fresh juice function as components of nerve cells, cellular membranes, and hormonelike substances called prostaglandins. They are also required for energy production.

Vitamins

Fresh juice is loaded with vitamins. Vitamins take part, along with minerals and enzymes, in chemical reactions. For example, vitamin C participates in the production of collagen, one of the main types of protein found in the body. Fresh juices are excellent sources of water-soluble vitamins such as C; many of the B vitamins and some fat-soluble vitamins such as vitamin E; the carotenes, known as provitamin A (they are converted to vitamin A as needed by the body); and vitamin K. They also come packaged with cofactors, such as vitamin C with bioflavonoids. The cofactors and vitamins help each other be more effective.

Minerals

Fresh juice is loaded with minerals. There are about two dozen minerals that your body needs to function well. Minerals, along with vitamins, are components of enzymes. They make up part of bones, teeth, and blood tissue, and they help maintain normal cellular function.

The major minerals include calcium, chloride, magnesium, phosphorus, potassium, sodium, and sulfur. Trace minerals are those needed in very small amounts, which include boron, chromium, cobalt, copper, fluoride, manganese, nickel, selenium, vanadium, and zinc.

Minerals occur in inorganic forms in the soil, and plants incorporate them into their tissues. As a part of this process, the minerals are combined with organic molecules into easily absorbable forms, which make plant food an excellent dietary source of minerals. Juicing is believed to provide even better mineral absorption than whole vegetables because the process of juicing liberates minerals into a highly absorbable, easily digestible form.

Enzymes

Fresh juices are chock-full of enzymes—those "living" molecules that work with vitamins and minerals to speed up reactions necessary for vital functions in the body. Without enzymes we would not have life in our cells. Enzymes are prevalent in raw foods, but heat such as cooking and pasteurization destroys them. All juices that are bottled, even if kept in store refrigerators, have to be pasteurized. Heat temperatures for pasteurization are required to be far above the limit of what would preserve the enzymes and vitamins.

When you eat and drink enzyme-rich foods, these little proteins help break down food in the digestive tract, thereby sparing the pancreas, small intestine, and stomach—the body's enzyme producers—from overwork. This sparing action is known as the "law of adaptive secretion of digestive enzymes." According to this law, when a portion of the food you eat is digested by enzymes present in the food, the body will secrete less of its own enzymes. This allows the body's energy to be shifted from digestion to other functions such as repair and rejuvenation. Fresh juices require very little energy expenditure to digest, and that is one reason people who start consistently drinking fresh juice often report that they feel better and more energized right away.

Phytochemicals

Plants contain substances that protect them from disease, injury, and pollution. These substances are known as phytochemicals. *Phyto* means "plant," and chemical in this context means "nutrient." There are tens of thousands of phytochemicals in the foods we eat. For example, the average tomato may contain up to ten thousand different types of phytochemicals, the most famous being lycopene.

Phytochemicals give plants their color, odor, and flavor. Unlike vitamins and enzymes, they are heat stable and can withstand cooking. Researchers have found that people who eat the most fruits and vegetables, which are the best sources of phytochemicals, have the lowest incidence of cancer and other diseases. Drinking freshly made vegetable juices gives you these vital substances in a concentrated form.

Biophotons

There's one more substance, more difficult to measure than the others, that's present in raw foods. It is being studied scientifically in tubes and is named bio-photons. It's light energy that the plants absorb from the sun, and it is found in the living cells of raw foods such as fruits and vegetables. Photons have been shown to emit coherent light energy when uniquely photographed (using Kirlian photography). This light energy is believed to have many benefits when consumed; one in particular is thought to aid cellular communication. Biophotons feed the mitochondria of the cells, which produce ATP—our body's energy fuel. Biophotons are also believed to contribute to our energy, vitality, and a feeling of vibrancy and well-being.

Frequently Asked Questions

Now that you know why juice is so effective for good health, you may have some questions about juicing. Below I will address some of the questions I am most commonly asked about juicing.

Why juice? Why not just eat the fruits and vegetables?

Though I always tell people to eat their vegetables and fruit, there are at least three reasons juice is important and should also be included in the diet.

First, we can juice far more produce than we would probably eat in a day. It takes a long time to chew raw veggies. Chewing is a very good thing. I highly encourage it. However, we have only so much time for chewing raw foods. One day I timed how long it would take for me to eat five medium-size carrots. (That's what I often juice along with cucumber, lemon, ginger root, beet, kale, and celery.) It was about fifty minutes of chewing. Not only do I not have that kind of time every day, but also my jaw was so tired afterward that I could hardly move it.

Secondly, we can juice parts of the plant we would not normally eat, such as stems, leaves, and seeds. I juice things I know I would rarely or never eat, such as beet stems and leaves, celery leaves, the white pithy part of the lemon with the seeds, asparagus stems, broccoli stems, the base of cauliflower, kohlrabi leaves, radish leaves, and ribs of kale.

Thirdly, juice is broken down, so it spares digestion. It is estimated that juice is at work in the system in about twenty to thirty minutes after it is consumed. When we have ailments, juice is therapy for this very reason. When the body has to work hard to break down veggies, for example, it can spend a lot of energy on the digestive process.

Juicing does the work for you. So when you drink a glass of fresh juice, all those life-giving nutrients can go to work right away to heal and repair your body, giving it energy for its work of rejuvenation.

JUICING RECOMMENDATIONS FOR DIABETICS AND PREDIABETICS

I've often heard people say they can't juice because they have diabetes. You can juice vegetables if you have sugar metabolism problems, but you should choose low-sugar veggies and only low-sugar fruits such as lemons, limes, and cranberries. Carrots and beets would be too high in sugar. You could add one or two carrots to a juice recipe or a very small beet or part of a beet, but they should be diluted with cucumber juice and dark leafy greens. You may use cranberries, lemons, and limes, but other fruits are higher in sugar and should be avoided. Berries are low in sugar, especially blueberries, and can be added to juice recipes.

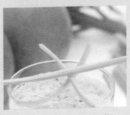

Green apples are lower in sugar than yellow or red apples. But I don't recommend that you use even green apples unless you have your blood sugar under control. Keep your juices very low in sugar.

I've worked with people who have reversed their diabetes by juicing low-sugar vegetables and eating many more living foods, along with a low-glycemic, high-fiber diet.

SPRINKLE CINNAMON IN YOUR JUICE

Researchers have suggested that people with diabetes may see improvements by adding ¼ to 1 teaspoon of cinnamon to their food. A twelve-week London study involved fifty-eight type 2 diabetics. After twelve weeks on 2 grams (about ½ teaspoon) of cinnamon per day, study subjects had significantly lowered blood sugar levels, as well as significantly reduced blood pressures.[1]

Don't we need the fiber that's lost in juicing?

It's true that we need to eat whole vegetables, fruit, sprouts, legumes, and whole grains for fiber. We drink juice for the extra nutrients; it's better than any vitamin pill. And for weight loss I recommend vegetable juices for appetite control. I also recommend juice as therapy. I cover more than fifty different ailments in my book *The Juice Lady's Guide to Juicing for Health* that can be improved with juice therapy, diet, and nutrients. Whole fruits and vegetables have insoluble and soluble fiber. Both types of fiber are very important for colon health. It's true that the insoluble fiber is lost when you juice. However, soluble fiber is present in juice in the form of gums and pectins. Soluble fiber is excellent for the digestive tract. It also helps to lower blood cholesterol, stabilize blood sugar, and improve good bowel bacteria. Don't worry about the fiber that is lost when you juice. Think about all the extra nutrition you are getting. Fresh juice is one of the best vitamin-mineral cocktails you could drink. You may not need as many nutritional supplements when you juice, so that could save you money in the long run. Drink your juice as a smart addition to your high-fiber diet.

Are most of the nutrients lost with the fiber?

In the past some groups have thought that a significant amount of nutrients remained in the fiber after juicing, but that theory has been disproved. The US Department of Agriculture analyzed twelve fruits and found that 90 percent of the antioxidant nutrients they measured was in the juice rather than the fiber.[2] This makes fresh juice a great supplement in the diet.

Is fresh juice better than commercially processed juice?

Fresh juice is "live food" with a full complement of vitamins, minerals, phytochemicals, and enzymes. It also contains biophotons that revitalize the body. You feel better when you drink fresh juice! In contrast, commercially processed canned, bottled, frozen, or packaged juices have been pasteurized, which means the juice has been heated and many of the vitamins and enzymes have been killed or removed. And the light energy is virtually gone. If you look at a Kirlian photograph of a cooked vegetable or a pasteurized glass of juice, you'll see very little "light" or no light emanating from them. This means the juice will have a longer shelf life, but it won't give your body life.

Making your own juice also allows you to use a wider variety of vegetables and fruit you might not otherwise eat, such as kale, beets with leaves and stems, lemon with the white part, stems, seeds, and chunks of ginger root. Some of my recipes include Jerusalem artichokes, jicama, green cabbage, celery leaves, asparagus stems, broccoli stems, kale, and parsley. These sweet, crisp tubers and healthy greens are not found in most processed juices.

How long can fresh juice be stored?

The sooner you drink fresh juice after you make it, the more nutrients you'll get. However, you can store juice and not lose too many nutrients by keeping it cold in an insulated container or covered in the refrigerator. You can also freeze it. Many busy moms are choosing to make a large batch of juice on the weekends and freeze it in individual containers.

On a personal note, when I had chronic fatigue syndrome, I would juice in the afternoons when I had the most energy and store the juice covered in the refrigerator and drink it for the next twenty-four hours until I juiced my next batch. I got well doing that.

How much produce is needed to make a glass of juice?

People often ask me if it takes a basket of produce to make a glass of juice. Actually, if you're using a good juicer, it takes a surprisingly small amount. For example, the following items yield about one 8-ounce glass of juice: five to seven large carrots or one large cucumber. The following each yield about 4 ounces of juice: one large apple, three to four large (13-inch) ribs of celery, or one large orange. The key is to get a good juicer that yields a dry pulp. I've used juicers, even expensive models, that ejected very wet pulp.

When I ran the pulp through the juicer again, I got more juice and the pulp was still wet. If the rotation speed (RPM) is too high or the juicer is not efficient in other ways, you will waste a lot of produce.

Will juicing cost lots of money?

If you were to crunch the numbers, you would find that the cost of a glass of juice is less than a latte. With three or four carrots, half a lemon, a chunk of ginger root, two ribs of celery, three or four green leaves, and half a cucumber, you will probably spend two dollars to three and a half dollars, depending on the season, the area of the country you live in, and the store where you purchase your produce. But wait—there are also hidden savings. You may not need as many vitamin supplements.

What's that worth? And you'll probably need far fewer over-the-counter medications such as pain-killers; sleeping aids; antacids; laxatives; and cold, cough, and flu medications. That's a whopping savings! And then there's time not lost from work. What happens when you run out of sick days? Or if you're self-employed, you've missed out on income each day you're sick. With the immune-building, disease-fighting properties of fresh juice, you should stay well all year long.

The Basics of Juicing

Juicing is a very simple process. Simple as the procedure is, though, it helps to keep a few guidelines in mind to obtain the best results.

- *Wash all produce before juicing.* Fruit and vegetable washes are available at many grocery and health food stores. Or you can use hydrogen peroxide and then rinse. Cut away all moldy, bruised, or damaged areas of the produce.

- *Always peel oranges, tangerines, tangelos, and grapefruit* before juicing, because the skins of these citrus fruit contain volatile oils that can cause digestive problems such as stomachaches. Lemon and lime peels can be juiced, if organic, but they do add a distinct flavor that is not one of my favorites for most recipes. I usually peel them. Leave as much of the white pithy part on the citrus fruit as possible, though, since it contains the most vitamin C and bioflavonoids. Bioflavonoids work with vitamin C; they need each other to create the best uptake for your immune cells. Always peel

91

mangoes and papayas since their skins contain an irritant that is harmful when eaten in quantity.

I also recommend that you peel all produce that is not labeled organic even though the largest concentration of nutrients is in and next to the skin. For example, nonorganic cucumbers are often waxed, trapping the pesticides. You don't want the wax or pesticides in your juice. The peels and skins of sprayed fruits and vegetables contain the largest concentration of pesticides.

- *Remove pits, stones, and hard seeds* from fruits such as peaches, plums, apricots, cherries, and mangoes. Softer seeds from cucumbers, oranges, lemons, limes, watermelons, cantaloupes, grapes, papayas, and apples can be juiced without a problem. Because of their chemical composition, large quantities of apple seeds should not be juiced for young children under the age of two, but they should not cause problems for older children and adults.

- *The stems and leaves of most produce can be juiced.* Beet stems and leaves, strawberry caps, celery leaves, radish leaves, and small grape stems are all fine to juice, and they offer nutrients. Discard larger grape stems, as they can dull the juicer blade. Also remove carrot tops and rhubarb greens because they contain toxic substances. Cut off the ends of carrots since this is the part that molds first.

- *Cut fruits and vegetables into sections or chunks* that will fit into your juicer's feed tube. You'll learn from experience what can be added whole and what size chunks work best for your machine. If you have a large feed tube, you won't have to cut up a lot of produce.

- *Some fruits and vegetables don't juice well.* Most produce contains a lot of water, which is ideal for juicing. The vegetables and fruits that contain less water, such as bananas and avocados, will not juice well. They can be used in smoothies and cold soups by first juicing other produce, then pouring the juice into a blender and adding the avocado, for example, to make a raw soup or green smoothie. Mangoes and papayas will juice but make a thicker juice.

- *Drink your juice as soon as you can* after it's made. If you can't drink the juice right away, store it in an insulated container such as a thermos or another airtight, opaque container and in the refrigerator if possible. You can store juice for up to twenty-four hours. Light, heat, and air will destroy nutrients quickly. Be aware that the longer juice sits before you drink it, the more nutrients are lost. You can also freeze the juice. If juice turns brown, it has oxidized and lost a large amount of its nutritional value; it is not good to drink it at this point as it may be spoiled. Melon and cabbage juice do not store well; drink them soon after they've been juiced.

- When I was very sick with chronic fatigue syndrome, I had only enough energy to juice once a day. I would store some of the juice for up to twenty-four hours. I got well doing that, so I know the juice had plenty of nutrients even in the stored amount.

LIVING FOODS INCREASE VITALITY and BETTER HEALTH

L IVING FOODS ARE a great weapon against the ravages of allergies and asthma. Unlike those prepackaged, nutrient-depleted snacks, living foods "love you back" by giving you a plethora of life-giving nutrients. That equates to higher energy levels, weight loss, detoxification, mental clarity, increased vitality, and fewer allergic or asthmatic episodes. Eating a wide variety of produce gives you a power-house of vitamins, minerals, enzymes, phytonutrients, and biophotons. Raw foods, which are rich in antioxidants, also help the body remove toxins, thus helping to keep you from getting ill.

A diet that is made up of 60 to 80 percent raw foods is a live foods diet, because the majority of the foods are eaten in their natural state. Eating living foods, especially vegetables, sprouts, wild greens, fruits, nuts, and seeds, is the healthiest for the human body. Truly they can transform you from the inside out.

Raw juices and living foods are packed with a cornucopia of nutrients, including biophotons—those light rays of energy the plants get from the sun. When we cook food, those beautiful rays of energy are destroyed or shrink way down. Professor Fritz-Albert Popp and Dr. H. Niggli are two researchers who have found that the light energy in biophotons is an important aspect of food. The more *light* a food is able to store, the more beneficial the food is to your body. Naturally grown fruits and vegetables that are ripened in the sun are strong sources of light energy. Numerous minute particles of light—biophotons, the smallest units of light—make their way into our cells when we eat these foods. They provide our bodies with important information and they control complex processes such as ordering and regulating our cells.[1]

Biophotons help to fix errors that have taken place within the body,[2] causing you to start feeling better, lighter, and more energized as time goes on. Your sleep improves, and you may need less of it. Your mind becomes more alert and creative, and your body comes to life. Your metabolism also ramps up, and you burn more calories helping you get fit with greater ease. In the process your overall health improves. Symptoms of poor health, ailments, allergies, asthma, and other chronic diseases begin to heal. Your whole life changes!

How Living Foods Love You Back

1. *Alkalinity:* Most Americans are slightly acidic because most of the American diet (animal products, grains, sugar and sweets of all kinds, coffee, black tea, sodas, sports drinks, and junk food) is acidic or turns acidic when it's digested. This causes a host of problems from weight gain to joint pain. The body tends to store acid in fat cells to protect delicate organs and tissues. It will hold on to fat cells; it will even make more fat cells to protect you. But a living foods diet, which is dominated with fresh vegetables, vegetable juices, fruit, sprouts, seeds, and nuts, provides an abundance of alkalinity. This neutralizes the acids, and the body can let go of fat cells. Many people report that their bodies also got rid of pain—all sorts of pain throughout the

body—when they began juicing and eating a living foods diet.

2. *Hydration:* One of the things lost when you cook food is the water content. Our bodies are about 70 percent water. Live foods contain plenty of water. Approximately 85 percent of many fruits and vegetables is water, so eating raw fresh produce is a wonderful way to obtain water. Plenty of water in our system equates to enzymes being able to carry out their metabolic work, and the easier it is for vitamins and minerals to be assimilated into our cells. The more live energy the water holds in the form of biophotons, the better the individual cells function and the higher the quality of your health.

3. *Superior protein:* Though not a complete protein, raw plants offer quality amino acids. Cooking denatures the proteins in our food—they coagulate, making them difficult to assimilate. The heat disorganizes their structure, leading to deficiencies of some of the essential amino acids, whereas

eating live foods offers amino acids in their best state.

4. *Abundant vitamins:* Many vitamins are destroyed when food is cooked or processed.

5. *Biophotons:* Plants release biophotons, which can only be measured by special equipment developed by German researchers.[3] These light rays of energy that plants take in from the sun energize our bodies and help our cells communicate more effectively.

6. *Greater strength, energy, and stamina:* Dr. Karl Elmer experimented with a raw food diet for top athletes in Germany. He saw improvement in their performance when they changed to an entirely raw food diet.[4] After eating raw food, rather than feeling fatigued or sleepy, most people feel energized. Also, most people eating a high raw food diet experience a more restful sleep and require less of it.

7. *Better mental performance:* Your memory and concentration should be clearer. You

should be more alert, more creative, and think more logically.

8. *Improved digestion due to more enzymes:* Enzymes are important because they are the catalysts of nearly every chemical reaction in our bodies. Vitamins and hormones need enzymes to do optimal work. Live foods contain a good mix of food enzymes. But when food is heated above 118 degrees, enzymes are destroyed, which forces our digestive system to work harder than it should. This can result in partially digested fats, proteins, and starches. When our diet is rich in enzymes, it spares our enzyme-producing organs extra work. That equates to better digestion and more energy.

9. *Reduced risk of disease:* A diet rich in raw vegetables and fruit has been shown to lower your risk of cancer and other diseases. Also, according to a study published in the *British Medical Journal*, eating fresh produce on a daily basis has been shown to reduce your chance of death from heart

attacks and related problems by as much as 24 percent.[5]

How to Shop for Living Foods

1. *Choose real, whole food.* These are the foods that are closest to their natural form and, therefore, retain the most nutrient value and deliver the highest health benefits. They are picked after they've ripened, and they are rich in flavor. They retain natural diversity of taste. They have full nutrient and antioxidant content. And if they are organically grown, seasonal, and local foods, they are the healthiest choices possible.

2. *Opt for the freshest fruit, vegetables, and legumes you can find.* Choose food items that have been grown organically to avoid toxic pesticides and to get increased nutrition. Buy from local growers whenever possible, because that produce is fresher than anything trucked in from other locations.

3. *Choose organic produce.* Organic produce doesn't have the many pesticides known or suspected to cause brain and nervous

system damage, cancer, disruption of the endocrine and immune systems, and a host of other toxic effects resulting from pesticides that are in our food supply. Studies have also shown that organic produce completely surpasses conventional produce in nutritional content.[6] When choosing organically grown foods, look for labels that are marked *certified organic*. This means the produce has been cultivated according to strict uniform standards that are verified by independent state or private organizations. Certification includes inspection of farms and processing facilities, detailed record keeping, and pesticide testing of soil and water to ensure that growers and handlers are meeting government standards.

4. *Support your local farms and farmers who sell their produce at farmers markets, local markets, and home deliveries.* Many of the smaller farms can't promote their wares as "organic," but if you talk with them, you'll learn that they don't use pesticides or chemical fertilizers; they just can't afford to get certified as organic. Buying your

produce from a local source is also the best way to insure freshness. The fresher the vegetables and fruit, the more biophotons you'll be receiving.

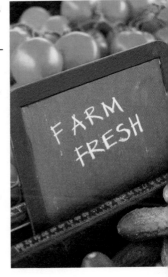

5. *Completely avoid irradiated foods.* Nonorganic vegetables, meats, and other products have been irradiated for years. Irradiation (exposure to radiation in very high levels) kills insects and other bugs that may have crawled into foods before being shipped to the grocery store. Irradiation has been shown to produce chromosome damage, and causes nutrient destruction.[7] Food growers and manufacturers must put the irradiation symbol (radura, which is a green flower within a circle) on the label that the food is irradiated, so avoidance of irradiated foods is possible if you shop carefully.

6. *Say no to genetically modified (GM) plant varieties that have been modified for*

herbicide tolerance and pest tolerance.[8] When trying to avoid the top GM crops, you'll need to watch out for maltodextrin, soy lecithin, soy oil, textured vegetable protein (soy), canola oil, corn products, and high-fructose corn syrup. Other GM crops to avoid include some varieties of zucchini, crookneck squash, papayas from Hawaii, aspartame (NutraSweet), milk containing rbGH, and rennet (containing genetically modified enzymes) used to make hard cheeses. We must become informed consumers and careful shoppers. We can look at the labels of packaged products to see if they contain corn flour or cornmeal, soy flour, cornstarch, textured vegetable protein (TVP), corn syrup, or modified food starch. Check labels of soy sauce, tofu, soy beverages, soy protein isolate, soy milk, soy ice cream, soy cheese, margarine, and soy lecithin, among dozens of other products. Another hidden danger regarding GMO foods is the splicing of different genes into foods. You might have a peanut gene with a tomato. The unsuspecting consumer could have an attack by eating a food that never posed a problem before. If it doesn't say organic or non-GMO, don't buy it; the chances are strong that they are GMO. To shop smart, see the Non-GMO Shopping Guide, created by the Institute for Responsible Technology, at www.nongmo shoppingguide.com.

7. *Wise up about red meat.* Not all red meat is created equal. In addition to being higher in omega-3 fats and CLA, meat from grass-fed animals is also higher in vitamin E. In fact, studies show the meat from pastured cattle is four times higher in vitamin E than meat from feedlot cattle and, interestingly, almost twice as high as the meat from feedlot cattle given vitamin E supplements. That's beneficial, in that vitamin E is linked with a lower risk of heart disease, asthma, and cancer.[9] Grass-fed beef is also lower in total fat and particularly the saturated fats linked to heart disease. It's also higher in beta-carotene, the B vitamins thiamine and riboflavin, and the minerals calcium, magnesium, and potassium.

8. *Know the difference between pastured poultry versus free-range or commercial fowl.* Pasture-raised poultry are far healthier than commercial-raised fowl. Pastured poultry are chickens, turkey, ducks, and geese that are raised in bottomless cages or pens outside or on grass where they can peck and scratch at the ground and hunt for bugs and seeds along with their grain. Sometimes they are mistakenly called free-range chickens, but free-range birds are still kept in confinement; they are just allowed to move about inside their buildings, which are often very crowded so "roaming" is not really possible. When you choose pasture-raised chicken, you avoid hormones, antibiotics, and drugs, which may pose immunological effects and cancer risks for consumers.[10] Commercial poultry are also often fed trace amounts of arsenic in their feed to stimulate their appetites so they'll fatten quickly for market. Traces of arsenic can be found in the meat we buy.[11]

9. *Look for eggs from chickens that are raised cage-free on pasture, without hormones,*

and fed an organic diet that includes green grass. Eggs from pastured hens contain all eight essential amino acids and are a rich source of essential fatty acids. They also contain considerably more lecithin (a fat emulsifier) than cholesterol. Additionally, eggs from hens bred outdoors have four to six times more vitamin D than eggs from hens bred in confinement.[12] Pastured hens are exposed to direct sunlight, which is converted to vitamin D and passed on to the eggs. And the eggs are rich in sulfur and glutathione as well. For organic pastured eggs, look to co-ops and natural food markets; also seek out local producers, farmers, and homesteaders who pasture their poultry in movable pens or let them roam free.

10. *Buy only wild-caught fish—meaning caught with a boat and hook or net.* The other option is ranched or farm-raised fish, which you should avoid. Farm-raised fish are housed within small pens that are set up in the ocean or in small ponds. The fish are often kept in overcrowded conditions

that increase their risk of infection and disease. Farm-raised fish do not have the essential fatty acids that wild-caught fish offer and that are so important for our health. When it comes to animal fat, wild-caught fish are a good source of the healthy omega-3 fatty acids, especially cold-water fish such as salmon, mackerel, and trout. Also, the smaller the fish, the less mercury and other heavy metals that will be stored in the flesh and fat.

How to Cook Living Foods to Reduce Allergies and Asthma

It has been found that radiation exposure can weaken the immune system and cause health-related problems such as cancer and degenerative diseases. It may also cause ailments such as "persistent cough, headaches, sleep disturbances, and gastrointestinal dysfunction," notes Dr. J. D. Decuypere. She has observed that respiratory illnesses such as asthma, bronchitis, chronic cough, and allergies have been increasing since the late 1970s, which prompted her to do her own investigation on radiation in our food.[13]

Though there are numerous ways that we are

exposed to radiation, there are two ways that it enters our food—microwave ovens and irradiation of food. Radiating food in a microwave oven is convenient, and many people use their microwave daily. But studies have shown that it may negatively impact the nutrition of the food, and it may be harmful to the people who eat it.

While the dangers of using microwave ovens are still embroiled in battle and controversy, it is highly recommended that you not use a microwave at all—even for heating water. I recommend that you only use your stovetop, oven, toaster oven, countertop grill, or convection oven. Recently a friend sent an e-mail to me about a woman who conducted a home experiment with two similar plants. She watered one with cooled microwaved water and the other with tap water. The microwave-watered plant died rather quickly.

Choosing organic living foods, which means raw or dehydrated and whole foods, feeds the body superior nutrition and does not stress the body with toxins from preservatives, pesticides, and fillers. The nutrients they provide support the immune system, adrenal glands, and nervous system, all of which affect a person's allergic and asthmatic responses. Also avoiding foods you are sensitive to, such as wheat, dairy, soy, sweets, and corn will remove stress from your body and allow your immune system to function more effectively. Purchase high-quality whole foods, and you will be investing in your health—one of the best investments you can make.

JUICE, SMOOTHIE, and LIVING FOOD RECIPES to ALLEVIATE ALLERGIES and ASTHMA

Juices

Allergy Relief

Parsley is a traditional remedy for allergic reactions. You need to juice a bunch as soon as possible after a reaction occurs. It can help open airways when sipped.

1 bunch parsley
2 celery stalks
1–2 carrots, scrubbed well, tops removed, ends trimmed
1 lemon, peeled if not organic
½ cucumber, peeled if not organic

Cut produce to fit your juicer's feed tube. Juice all ingredients and stir. Pour into a glass and drink as soon as possible. Serves 1.

Asthma Helper

Radish is a traditional remedy for asthma.

5 carrots, scrubbed well, tops removed, ends trimmed
5–6 radishes with leaves
1 green apple
½ lemon, peeled if not organic

Cut produce to fit your juicer's feed tube. Juice all ingredients. Stir and pour into a glass. Serve at room temperature or chilled, as desired. Serves 1.

Congestion Helper

In Chinese medicine, mustard greens provide what's known as "hot energy," which is good for congestion and poor circulation.

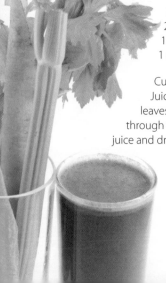

3 carrots, scrubbed well, tops removed, ends trimmed
2 ribs of celery with leaves
2–3 mustard leaves
1 cucumber, peeled if not organic
1 apple (green is lower in sugar)

Cut produce to fit your juicer's feed tube. Juice carrots and celery. Roll mustard leaves and place in juicer. Push the greens through with the cucumber and apple. Stir the juice and drink as soon as possible. Serves 1–2.

Healthy Sinus Solution

Radish juice is a traditional remedy to open up the sinuses and support mucous membranes. The best sinus healer is a liver cleanse.

2 tomatoes
6 radishes
1 lime, peeled if not organic
½ cucumber, peeled if not organic

Cut produce to fit your juicer's feed tube. Juice all ingredients and stir. Pour into a glass and drink as soon as possible. Serves 1.

Immune Builder

Studies show that garlic has a compound that has a natural antibiotic-like effect. It is antibacterial, antifungal, antiparasitic, and antiviral, but it must be consumed raw to have this effect. So juice it up for your immune system.

1 handful watercress
1 turnip, scrubbed, tops removed, and ends trimmed
3 carrots, scrubbed well, tops removed, and ends trimmed
1 to 2 garlic cloves
½ green apple such as Granny Smith or pippin

Bunch up the watercress. Cut produce to fit your juicer's feed tube. Tuck the watercress in the feed tube and push through with the turnip. Juice the remaining ingredients, finishing with a carrot. Stir the juice, pour into a glass, and drink as soon as possible. Serves 1.

Liver Life Tonic

Dandelion juice is a traditional remedy for cleansing the liver.

1 handful of dandelion greens
3–4 carrots, scrubbed well, tops removed, ends trimmed
1 cucumber, peeled
1 lemon, peeled

Bunch up dandelion greens. Cut produce to fit your juicer's feed tube. Tuck the greens in the feed tube and push through with a carrot. Juice the remaining ingredients. Stir the juice, pour into a glass, and drink as soon as possible. Serves 1.

Lung Rejuvenator

Turnip juice has been used as a traditional remedy to strengthen lung tissue.

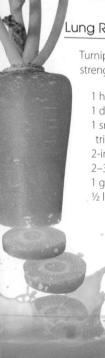

1 handful of watercress
1 dark green lettuce leaf
1 small turnip, scrubbed well, tops removed, ends trimmed
2-inch-thick chunk of jicama, scrubbed well or peeled
2–3 carrots, scrubbed well, tops removed, ends trimmed
1 garlic clove with peel
½ lemon, peeled if not organic

Bunch up watercress and roll in lettuce leaf; push through juicer slowly. Cut produce to fit your juicer's feed tube. Juice all remaining ingredients. Stir the juice, pour into a glass, and drink as soon as possible. Serves 1.

Perky Parsley

1 bunch of parsley
2 dark green lettuce leaves
3 carrots, scrubbed well, tops removed, ends trimmed
2 ribs of celery with leaves
1 cucumber, peeled if not organic
1 lemon, peeled if not organic

Cut produce to fit your juicer's feed tube. Wrap parsley in lettuce leaves and push through juicer slowly. Juice remaining ingredients and stir. Pour into a glass and drink as soon as possible. Serves 1–2.

Spinach Power Up

½ cucumber, peeled if not organic
1 small handful of parsley
1 green lettuce leaf
3 carrots, scrubbed well, tops removed, ends trimmed
2 ribs of celery with leaves
½ beet, scrubbed well, with stem and leaves
½ lemon, peeled if not organic

Cut produce to fit your juicer's feed tube. Start with cucumber; then wrap parsley in lettuce leaf and push through the machine slowly. Juice all remaining ingredients and stir. Pour into a glass and drink as soon as possible. Serves 1–2.

Spring Veggie Tonic

Asparagus is a natural diuretic that helps flush toxins from the body and promotes kidney cleansing. This juice is a great tonic for the kidneys, and it is a great way to use up asparagus stems.

1 tomato
1 cucumber, peeled if not organic
8 asparagus stems
1 lemon, peeled if not organic

Cut produce to fit your juicer's feed tube. Juice all ingredients and stir. Pour into a glass and drink as soon as possible. Serves 1–2.

The Morning Energizer

3–4 carrots, scrubbed well, tops removed, ends trimmed
1 cucumber, peeled if not organic
1 small beet, scrubbed well, with stems and leaves
1 lemon, peeled
1-inch chunk ginger root, peeled
½ green apple

Cut the produce to fit your juicer's feed tube. Juice all ingredients and stir. Pour into a glass and drink as soon as possible. Serves 1–2.

Twisted Ginger

4 carrots, scrubbed well, green tops removed, ends trimmed
1 handful parsley
1 lemon, peeled
1 apple
2-inch piece fresh ginger root, peeled

Cut produce to fit your juicer's feed tube. Juice ingredients
and stir. Pour into a glass and drink as soon as possible.
Serves 1–2.

Wheatgrass Light

1 green apple, washed
1 handful wheatgrass, rinsed
½ lemon, peeled
2–3 sprigs mint, rinsed (optional)

Cut produce to fit your juicer's feed tube. Start with the
apple and juice all the ingredients and stir. Pour into a
glass and drink as soon as possible. Serves 1.

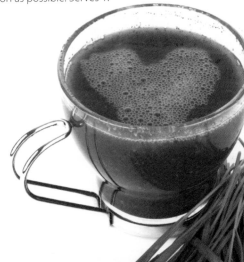

Teas

Healing Tea

This tea is very good for sore throat, cold, flu, and infections.

2-inch-chunk fresh ginger root, juiced
Juice of ½ medium lemon, peeled if not organic
2 cups purified water
1 Tbsp. loose licorice tea or 1 licorice herbal tea bag
    (optional)
4–5 whole cloves
1 cinnamon stick, broken
Dash cardamom
Dash nutmeg

Place all ingredients in a saucepan and simmer for about ten minutes. Strain and drink while warm. Serves 1.

Harmonize Energy Tea

1 Tbsp. rose hips
1 Tbsp. chicory root
1 Tbsp. chamomile
1 Tbsp. red clover
1 Tbsp. rose buds

Bring three cups of water to boil in a pot. Place the roots and berries in first, reduce the heat and simmer, covered, for 10 min. Add the leaves and flowers, turn the heat off, and let steep, covered, for another 10 min. Strain and drink through the day. Each tea blend can be used twice.

Smoothies

Calcium Booster

Kale is packed with calcium in a form that is assimilated by the body far better than the calcium in dairy products— and that's a great bonus for your bones!

1 cucumber, peeled if not organic
1 cup chopped kale
2 pears (Asian or Bartlett)
1 avocado
6 ice cubes

Chop cucumber, kale, and pear. Place in the blender and process until smooth. Add the avocado and ice, and blend until creamy. Serves 2.

Cherie's Green Morning Blend

½ English cucumber, peeled if not organic and cut in chunks
1 avocado, peeled, seeded, and cut in quarters
1 cup loosely packed baby spinach
Juice of 1 lime
1 Tbsp. green powder of choice (optional)
2–3 Tbsp. ground almonds (optional)

Combine all ingredients in a blender and blend well. Sprinkle ground almonds on top, as desired. Serves 1.

Coconut Green Delight

Coconut oil is an ally in breaking the yeast-fat cycle. It is very effective at killing Candida albicans. Its medium-chain fatty acids split open the protective outer coating of yeast cells, thus killing the yeast.

1 cucumber, cut in chunks
1 cup raw spinach, kale, or chard, chopped
1 avocado, peeled, seeded, and cut in quarters
½ cup coconut milk
1 Tbsp. organic virgin coconut oil
Juice of 1 lime or lemon

Combine all ingredients in a blender and process until smooth. Serves 2.

Green Berry Delight

1 cucumber, peeled if not organic
½ apple
1 cup berries (blueberries, raspberries, or blackberries), fresh or thawed if frozen
3–4 dark green leaves (collards, Swiss chard, or kale)
1-inch chunk ginger root
Juice of ½ lemon
1 avocado, peeled, seeded, and cut in chunks

Cut the cucumber and apple in chunks. Place the cucumber, berries, and apple in a blender and process until smooth. Chop the greens and ginger and add to the blender along with the lemon juice and avocado. Process until well blended. Serves 2.

Sweet Green Tahini

1 apple, washed and juiced (about ½ cup juice)
1 stalk of celery with leaves, juiced
1 Tbsp. tahini (sesame butter)
1 banana, peeled and cut in chunks
½ cup packed baby spinach
6 ice cubes

Combine all ingredients in blender and process until creamy and smooth. Serve chilled. Serves 1.

Green Smoothie Supreme

1 broccoli stem (save the florets for steaming, if you like)
1 apple
1 lemon
½ cucumber, peeled if not organic, cut in chunks
1 handful of spinach
1 small handful of parsley
1 cup blueberries (fresh or frozen)
1 kiwifruit
1 avocado, peeled, seeded, and cut into chunks
2–3 drops stevia
4–6 ice cubes, as desired

Juice the broccoli stem, apple, and lemon. Pour the juice in the blender, and add the cucumber, spinach, parsley, blueberries, kiwi, and avocado. Add stevia if you like it sweeter and ice cubes if you like it cold. Blend until the mixture is smooth and creamy. Serves 2.

Dr. Nina's Green Vitality Smoothie

1 bunch of spinach
1 pear
3 pineapple guavas (optional)
½ tsp. raw honey
5-10 stems Italian parsley
1 Tbsp. goji berries
1 cup purified water
¼ cup organic coconut milk

Place all ingredients in a blender and blend until smooth. Serves 2.

Dr. Nina's Sweet Dandelion Smoothie

1 pear, Bartlett or Asian
1 apple (green has less sugar)
1 large handful dandelion greens
1 cup coconut milk
Juice of ½ lemon
¼ cup flaxseeds
6 ice cubes (optional)

Place all ingredients in a blender and process until a creamy shake. Serves 2.

Living Foods

Walnut Zucchini Greens

1 head of broccoli, lightly blanch broccoli florets under hot tap water until it turns bright green
2 small zucchini, finely shredded in food processor
1 red pepper, finely chopped

2 cups torn romaine or green leaf lettuce
½ cup walnuts, chopped (optional)

Ginger Lime Dressing

¼ cup fresh lime juice
¼ cup sesame oil
¼ cup purified water
2 Tbsp. tamari
2 Tbsp. fresh mint
1 Tbsp. fresh cilantro
1 tsp. ginger root
1 thin slice red chili pepper or dash of cayenne pepper
1 Tbsp. pure maple syrup
1 tsp. Celtic sea salt

Mix first 3 ingredients in bowl. Place veggies on the bed of greens. Sprinkle walnuts over top. Drizzle dressing over salad. Serves 4.

Apple Fennel Salad With Lemon Zest

2 cups fennel, sliced julienne thin
2 cups apple, sliced julienne thin
2 Tbsp. fresh lemon juice
2 Tbsp. lemon zest
2 Tbsp. extra-virgin olive oil
2 Tbsp. fresh, minced thyme
1 sliver of jalapeño, minced
1 tsp. Celtic sea salt

Place the fennel and apple sliced in a bowl; set aside. In a small bowl, whisk together lemon juice, zest, olive oil, thyme, jalapeño, and salt. Pour dressing over fennel-apple mixture and toss. Serves 4.

Nan's Sunflower Pate

Sunflower seeds are an excellent source of vitamin E, the body's primary fat-soluble antioxidant. Vitamin E has significant anti-inflammatory effects that result in the reduction of symptoms in asthma, osteoarthritis, and rheumatoid arthritis, conditions where free radicals and inflammation play a big role.

3 cups sunflower seeds, soaked 8–12 hours, rinse and sprout about 4 hours
1 cup fresh lemon juice
½ cup chopped scallion
¼–½ cup raw tahini
¼ cup liquid aminos or shoyu
2–4 slices red onion, cut into chunks
4–6 Tbsp. chopped parsley
2–3 medium cloves garlic
½ tsp. cayenne pepper
1–2 Tbsp. chopped ginger
1 tsp. cumin

Blend all ingredients in food processor until all the ingredients are smooth and creamy. This mixture should be on the thick side rather than thin. Add a bit of water as needed. Makes 7–8 cups.

Almond Roulade

Collard leaves are an excellent source of calcium and a fairly good source of magnesium and vitamin K, making this dish outstanding for healthy bones.

Almond Filling

2 cups almonds, soaked 7–8 hours, rinsed well
2 stalks celery, cut ends, finely minced
1 medium red pepper, with seeds and ribs removed, finely diced
1 carrot, cut ends and peel (and chop, if using food processor)
1 small onion, finely minced

Using a juicer with a blank blade such as the Champion or the Omega, or a food processor, homogenize the almonds and carrot, catching them in a large bowl. Or place the soaked almonds and carrot in a food processor and blend until homogenized. To this mixture add celery, red pepper, and onion. Thoroughly knead, integrating all ingredients with your hands. Makes about 3 cups.

Marinated Collard Greens

1 bunch fresh collard greens, wash; remove tough stems and trim out center vein
4 Tbsp. extra-virgin olive oil
Juice of 1 to 2 lemons
1–2 cloves garlic, finely minced

Place extra-virgin olive oil, lemon juice, and garlic in a small bowl and whisk together. Set aside. Place collard leaves in large rectangular dish, alternating the direction of the leaves as you overlap and stack them. Pour in olive oil mixture, coating all leaves. Set aside for 3 hours before serving.

Take collard greens and spread 2–3 tablespoons Almond Filling on one side of each leaf. Roll each collard leaf, forming a roulade. Repeat this process, using up all the Almond Filling and collard greens. Cut each roulade in half or thirds and serve one or two per person. Serves 10–12.

Dr. Nina's Russian Cabbage Slaw

4 cups shredded cabbage
1 cup grated carrot
½ cup dandelion greens or watercress, chopped
4 cloves garlic, minced
Juice of ½ lemon
¼ cup extra-virgin olive oil

Place the cabbage, carrot, greens, and garlic in a bowl; set aside. In a small bowl, whisk together lemon juice and olive oil. Pour over the cabbage mixture and toss well. Serves 4.

Cooked Food Recipes With Raw Foods

I've included some of my favorite cooked food recipes to give you an idea of how to include raw foods with cooked and increase your living foods intake.

Squash and Arugula Enchiladas

Delicata squash is my favorite in this recipe. It features yellow skin with green stripes on an oblong shape. A ¾-cup portion contains just 30 calories, so it's a great choice if you're wanting to lose weight. It's a good source of vitamin C and carotenes. Adding arugula or watercress gives you an example of combining cooked and living foods.

2 delicata squash or 1 acorn, or about ¼ butternut (other winter squash, sweet potatoes, or yams can be substituted)
1 cup brown rice, cooked
½–1 cup chopped arugula

4–6 tortillas (sprouted whole grain, spelt, or gluten free)
1 Tbsp. virgin coconut oil
Salt and pepper to taste

Bake the delicata squash in a preheated oven set at 400 degrees for 30 minutes or until tender but not soft. Add water about an inch deep to the baking pan and they cook faster.

While the squash is baking, cook the rice. (If you want meat in this dish, you can reduce the rice to ½ cup and add ½ pound of ground meat, cooked.)

When the squash is tender, remove from the oven and cut in half. Scoop out the seeds and peel, but if you are using delicata and the skin is tender, you don't need to peel. Cut the squash in chunks and mix with rice; add seasoning to taste and set aside, keep warm.

In a large skillet, heat the oil. Heat the tortillas one at a time until warm and slightly browned, but be careful not to overcook or they will get crisp and won't roll into an enchilada.

Spoon 2–3 tablespoons of the squash-rice mixture into the center of each tortilla and spread from one end to the other. Add arugula to the top of that mixture and roll each side toward the center. Serve hot. Serves 4–6.

Carrot Sauce With Asparagus and Fresh Peas Over Rice

1 cup brown rice or quinoa
1½ cups carrot juice (about 8–11 carrots)
½ cup raw cashews
2 Tbsp. white or yellow miso
1 pound fresh asparagus
½ cup fresh or frozen peas
2 scallions, chopped
¼ cup marinated sun-dried tomato halves, thinly sliced
2 cloves garlic, pressed
3 Tbsp. finely chopped fresh basil

Cook brown rice or quinoa according to directions.

While rice is cooking, combine the carrot juice, cashews, and miso in a blender or food processor, blending on high until the cashews are no longer gritty and the mixture is smooth and creamy.

Snap off the tops of the asparagus. Cut the tender upper portion into 1-inch pieces.

In a medium-size skillet, combine the carrot juice mixture and asparagus. Bring to a boil and then reduce the heat to simmer, stirring occasionally for 2–3 minutes. Add the peas and simmer until the asparagus is just tender, about 2 minutes. Add the scallions, sun-dried tomatoes, and garlic, mixing well; simmer for 1–2 minutes. Remove the sauce from the heat.

Divide the rice or quinoa in 4 portions. Top each portion with about ¼ of the sauce and sprinkle chopped basil on top of each portion. Serves 4.

NOTES

Chapter 2—Allergies: When Good Immune Systems Go Bad

1. A. Blair, S. H. Zahm, N. E. Pearce, E. F. Heineman, and J. F. Fraumeni Jr., "Clues to Cancer Eitology From Studies of Farmers," *Scandinavian Journal of Work, Environment and Health* (Helsinki) 18, no. 4 (1992): 209–215.

2. Environmental Working Group, "EWG's 2013 Shopper's Guide to Pesticides in Produce," http://www.ewg.org/foodnews/summary.php (accessed January 14, 2014).

3. Ibid.

Chapter 3—Food Allergies: The Dangers in Your Dinner

1. G. Roberts, N. Patel, F. Levi-Schaffer, P. Habibi, and G. Lack, "Food Allergy as a Risk Factor for Life-Threatening Asthma in Childhood," *Journal of Allergy and Clinical Immunology* 112 (2003).

2. Yager, *The Doctor's Book of Food Remedies*, 268.

3. Ibid.

4. Ibid., 269.

5. Mehmet Oz and Mike Roizen, "Give Your Liver a Break: Avoid Toxins," *Wichita Eagle*, November 9, 2010, http://www.kansas.com/2010/11/09/1580014/give-your-liver-a-break-avoid.html#ixzz1CNfMO7Ov (accessed January 20, 2014).

6. Dr. Nina Walsh is a naturopathic physician and practitioner of Eastern medicine. Her love of medicine was born growing up in Russia in a family of physicians, artists, and herbalists. In her own journey to wellness she traveled extensively in Europe, Asia, and the US,

studying traditional healing approaches and later completed a formal study of naturopathy and East Asian Medicine at Bastyr University in Kenmore, WA, and Shanghai, China. She is also one of the leaders of the Juice Lady's Raw Foods and Juice Cleanse Retreats.

7. L. Kotze, R. Nisihara, S. Utiyama, G. Custodio Piovezan, and L. R. Kotze, "Thyroid Disorders in Brazilian Patients With Celiac Disease," *Journal of Clinical Gastroenterology* 40, no. 1 (January 2006): 33–36.

Chapter 4—Asthma: Learning to Catch Your Breath

1. Jacob Teitelbaum, *Real Cause, Real Cure* (New York: Rodale, 2013), 213.

2. Ibid.

3. Murdoc Khaleghi and Colleen Totz Diamond, *The Complete Idiot's Guide to Boosting Your Immunity* (New York, Penguin Books Group [USA] Inc., 2013).

4. Selene Yager, *The Doctor's Book of Food Remedies* (New York, Rodale, 2007), 62.

5. Ibid., 63.

6. Ibid.

7. Ibid.

8. Ibid., 64.

Chapter 5—Best Tips for Making Fresh Juices and Smoothies

1. R. Akilen, A. Tsiami, D. Devendra, and N. Robinson, "Glycated Haemoglobin and Blood Pressure-Lowering Effect of Cinnamon in Multi-Ethnic Type 2 Diabetic Patients in the UK: A Randomized, Placebo-Controlled, Double-Blind Clinical Trial," *Diabetic Medicine* 27, no. 10 (October 2010): 1159–1167.

2. Hong Wang, Guohua Cao, and Ronald L. Prior, "Total Antioxidant Capacity of Fruits," *Journal of Agricultural and Food Chemistry* 44, no. 3 (March 19, 1996): 701–705.

Chapter 6—Living Foods Increase Vitality and Better Health

1. Joseph Mercola, "McDonald's and Biophoton Deficiency," Mercola.com, August 21, 2002, http://articles.mercola.com/sites/articles/archive/2002/08/21/biophoton.aspx (accessed January 14, 2014).

2. John Switzer, "Bio-Photon Nutrition and Wild Green Energy Cocktails for Optimal Health (English)," May 21, 2009, http://tinyurl.com/lkxqve4 (accessed January 14, 2014).

3. Marco Bischof, "Humans Emit Biophotons—the Light of Our Cells," HeartSpring.net, January 30, 2011, http://heartspring.net/biophoton_meditation.html (accessed January 14, 2014).

4. Arthur M. Baker, "Raw Fresh Produce vs. Cooked Food," RawFoodHowTo.com, http://rawfoodhowto.com/raw-fresh-produce-vs-cooked.cfm (accessed January 14, 2014).

5. Timothy J. A. Key, Margaret Thorogood, Paul N. Appleby, and Michael L. Burr, "Dietary Habits and Mortality in 11,000 Vegetarians and Health Conscious People: Results of a 17-Year Follow Up," *British Medical Journal* 313, no. 7060 (September 28, 1996): 775.

6. Jon Ungoed-Thomas, "Official: Organic Really Is Better," *Sunday Times*, October 28, 2007.

7. J. D. Decuypere, "Radiation, Irradiation, and Our Food Supply," *The Decuypere Report*, http://www.

healthalternatives2000.com/food-supply-report.html (accessed January 14, 2014).

8. US Food and Drug Administration, "Regulation of Foods Derived from Plants," statement of Lester M. Crawford before the Subcommittee on Conservation, Rural Development, and Research House Committee on Agriculture, June 17, 2003.

9. G. C. Smith, "Dietary Supplementation of Vitamin E to Cattle to Improve Shelf Life and Case Life of Beef for Domestic and International Markets," Colorado State University, referenced in EatWild.com, "Summary of Important Health Benefits of Grassfed Meats, Eggs, and Dairy," http://www.eatwild.com/healthbenefits.htm (accessed January 14, 2014).

10. World-wire.com, "American Public Health Association Supports Ban on Hormonal Milk and Meat," news release, November 13, 2009, http://www.world-wire.com/news/0911130001.html (accessed January 14, 2014).

11. Consumer Reports, "Chicken: Arsenic and Antibiotics," July 2007.

12. Tabitha Alterman, "Eggciting News!" MotherEarthNews.com, October 15, 2008, http://www.motherearthnews.com/Relish/Pastured-Eggs-Vitamin-D-Content.aspx (accessed January 14, 2014).

13. J. D. Decuypere, "Radiation, Irradiation, and Our Food Supply," *The Decuypere Report*, http://www.healthalternatives2000.com/food-supply-report.html (accessed March 11, 2011).

FOR MORE INFORMATION

S IGN UP FOR the Juice Lady's free Juice News-letter at www.juiceladycherie.com.

Cherie's website

- www.juiceladycherie.com—information on juicing and weight loss

The Juice Lady's health and wellness juice retreats

I invite you to join us for a week that can change your life! Our retreats offer gourmet organic raw foods with a three-day juice fast midweek. We offer interesting, informative classes in a beautiful, peaceful setting where you can experience healing and restoration of body and soul. For more information, a brochure, and dates for the retreats, call 866-843-8935.

Schedule a nutrition consultation with the Juice Lady

Call 866-843-8935.

Dr. Nina Walsh, ND

Flow Natural Medicine & Acupuncture
10838 Main street
Bellevue, WA 98004
www.flowmedicine.net
e-mail: ninawalshnd@yahoo.com
206-384-2414

Don't let stress ruin your health.

FIGHT BACK WITH THESE ALL-NATURAL REMEDIES.

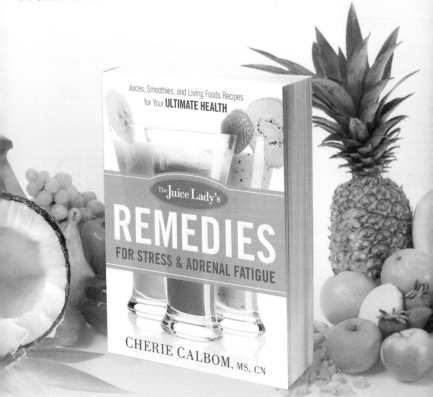

Juices, Smoothies, and Living Foods Recipes
for Your **ULTIMATE HEALTH**

The Juice Lady's

REMEDIES

FOR STRESS & ADRENAL FATIGUE

CHERIE CALBOM, MS, CN

YOU DON'T HAVE TO SUFFER with the effects of stress and exhaustion. This quick-reference guide helps you naturally repair, rejuvenate, and reclaim your health with valuable tips on stopping stress and adrenal fatigue at the source, including:

- Practical ways to lower your stress levels
- Nine common symptoms of adrenal fatigue
- Seven steps you can take to combat stress eating, and more!

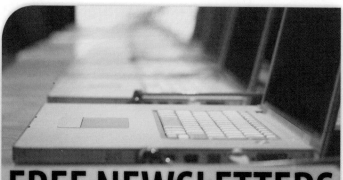

VIII. *The dilemma*

Population historians are not yet agreed about the causes of population growth, whether it was primarily the decline of diseases (such as smallpox) or the improvement of food supply and living conditions as they affected both the death and birth rates.[51] But the consequences of the great population expansion for every region of Britain (and indeed the rest of humanity) were startlingly obvious: these extra people had to be fed and clothed and employed.

The old economies of the British Isles were incapable of accommodating the new scale of population. The economies had to change or the people would not survive. The dilemma was barely perceptible until 1801, and so the reaction was unplanned. But as the world responded spontaneously to the new demands, structural changes were forced up in every corner of the country. The Highlands, despite changes before and after Culloden, were not well prepared for the challenge.

Some contemporaries soon came to the view that the role of the Highlands was predetermined: it was intended to supply raw materials to the rest of the kingdom. The people should disperse.

Notes

1 See Eric Richards, 'Margins of the Industrial Revolution', in *The Industrial Revolution and British Society* edited by Patrick O'Brien and R. Quinault (Cambridge, 1993), pp. 203–28.

2 Joseph Mitchell, *Reminiscences of my Life in the Highlands* (2 vols., originally published privately in 1883 and 1884, reprinted in 1971) I, pp. 13–14.

3 Ibid., II, p. 81.

4 Leah Leneman, 'A new role for a lost cause: Lowland romanticisation of the Jacobite Highlander' in Leah Leneman (ed.), *Perspectives on Scottish Social History* (Aberdeen, 1988), pp. 114–15.

5 Hunter, op. cit, pp. 31, 38, 196.

6 See Devine, op. cit., pp. 11, 37.

7 Robert A. Dodgshon, *From Chiefs to Landlords: Social and Economic Change in the Western Highlands and Islands, c. 1493–1820* (Edinburgh, 1998), Chapter 1; Devine, op. cit., pp. 214-15.

8 See Hunter, op. cit., p. 102.

9 I.F. Grant, *Everyday Life*, pp. 23–4, 123; another detailed pre-clearance portrait set in the southern Highlands is found in Leneman, *Living in Atholl*, op. cit.

10 E.R. Cregeen, review of T.C. Smout, *History of the Scottish People* in *Scottish Studies* (hereafter *SS*), vol. 14 (1970), p. 157.

11 Quoted by the Duke of Argyll in 'On the economic condition of the Highlands of Scotland', *Nineteenth Century*, vol. XIII (1883), p. 186.

12 Dodgshon, op. cit., p. 152.

13 Ibid., p. 116.

14 See Macinnes, op. cit., p. 75; cf. Dodgshon, op. cit., pp. 21–7.

15 Allan I. Macinnes, 'Social mobility in medieval and early modern Scottish Gaeldom: the controvertible evidence', *Transactions of the Gaelic Society of Inverness*, LVIII, 1993–4, p. 400.

16 Devine, 'New élites', in *Clanship*, op. cit., p. 117.

17 A. Macinnes, *Clanship, Commerce and the House of Stuart, 1603–1788* (1991), p. 73.

18 Macinnes, *Clanship*, p. 210.

19 Dodgshon, op. cit., p. 94.

20 Ibid., p. 55.

21 See especially Leneman, *Atholl*, pp. 58–9 and Dodgshon, op. cit., p. 47.

22 See R.A. Dodgshon, 'West Highland and Hebridean settlement prior to crofting and the Clearances: a study in stability or change?' *Proc Soc Antq Scot* 123 (1993) pp. 419–38.

23 See Dodgshon, *Chiefs to Landlords*.

24 Dodgshon, op. cit., pp. 3–4, 27, 118.

25 Macinnes, *Clanship*, p. 210.

26 Ibid., pp. 211–2.

27 See Bob Harris, 'Patriotic commerce and national revival: The Free British Fishery Society and British politics, c.1749–58', *English Historical Review*, 114 (1999), pp. 285–313.

28 *The Letters of Sir Walter Scott*, edited by H.J.C. Grierson (1932) 3, p. 23.

29 See Harris, art. cit.

30 Macinnes, op. cit., pp. 228–32.

31 See A.J.G. Cummings, 'Industry and investment in the eighteenth century Highlands: the York Buildings Company of London', in A.J.G. Cummings and T.M. Devine, *Industry, Business and Society in Scotland since 1700* (Edinburgh, 1994).

32 Virginia Wills, 'The gentleman farmer and the annexed estates:

agrarian change in the Highlands in the second half of the 18th century', in T.M. Devine (ed.), *Lairds and Improvement in the Scotland of the Enlightenment* (Dundee, 1979).

33 See Devine, op. cit., p. 15, and Dodgshon, op. cit., pp. 47, 137, 240, 237, 239.

34 Dodgshon, op. cit.

35 Robert A. Dodgshon, 'Livestock production in the Scottish Highlands before and after the Clearances', *Rural History*, 9 (1998) pp. 19–42. See also review of Dodgshon, *From Chief to Landlords*, by Bangor-Jones, *Scottish Historical Review* (hereafter *SHR*) Vol. 79, 2000.

36 See R. H. Campbell and T. M. Devine, 'The rural experience' in *People and Society in Scotland. II 1830–1914*, edited by W. Hamish Fraser and R.J. Morris.

37 Dodgshon, ibid., p. 137.

38 Dodgshon, ibid., pp. 196, 244.

39 Robert A. Dodgshon, *From Chiefs*, p. 50.

40 Dodgshon, ibid., p. 319.

41 Campbell and Devine, 'The rural experience', p. 50.

42 Dodgshon, *From Chiefs*, p. 242.

43 On the early emigrations see Anthony W. Parker, *Scottish Highlanders in Colonial Georgia* (Athens, Georgia, 1997).

44 Cregeen, *Argyll Estate Instructions*, pp. xxvii i–xxix.

45 See R.E. Tyson, 'Contrasting regimes: population growth in Ireland and Scotland during the eighteenth century', in S.J. Connolly, R.A. Houston, R.J. Morris (eds.), *Conflict, Identity and Economic Development: Ireland and Scotland, 1600–1939* (Preston: Carnegie Publishing, 1995), pp. 64–76.

46 Macinnes, op. cit., p. 83.

47 Cregeen, *Argyll Estate Instructions*, pp. xxviii–xxix.

48 Quoted in Grant, *Everyday Life*, p. 98.

49 Anderson, *Hebrides*, pp. 168–9.

50 Macdonald, *General View of the Hebrides*, pp. 102–7.

51 See Peter Razzell, *Essays in English Population History* (1994).

4

Parallels and Precedents

I. Beginnings

THE HIGHLAND CLEARANCES BECAME a Scottish quarrel about the responsibility for the depopulation of the region. It has persisted for two centuries.[1] It is a quarrel from which current landowners and the modern descendants of the clearers wish to dissociate themselves. This must be a vain hope, but as the historian Herbert Butterfield observed:

> Studying the quarrels of an ancient day . . . [the historian] can at least seek to understand both parties to the struggle and he must want to understand them better than themselves; watching them entangled in the net of time and circumstances he can take pity on them – these men who perhaps had no pity for one another.[2]

The Scottish Highlands was part of a 'net of time and circumstances' which extended across Europe. Evictions and changing land use are universal elements in virtually every agrarian society. In the Highlands there was always a substantial turnover of tenantry, even on an annual basis, long before the introduction of sheep. The security of landholding in the old Highlands was possibly no greater than in the rest of the British Isles. In a detailed local study in the period 1735–66, R.A. Gailey found 'a minimum of forty-seven changes over a period of thirty-two years [which] cannot be explained solely in terms of normal family succession'.[3] Such shifting tenancies suggest that the people possessed a precarious relationship with the land. This insecurity was greatly intensified after 1750 under the impact of commercialisation and population growth, and the extension of cattle and sheep production, both of which tended to reduce the labour requirements in the Highland economy.

There were precedents within the Highlands for eviction and a sharper attitude to land usage, as we have seen. At Glen Lui, on the estate of the Earl of Mar in 1726, Lord Grange conducted an eviction to increase his deer stock which caused a reduction of population, and there was a less successful clearance attempted at Baddoch in 1733.[4] The Highlands were distinctive because a large number of small tenantry with tenuous rights occupied land from landlords: it was a true peasantry and differed from other parts of mainland Britain because the tenantry had not been rationalised into compact farms typical of England and central Scotland. In the Highlands there existed a greater legacy of feudalism hanging over into the eighteenth century – there was more catching up to be done: when the rural revolution arrived it was in a greater hurry than elsewhere.[5]

II. Parallels

Agrarian people, with or without the oppression of landlords, have been subject to shifting conditions throughout history. Peasantries are commonly ousted when the demands upon the land have changed beneath their feet. Some of the circumstances associated with the clearances were very particular to the Scottish Highlands: notably the conditions of clan decline, of political and social humiliation after the defeat of the Jacobite Rebellion, and especially the radiating effects of industrialisation of the British economy in the south. But some elements of the clearances were replicated in many other scenes of capitalist change which have usually included land hunger, overpopulation, landlordism, peasant recalcitrance, famine and the effects of modernising forces pitted against the remnants of a feudal system. Karl Marx was adamant that the Highland Clearances were the culmination of a general process which began in Britain in the fifteenth century, was accelerated by the Reformation, and reached its climax with the enclosures of the eighteenth century. First there was the 'Expropriation of the Agricultural Population from the Land', followed by 'Bloody Legislation against the Expropriated' and then the 'Genesis of the Capitalist Farmer'.[6]

Across the history of agrarian Europe there have been repeated shifts in the use of land, whereby the weaker have been pushed out by the stronger, under the influence of land hunger, technological change and market forces. Land use has been constantly restructured and one system substituted for another. Such changes sometimes took centuries: sometimes they occurred with cataclysmic violence. The Clearances are located towards the latter end of the spectrum of agrarian transformation.[7]

The greatest single force acting upon all European agriculture in the eighteenth century was the population upsurge which occurred over almost all of Europe about 1750. This demanded dramatic agrarian adjustments – in effect the widespread restructuring of agriculture across Europe in the following century. The unforeseen rise in population bewildered contemporaries, who were realistically afraid it would end in disastrous famine. In truth this might well have happened if new ways of increasing agricultural production and greatly expanding industry had not been discovered.[8]

The Scottish Highlands were located on the periphery of these epochal changes, caught in the demographic upsurge and faced with the ubiquitous pressures for agricultural, industrial and social change. The Highland experience was a regional variant of the European pattern. But there was a key difference: under the impact of population growth, cereal and dairy prices rose faster than meat prices throughout Europe after 1750, and almost everywhere there was a great expansion of labour-intensive arable production at the expense of pasture, and it was associated with the internal colonisation of much territory within Europe. From England to Spain, from East Friesland to Silesia, there was more extensive and intensive agricultural production under the pressure of population growth. The Irish case, so often especially relevant for comparison with the Scottish Highlands, witnessed the ploughing of pastures for both potato and wheat production. The pace and timing of the transition varied across Europe, but the consequences were remarkably uniform. The general switch to arable was only halted after Waterloo, when cereal prices fell and there was a reversion to pasture, even in England. Against these trends the Highland economy was an exceptional case: cattle and sheep farming expanded throughout the eighteenth century. The population growth was mainly accommodated by the intensive cultivation of potatoes on the margins of the region, and by increased dependence on meal imports into the region.

The second response of European agriculture to the pressures of the eighteenth century was in the widespread reorganisation of the tenurial basis of landholding. In other words the old peasantries, the old ways of holding land, and the old obligations between landlords and people, were transformed with remarkable speed across most of Europe. There was a rapid erosion of older types of communal agriculture. At the end of the eighteenth century

> each country began to develop its agriculture along individual lines . . . [for instance] in England the redistribution of the open fields, the enclosure and partition of the common lands; in France the confiscation of church property and the estates of the émigrés; in Germany the east German Gutszitz and the peasants' release from serfdom.[9]

The older feudal ways were in retreat all over Europe (even in Russia), and the Scottish Highlands were no exception. There can be no doubt about the direction of the transformation towards modern forms of individualistic occupation and use of land. This made Europe's ability to meet the inescapable challenge of unprecedented population growth much more effective, though it did not prevent appalling famines in Ireland and Russia. Mostly, though, it was a stunning achievement in the face of potential demographic disaster.

The liberalisation of agrarian structures was a two-edged sword. The Gordian knot of the old systems was severed and individuals were freed from ancient seigneurial obligations, even from serfdom itself. The release of individual energy and the emergence of individual freedoms were positive achievements for the evolution of modern Europe, but there was also the loss of the elements of protection in the paternalist framework of the older system and the social cohesion of a communal life. The benefits and losses, in terms of collective social welfare, depended upon measures of the oppression and benevolence in the old regimes in relation to the freedom and insecurity of the new. In some places the changes were resisted by the people, and in some rare cases the popular pressure forced the transformation into particular channels – for instance, the triumphs of peasant agriculture in France after the Revolution of 1789. In the Scottish Highlands the transformation mainly took the form of the clearances, and the ordinary Highlanders, as we shall see, expressed little other than revulsion from the entire process.

In the general European context the response of agriculture was partly contingent on the degree to which the old seigneurial grip on the land had been loosened. The decline of serfdom and other servile obligations did not prevent the proprietors from exercising 'the right to cream off a considerable sum in money payments from the peasants' production'. In many places, including the Scottish Highlands, the rights of the land users were extremely tenuous, and often useless against the legal power of the landlords. By contrast in Sweden and Norway peasant rights emerged with an extraordinary independence, into virtually absolute control of the land.[10]

Some parts of Europe, such as England and Prussia, pursued the full logic of consolidation and concentration of ownership and there emerged a pattern of large estates and great farms devoted to commercial farming. The termination of peasant farming was effectively completed. In France the peasantry successfully resisted much of the change and confirmed their hold on the land, often in a more individualistic form.[11] In Denmark the entire society was reorganised; the open-field system was terminated, feudal relationships were dissolved, the old village community was summarily destroyed and an individualist agriculture erected in its place but it eventually evolved towards co-operative arrangements which gained the advantages of both communal and individualist modes of production.[12] In reality, therefore, though there were universal forces demanding change in European agricultures after 1750, the responses varied significantly. The Highland experience was not entirely exceptional but the ousting of its resident peasantry was certainly one of the more aggravated versions of adjustment to be found in the litany of agrarian change.

III. British precursors

Within the British Isles the Highland Clearances were a particularly severe type of enclosure, one of the last and most turbulent acts in the transformation of British agriculture. In England there had been accelerated enclosure in the Tudor period when it was feared that the international division of labour would turn the entire country into a sheep walk. According to Thirsk, 'The ultimate stimulus was a rising population, compelling individuals and whole communities to devise more economical ways of using their land'. In pastoral areas, entire settlements were swept away. 'The deserted village,' said Maurice Beresford, 'is a sign of men changing their view of the most profitable use to which land could be put . . . It is the sign of a class of men who were able to pursue their own advantage to the point of the annihilation of communities.'[13] About three-quarters of England was already enclosed by 1760 and there was never much doubt that in commercial terms enclosure increased production greatly, though at considerable social cost to the community.

The second great round of English enclosures was concentrated in the 1760s and 1770s and during the Napoleonic Wars until about 1815, coinciding with the earlier sweeps of the Highland Clearances. It was the final decline of the small owners and occupiers, and the imposition of a highly concentrated pattern of landownership. In his classic indictment Marx speaks of the 'systematic robbery of the communal lands' of the people, and the creation of a large capitalist farming industry which, no less importantly, set free the agricultural population for the uses of modern manufacturing industry. Historical controversy over enclosures is far from extinct, and the condemnation of the English gentry is similar to the charges made against the clearing landlords of the Highlands. The elimination of the small landowner became a symbol of the social and human costs of the rise of industrial bourgeois capitalism. About six million acres of waste, commons and open fields were enclosed in this phase, much expedited by the employment of about 4000 enclosure Acts of Parliament, though much was accomplished by agreement. It was a final acceleration of the great drama of English rural change which had been in train for centuries.

The lowest strata of rural English society – the cottagers and squatters – lost most by enclosure. They lost residual rights of access to commons and waste land on which much of their existence had depended. The actual implementation of enclosure did not diminish the demand for labour, and the new agriculture required, in absolute terms, larger amounts of labour than before. The number of families engaged in agriculture continued to increase throughout the period of enclosure. The census figures, notwithstanding Cobbett's infamous disbelief, allow no doubt on this question. Of itself enclosure did not cause unemployment and depopulation. Much more fundamental in determining the parallel drift from the land and the creation of the urban and industrial proletariat was the demographic trend: there was, after 1750, a general increase of population which neither the old nor the new agriculture could accommodate. The evidence on this question is unequivocal; as J.D. Chambers put it, 'the effect of population growth in both open and closed villages was to create a surplus of rural labour that agriculture, although expanding, could not absorb; it was from this surplus that the industrial labour force grew.' Moreover, in terms of efficiency and the national economy, enclosures 'meant more food for the growing population, more land under cultivation and, on balance, more employment in the countryside; and enclosed farms provided the framework for the new advances of the nineteenth century'.[14]

The most potent cause of the decay of the small landholder was the collapse of cereal prices after 1813. Economic circumstances in agriculture deteriorated rapidly and the least efficient and competitive were unable to survive. It was general economic circumstances, rather than oppressive landlordism, that rang the death-knell of the small owner. The combined effects of rising population, the post-war depression in agriculture, and the higher wages in towns, induced the flight from the land after 1815. All of these adverse circumstances operated concurrently in the Scottish Highlands, a region much less favourably placed to retain its swollen numbers of people. Equally germane for the comparison with the Highlands was the response of the English smallholders to their relegation from so much of the land. It is now generally accepted that the enclosures were forced through against the will of the people but with relatively muted protest and little active or physical protest, though there may have been 'long wars of attrition' waged by the villagers of England.[15]

The Highland Clearances were an important regional variant of the enclosure movement and the associated changes in British agriculture. Clearances, however, were executed with fewer legal restraints. There was no bucolic umpire in the form of an Enclosure Commissioner: Highland landlords had much more absolute command over the land. The clearances represented the shifting of tenants rather than independent small proprietors. Left in the hands of unrestrained landlords, the change in land use, therefore, was much harsher than in England. There was no requirement for parliamentary approval or the co-operation of the tenantry. Where arable land was reorganised and extended, particularly on the fringes of the Highlands, the process bore many similarities to English enclosure, in terms of labour requirements, the extension of acreage and the creation of consolidated farms. But, mostly, the clearances were devoted to the advancement of pastoral farming, and the amount of arable production, in aggregate, may have declined. Sheep farming in the cleared territories required less labour, and this change exacerbated the impact of demographic forces. And although some resettlement provision was made on various estates, the clearances increased land hunger in the Highlands and accelerated the migration of the people.

IV. Uplands and Ireland

The clearances were also about regional differentiation within the British economy. This was new only in terms of its intensity at the end of the eighteenth century. The growth of inter-regional trade was related to a much enhanced articulation of regional comparative advantages. It was a course which had profoundly influenced the Scottish Highlands, first with the rise of the cattle trade by the end of the seventeenth century. At the other end of the island, on Dartmoor, a similar concentration on livestock output was prompted in association with a diminution of subsistence corn production.[16] No region in Britain was immune from these influences, and the adjustments in higher areas naturally bore greatest similarity to those in the Scottish Highlands.[17]

On the Scottish borders in Tudor times there were scenes which bring the clearances to mind: the conversion of arable to pasture, the emparking of estates and the eviction of tenants such as those of Sir Thomas Grey of Chillingham who 'expelled seventeen score men and women and children, all upon one day as the reports of the inhabitants have it'. The dispossession of runrig tenants in Berwickshire about 1739–40 heralded a stronger trend to consolidated farms and the loss of common rights: landlords replaced the old townships by model villages for the settlement of estate workers. The great sheep walks of the Cheviot Hills were also created at this time – saving labour, increasing profits and marked in long, straight, stone dykes.[18]

The Welsh uplands passed through bewilderingly rapid agrarian changes at the time of the clearances.[19] As in Scotland, it was the Welsh border counties which led the attack on the inefficiency of the old agriculture, and the period of greatest acceleration coincided with the Napoleonic Wars. The rising price of wool and greater demand for horses reinforced the pressure for more rational uses of the pastoral lands. Added to this, in A.H. Dodd's spirited phrases, was 'the growing prejudice among the governing classes against anything that savoured of communal ownership, and the almost idolatrous belief in the magic of private property (in the right hands, of course)'.[20] Acts of Parliament enclosed 200 000 acres of Wales during the wars, and large areas of mountain grazing became private property, enclosed by drystone walls. There were productivity benefits in the control of pasturing, but there was an over-expansion of capital expenditure which could not reap adequate returns in the post-war years. Labourers, cottagers and squatters suffered from the denial of cheap fuel and potato patches and by the loss of employment.

The elbowing aside of the resident population by powerful

Welsh landowners was very similar to the story in the Highlands. The main difference concerned the marginally restrictive character of the law as it applied to the Welsh landowner: his Scottish counterpart was even less restrained. The response of the Welsh by way of emigration, religious stoicism and sporadic violence, as we will see, bears a close resemblance to that of the common Highlanders during the clearances.

For the Scottish Highlands there was always a more powerful and immediate parallel to all the problems of landlordism, population pressure and social protest. In Ireland the tragedy of the peasant periphery was presented in the darkest colours; it was an awful warning to the rest of Britain but especially to the Scottish Highlands. Without modern industry, dependent on an inefficient, under-capitalised and precarious agriculture, and grossly overpopulated, Ireland was the antithesis of the economic development that occurred in southern Britain. Ricardo wrote: 'Ireland is an oppressed country – not oppressed by England, but by the aristocracy which rules with a rod of iron within it.'[21] Their reputation was in much the same league as that of the Highland lairds. But, in the judgement of R.D.C. Black, 'the majority of landlords were either careless of their obligations as proprietors, or so handicapped by encumbrances and settlements as to be unable to discharge their obligations'.[22] They were condemned for allowing the continuous sub-division of holdings, which was the basic cause of the ultimate demographic tragedy of the famine in 1846–7; they were also condemned for evicting the people and creating a capitalistic agriculture. But one of the key historical problems in Irish history is that of defining realistically the possible range of effective landlord action; short of making the land over to the people (which may have been an answer), it is difficult to imagine exactly what a landlord should have done in the circumstances of nineteenth-century Ireland.

Nor, of course, did parallels cease with the nineteenth century. At the end of the following century economies, even in Europe, still entered a painful transformation under the tyranny of market demands. Polish farmers in 1999 might have thought of the Highland experience, when Poland entered the European market and they were told that only 160 000 farms out of two million were likely to be able to cope with the competition. As one observer remarked, 'the prospect of restructuring looms like distant thunder' and the countryside was emptying.[23]

V. *Within Scotland*

There were parallels enough within Scotland itself; as we have seen, clearances of a sort were occurring in the Highlands before Culloden; clearances of another sort had been taking place in the Lowlands in advance of the northern events of the late eighteenth century. Everyone knows that Scottish landlords were equipped with stronger legal powers than elsewhere. An Act of the Scottish Parliament in 1555 'Anent the Warning of Tenants' governed the occupation of all land and was confirmed in 1707 and subsequently modified by the Court of Session in 1756. It permitted much easier and swifter removal of tenants in Scotland than elsewhere and it empowered local sheriffs too.[24]

Devine, in his account of the transition from peasant to capitalist agriculture in four Lowland counties, emphasises the radical character of these changes. In a short space of time there was a marked alteration of the rural social structure which accompanied a great improvement in productivity. Lowland agriculture quickly caught up with England. Devine insists that these changes constituted 'Lowland Clearances' in which the cottar populations were seriously diminished. Often the change was not registered, especially where it affected the cottars, who barely counted as official people on the estates. As Devine says 'the Lowland Clearances still await their historian' and the arguments used to dislodge and reduce the cottar populations ran parallel with those employed in the Highlands: 'The cottar structure was in conflict with the new economic order.'[25] Moreover the 'cottar clearances' induced little agrarian revolt partly because the transition took place in the context of rising living standards before 1790. This was a critical difference with the Highlands which also had no equivalent to the rapid increase in the employment opportunities in the Lowlands.[26]

Parallels and precursors of the Highland Clearances were not, therefore, scarce. We can accept the argument that clearances of a sort occurred in the Lowlands; we can accept the idea that there were earlier phases of clearances even within the Highlands. But it is still vital to register a distinction. There were indeed preparatory changes in the Highlands before 1780 and even before Culloden. But the events after 1770 were a marked acceleration. The velocity and scale of the clearances was greater and more dislocating than anything that had gone before. While the origins are deep, the cataclysmic character of the events that followed remains a defining quality of the Clearances.

From the 1770s a much greater sense of urgency fell upon the Highlands. It was mediated by price trends in cattle and other marketable commodities. The returns on Highland exports rose rapidly at the beginning of a very long period of inflation which affected all prices and, most sensitively, food and rents, until 1813. Tenants were now bidding up the cost of occupying the land; there was continuously increasing competition for the resources of the region. Opportunities and pressures built upon each other: in kelp production, and in fishing also, in cattle production, in linen, in arable farming, but most of all in sheep production. The great engine of change was the price of wool which outstripped even the inflation of all other indicators. Moreover, the rents of land in the Highlands, though rising, remained much cheaper than in the south. This created a continuing lure to southern flockmasters seeking farms in the Highlands. Sheep farmers were drawn north by the magnetic cheapness of grazing land. Soon sheep in the Highlands were being denounced in the same language they had attracted in England two centuries earlier: in 1787 they were described as 'a most devouring Animal to the Human Race'.[27]

It was a spontaneously rationalising process by which more production was being wrung out of the region in response to the greater demands being made upon it internally and externally. And upon this were the accumulating effects of the great population explosion described in the last chapter. It was a recipe for tension and dislocation.

The symptoms of this change were ubiquitous. It was captured in the experience on the very southerly margin of the Highlands, the island of Arran. Here the owner, the Duke of Hamilton, decided on a substantial reorganisation of his estates in line with the current impulses of improvement farming. As early as 1773 he made a direct effort to abolish communal farming throughout the island in favour of enclosed agriculture with increased rents. The process was intermittent but all in the same direction: by 1829 the entire island was converted, apart from a few spots in the north and north-west. Parts of the island were completely cleared in favour of sheep, notably at Glenree in 1825. Then, in 1829, the rest was cleared, including Glen Sannox, for sheep. At this point the transformation was accompanied by an offer from the landlord to pay half the fares of the displaced tenantry to Upper Canada, together with the offer of 100 acres of colonial land from the government. Eventually seventeen families took advantage of this offer.[28]

Landlords reorganised their small tenantry along modern lines across Scotland, very often without the involvement of sheep. In the Highlands these rearrangements usually required the initial removal of hundreds of small tenants prior to their resettlement. This process was indeed the genesis of crofting, designed to eliminate the old runrig system and replace it with individualised holdings in compact settlements – increasing arable cultivation and raising rents into the bargain. Such developments can be detected certainly as early as the 1760s and were part of the response not only to improvement advocacy but also to the pressure of population and the need to extend the production of food in the region. It was a form of intensive development, of internal colonisation. The boom in kelp gave it special impetus. In North Uist, for example, plans were made by Lord Macdonald in 1799 to alter the entire basis of the small tenantry on the estate, in a pattern already established in Skye. Execution was delayed until 1814, for fear of precipitating emigration.[29]

Such changes penetrated the rest of the Highlands, but the timing depended on local conditions and the determination of the landlord, though generally proceeding northwards. The attendant turmoil manifested itself in a thousand ways. There was widespread disquiet about the rise of rents and the displacement of tenants. There was some low-level resistance. An early expression of popular feeling against the clearances was caught in a Gaelic poem of Duncan Ban Macintyre who had been removed from Glenorchy in 1766 – entitled 'Orain nam Balgairean'.[30] Internal migration was almost certainly accelerated, though it seems to have been greatest from those Highland regions least affected by clearances. It is well known that most internal migration from the Highlands came from the more prosperous parts, and least from the poorest; moreover the rate of emigration did not correlate unambiguously with the districts of sheep clearance.[31] The role of internal migration was even more complicated.

VI. Emigration

Emigration was rarely a simple response to poverty and eviction, and often occurred where living standards were rising. In the Highlands most emigration occurred in a context of changing expectations, often in a mood of estrangement from the rack-renting lairds. It was most fundamentally a symptom of the intensifying competition for the landed resources of the Highlands. The outflow from the west Highlands to America was very early by general British standards; outflows certainly predated Culloden and many were undertaken in the teeth of landlord opposition. Emigration was flowing as early as the 1730s and 40s, including the substantial emigration from Islay in 1738–40.[32] Between 1735 and 1754 small groups of Highlanders, led by gentry, were taken to America as labourers. The best-known group, mostly from Inverness-shire, comprised 170 men, women and children who were engaged in founding a settlement called Darien, south of Savannah, designed to defend Georgia as a barrier against the Spaniards. More were recruited in 1737 and 1741 and they proved to be hardy soldiery, good for the frontier. Alexander Murdoch points out that the Highlanders were in a geographical position 'on the periphery of Europe [which] put them at the centre of the Atlantic world and on the cusp of European expansion overseas'.[33]

Some of the early tacksman-led emigrations from the west Highlands were undertaken in an attitude of defiance and anger against landlords and expressed many of the religious, social and economic tensions in the post-Culloden society. Writing to his cousin in March 1772, John Macdonald contemplated emigration with more than 200 kinsfolk to Prince Edward Island. He noted that Skye had 'given' 274 souls to Carolina after the last harvest. He remarked with some satisfaction that 'emigrations are likely to demolish the Highland Lairds'.[34] Macinnes suggests that such emigration was 'a community movement led by tacksmen whose managerial function was usurped by the Clearances'.[35] Emigrants left the west Highlands very often in family and group formation, mainly self-financed, often carrying away considerable capital and in defiance of their increasingly demanding landlords. They were not directly forced out of the Highlands, but rebelled at the growing pressures on their leases and their status. Others departed more conventionally as indentured labour, common in that phase of British emigration.[36] In the intervals between the wars the exodus swelled and almost 20 000 Highland Scots emigrated to Cape Breton Island alone from 1802 to the early 1840s.

There was a growing awareness of networks of Highlanders in America. The rising pressure on land in the Highlands effectively shifted the propensities to emigration between the years 1754 and 1769.[37] The attractions of America increased markedly, so that in 1772 it was said that Highlanders in North Carolina

> live as happy as princes, they have liberty & property & no excise, no dread of their being turned out of their lands by tyrants, each has as good a charter as a D[uke] of Argyll to a Sir A. Macdonald and only pay half a Crown for 100 Acres they possess, in Short I never saw a people seemed to me to be so happy as our Countrymen there.[38]

But the great privations in the famine of 1772 were decisive, especially in districts close to Drummond, Lochaber, Badenoch and Strathcarron. The expelling force of poverty and rising rents, representing not only seasonal failure but also pressure on landed resources, and was evidently translated into emigration.[39] Added to this was also a religious dimension in some of the west Highland emigrations; Catholics felt the chill of landlord discrimination to such a degree that people of this faith left for North America in disproportionately large numbers, often effectively well stimulated by emigration agents perambulating the Highlands before the end of the century.

The pressures all worked in the same direction to induce emigration. Landlords tried to staunch the exoduses: every effort was made to retain population and there was fear of departures, as in June 1773, when there was a reported 'infectious frenzie of Emigration' from the Lovat and Cromartie estates. It was regarded as a 'disease' which better seasons would eradicate.[40] It was the greatest claim of Archibald Lord Lovat that he had 'repressed emigration and preserved in his country' the common people of his estates, and his achievement was carved upon his tombstone.[41]

The fear of emigration among Highland landlords is indisputable and they went to great lengths to prevent it. For this was still a mercantilist age; rents were regarded as dependent on the size of the population and landlords measured their importance in terms of their 'followers'. But people left in worryingly large numbers. Some historians argue that the impetus came from below, from the people themselves, rather than the landlords.[42] This is a tricky distinction because it is clear that landlords were simultaneously bemoaning emigration while also causing conditions (including eviction and rent increases) which prompted emigration. The landlords often wanted both increased rentals and the retention of population and this contradiction was common until about 1815, after which few Highland landlords attempted to hinder emigration.[43] More than 10 000 Highlanders left for North America in the period 1770–1815.

Whether or not the émigré Highlanders were victims or adventurers, their role in North America was diverse. Some were regarded as the shock troops of the frontier, pioneering the roughest margins of European incursion and clearing out the indigenous population in advance of more refined colonial commercialisation. The Highland Scots, forced off their ancestral lands in Scotland, were now robbing the American Indians of their own ancestral lands.[44] The ironies of the story multiplied throughout the age of the clearances, which mainly began after 1780.

Notes

1 See Charles W.J. Withers, *Urban Highlanders* (1998), pp. 15–16.

2 H. Butterfield, *The Whig Interpretation of History* (London, 1959), p. 3.

3 R.A. Gailey, 'Mobility of tenants on a Highland estate in the early nineteenth century', *SHR* 40 (1961), p. 143.

4 See Adam Watson and Elizabeth Allan, 'Depopulation by Clearances and non-enforced emigration in the north east Highlands', *Northern Scotland* 10 (1990), pp. 32–4.

5 Compare Alun Howkins, 'Agrarian histories and agricultural revolutions', in William Lamont (ed.), *Historical Controversies and Historians*, (1998), pp. 88–90.

6 See G.E. Mingay, introduction to E.C.K.Gonner, *Common Land and Enclosure* (2nd edn., London, 1966), p. xxxvii.

7 See Richards, *History*, op cit., I.

8 Ibid., p. 216 et seq.

9 Ibid., p. 318 et seq; and see also Devine, *Clanship*, op cit. pp. 38–9.

10 A.S. Milward and S.B. Saul, *Economic Development*, pp. 43–7, 60.

11 Ibid., p. 253.

12 K. Skovgaard, 'Consolidation of agricultural land in Denmark', *International Journal of Agrarian Affairs*, vol.1, no.4 (1952), p. 10.

13 Maurice Beresford, *The Lost Villages of England* (London, 1954), p. 23.

14 J.D. Chambers and G.E. Mingay, *The Agricultural Revolution, 1750–1880* (London, 1966), Chapter 4.

15 See J. Neeson, *The Commoners*, pp. 262–3.

16 Crispin Gill (ed.), *Dartmoor: A New Study* (Newton Abbott, 1970), p. 154.

17 See Richards, *History*, op. cit.

18 John Talbot White, *The Scottish Border and Northumberland* (London, 1973), pp. 120, 128. Other cases are documented in Thomas Johnston, *The History of the Working Classes in Scotland* (Glasgow, 1922), pp. 186–7.

19 David Thomas, *Agriculture in Wales during the Napoleonic Wars* (Cardiff, 1963), p. 3.

20 A.H. Dodd, *The Industrial Revolution in North Wales* (2nd edn., Cardiff, 1951), p. 56.

21 Ibid., p. 23.

22 Ibid., p. 240.

23 Peter Finn, 'Polish farms face being plowed under', *Guardian Weekly*, 1 November, 1998.

84 *The Highland Clearances*

24 Devine, *Great Highland Famine*, pp. 140, 184–5, *Clanship*, op. cit., pp. 39–40, and Malcolm Bangor-Jones, *The Assynt Clearances*, p. 3.

25 T.M. Devine *The Transformation of Rural Scotland* (Edinburgh, 1994), p. 144, 165.

26 Ibid., p. 150 and especially Chapter 8.

27 Quoted in Alex Murdoch, 'Emigration from the Scottish Highlands to America in the eighteenth century', *British Journal of Eighteenth-Century Studies*, 21 (1998) p. 169.

28 See Ronald I.M. Black, 'An emigrant's letter in Arran Gaelic, 1834', *SS* 31 (1992–3), pp. 62–87.

29 See James B. Caird, 'The creation of crofts and new settlement patterns in the Highlands and Islands of Scotland', *Scottish Geographical Magazine*, 103 (1987), pp. 67–75.

30 In *Modern Scottish History: 1707 to the Present*, vol. 5., (Dundee, 1998) p. 103.

31 See T.M. Devine 'Highland migration to Lowland Scotland, 1760–1860', *SHR*, LXII pp. 137–49, and Charles W.J. Withers, 'Highland–Lowland, migration and the making of the crofting community, 1755–1891', *SGM* 103 (1987).

32 See *Day Book of Daniel Campbell of Shawfield 1767*, edited by Freda Ramsay (Aberdeen, 1991), p. 21. Alexander Murdoch, 'A Scottish document concerning emigration to North Carolina in 1772', *The North Carolina Historical Review*, LXVII (1990), p. 438.

33 Ibid., p. 163.

34 Quoted in Iain R. Mackay, 'Glenalladale's settlement, Prince Edward Island', *Scottish Gaelic Studies*, 10 (1963) p. 20.

35 Allan Macinnes, 'Scottish Gaeldom: the first phase of clearance', in *People and Society in Scotland I 1760–1830*, p. 79.

36 See Marianne McLean, 'The People of Glengarry: Highlanders in Transition, 1745–1820' (Montreal, *Rural History 1991*) and J.M. Bumsted, *The People's Clearance* (Edinburgh, 1982).

37 This is documented in Barbara De Wolfe (ed.), *Discoveries of America* (Cambridge 1997), especially pp. 36–7, and 134 fn.

38 Quoted in Alex Murdoch, 'Emigration from the Scottish Highlands to America in the eighteenth century', *British Journal of Eighteenth-Century Studies*, 21 (1998), p. 172.

39 See Kathleen Toomey, 'Emigration from the Scottish Catholic bounds 1770–1810 and the role of the clergy'. (D.Phil. thesis, Edinburgh University, 1991) passim.

40 Virginia Wills, 'The gentleman farmer and the annexed estates:

agrarian change in the Highlands in the second half of the 18th century', in T.M. Devine (ed.), *Lairds and Improvement in the Scotland of the Enlightenment* (Dundee, 1979).

41 Monica Clough, unpublished paper entitled 'Ornaments in the rude North', with permission of the author.

42 See especially J.M. Bumsted, *The People's Clearance* (Edinburgh, 1982), but see the opposing view by Cowan in Rae Fleming (ed.), *The Lochaber Emigrants to Glengarry* (Toronto, 1994), pp. 60–2.

43 See for instance, J.L. Campbell, *Songs Remembered*, p. 20 ff.

44 James Roderick MacDonald, 'Cultural retention and adaptation among the Highland Scots of North Carolina' (D. Phil. thesis, Edinburgh, 1991), p. 239.

The Quiet March of the Sheep

I. Conquerors

THE SHEEP CLEARANCES CAME to the Highlands in a series of waves from several directions, but mainly from the south. They began slowly in the sixth decade of the eighteenth century. At times, the movement ran fast and overwhelmingly, covering great stretches of the north, sweeping most animal and human life before it. In some parts the invasion was resisted for many years: some proprietors withstood the temptation of sheep rents and the common people placed various obstructions in the way of the advance of the sheep farmers. For a long time the far north, beyond the Great Glen, seemed too far away to be at risk. But eventually the movement spread across the Highlands, almost inexorably, and resistance collapsed. The eastern rim was more profitable for arable, and therefore the sheep were held at bay; elsewhere a few islands of the old life remained as eccentric survivals – such as the limestone districts of Elphin and Knockan in west Sutherland, and Coigach in Wester Ross. Virtually everywhere else the sheep conquered. The old economy was transformed under the pressure of the sheep empire. The human population of the Highlands was either displaced altogether, or else deposited on the very fringe of the land mass.

II. Southern models

The sheep clearances were a northern extension of the shift long occurring in the south. Southern Scots farmers had been following the English pattern of enclosure, urged on by their landlords to straighten their rigs, to consolidate and enlarge their fields and farms. Larger farms were carved out for fewer tenants and there was regular dispossession and eviction.[1]

Opposition to enclosure in Scotland, as in England, was slight. The anti-enclosure disturbances in Galloway in the 1720s were the only recorded case of actual resistance, but there was minor discontent in other parts of the south, though the usual attitude of the common people was sullen and stoical.[2] In 1740 Clerk of Penicuik, who had more trouble than most improving landlords, complained:

> Hitherto I have found that our Scotch tenants are so far from understanding and encouraging Inclosures that they take all the pains in the world to destroy them.[3]

Agricultural improvement came in many shapes; the extension of cattle and sheep production both caused evictions in many parts of Scotland and long before the Highland Clearances. In the 1680s several landowners in the Forest of Ettrick, being bankrupt, signed over their estates to Edinburgh lawyers who rationalised the management and land use. As Douglas Young has said, 'They were not interested in having lots of able-bodied men around to enlist in regiments; so they evicted them and their families, to consolidate the holdings for lucrative sheep farming.'[4] Sheep farming in the southern uplands was certainly disruptive and preceded the process in the Highlands by at least half a century. In 1772 General Alexander Mackay predicted without hesitation that the Highlands must follow the revolution in land use that had overtaken the 'south sheep country about sixty or seventy years ago'. He also asserted that those districts were 'now happy and wealthy' as a consequence of the changes.[5]

Before 1770 cattle caused the greatest dislocation. Fattened for the English market, Scots cattle needed enlarged pasture lands at the expense of arable, which in its turn required the engrossment of holdings and evictions. The effects were widespread. After Culloden the Commissioners of the Forfeited Estates implemented such evictions at Rannoch.[6] The creation of large grazing farms in the district of Cowal drove people towards the towns on the Clyde. It was very similar in West Perthshire and Dunbartonshire. The pressure of large-scale cattle and sheep production developed on the Duke of Argyll's estate before the mid-century. The human population of various parts of the southern Highlands declined between 1755 and 1790 in districts which, according to John Walker, were 'in a great part laid out into large grazing farms to black cattle, soon after the year 1755, and many tenants were turned out of their possessions'.[7] These changes, much ahead of the main phase of sheep farming in the Highlands, were little publicised and hardly at all recorded.

Swift or slow, the rationalisation of agriculture spread its tentacles across Scotland. The essential model entailed the reduction in the number of tenants and an increase in farm size. The key factor in Scotland was the insecurity of tenants, who normally possessed no legally established position on the land. 'The Scots tenant never acquired the right to the hereditary tenure of a farm similar to that enjoyed by some of his English counterparts under the copyhold system.' Hence, any adjustment of landholding in Scotland was at the discretion of the landlord and required minimal legal process; enclosure and rearrangement were 'purely an internal estate affair'.[8] And throughout the age of the clearances 'the majority of tenants moved without much fuss'.[9]

The *Old Statistical Account* of the 1790s was full of ministerial complaint about the decline of the rural population and the drift to the villages in many parts of Scotland. For the most part black cattle production was accommodated within the quasi-communal economy of the old Highlands, and the common people remained the main agents of production. This contrasted with the later expansion of sheep production in which the people participated hardly at all and were replaced by interloping sheep farmers, many from the south, as well as home-grown capitalists. During the expansion of cattle grazing there were cases of clearance. John Walker observed that many parishes of Dunbartonshire, Perth and Argyll were 'in a great part laid out into large grazing farms for black cattle, soon after the year 1755, and many tenants were turned out of their possessions'.[10] In Eddrachillis in north-west Sutherland in the 1780s, where population was thought to have declined, 'One of the causes of this decrease has been the rise that has happened in the price of black cattle, which gave occasion to some gentlemen, not residing in the parish, to take leases of extensive grazings in it, which they manage by a few servants', who, presumably acting under orders, removed the old occupants.[11] Thomas Garnett also testified to the impact of rising cattle prices upon the agrarian structure: rents were driven up to a point at which small tenants, no longer able to afford their lands, as on the island of Mull, turned increasingly to seasonal employment in the lowlands.[12] These generalised pressures sometimes took the form of outright eviction, such as that at Aberarder in 1770.[13]

Cattle were not the only culprits. Even in the Highlands there were clearances for arable production. James Anderson, writing in 1785, identified lairds in the act of consolidating the lands of small tenants into large farms, eliminating whisky distilling and ejecting their people.[14] In the eastern Highlands the process proceeded rapidly. At Kilmorack in Easter Ross the old communal system had given way to individual holdings: 'The letting of large tracts of land to single individuals has occasioned the banishment of many of them who, for many generations, possessed the soil'. These people spilled out mainly into the neighbouring village of Beauly.[15] On the estate of Mackenzie of Allangrange, also in Easter Ross, on the very fringe of the pastoral country, the owner succeeded to a small property of 700 Scots acres in 1773, when it was mainly in the hands of small tenants 'who laboured there under the old system'. All efforts to persuade and cajole them to use modern agricultural practice failed. Mackenzie, frustrated by this obstructive ignorance, decided to cut the knot, ejecting his tenantry (who found asylum in the same neighbourhood) invested his capital in the land, and introduced Berwickshire and East Lothian men to act respectively as grieve (farm overseer) and principal ploughman. His efforts reaped a rich reward: rents quadrupled and he became a model for good farming in the district.[16]

The Duke of Atholl in Perthshire inaugurated great changes in the 1750s. Moray, on the north-east fringe of the Highlands, saw rationalisation in a relatively early and complete form and developed a very efficient agriculture on good soils. At Monymusk the growth of capitalist farming was accompanied by the displacement of small tenants but also by an extension of the area under cultivation.[17] In the Cowal district of Argyllshire removals had already forced migration to the towns of the Clyde even by 1745.[18]

Rural change in most of Scotland was gradual. The new commercial farming system which emerged was marked by a concentration of the rural population into villages with the new status of proletariat. The employment of labour in agriculture, in aggregate terms, probably did not decline. The rapid growth of population permitted both an efflux to the southern towns, and stability of numbers in the rural community. The new arable agriculture employed more rather than less labour, even into the middle decades of the nineteenth century. Pastoral changes, especially in the Highlands, were to provide the opposite case; the people displaced by the sheep could not easily transfer to the distant new industrial centres. Thus the agrarian transformation caused very large numbers in the population to become virtually redundant, depending on the numbers displaced, the availability of alternative employment opportunities, and the scale of ongoing population growth in the district. The further the district was from industrialisation in Central Scotland, the greater was the problem of adjustment.[19]

The contest for use of the land – between arable, cattle, sheep and later sport – was keen. Nor should it be assumed that, even in the Highlands, pastoralism was universally triumphant. On the marches between the Highlands and the Lowlands, along the Moray Firth for instance, arable encroached upon the land traditionally devoted to animal culture. In the arable districts of Aberdeenshire, along the low country by the Moray Firth, and in Angus and Fife, cereal and cattle production expanded at the expense of local sheep farming, which quickly ceased to dominate. The sheep stock of Aberdeenshire declined from 600 000 to 100 000 between 1690 and 1810, and in one parish the number fell from 4500 in 1778 to 141 in 1809.[20] The triumph of the sheep was therefore not universal, and was strictly contingent upon geographical conditions. It was clearly part of the endless inter-regional adjustment of specialisation in British agriculture.

III. Sheep in the Highlands

The most obvious difference between the Highland Clearances and similar events in other parts of upland Britain was the rapidity and lateness of the changes in the extreme north. The clearances frequently required the immediate removal of entire communities of peasants from the land in an age in which the public conscience was becoming more responsive to allegations of inequity and cruelty. There was undoubtedly more drama and more concentrated human suffering in the Highland Clearances than in other forms of enclosure. The rapidity of the change also exacerbated the chronic problems of absorbing the people displaced by the clearing landlords.

The timing of the clearances was largely a matter of the relative fortunes of cattle and sheep production, connected to a lesser extent with the chronology of population change in the Highlands. Sheep surged northwards into the Highlands in the late eighteenth century at the moment when population pressure reached a new intensity.

The ultimate victory of the sheep required the displacement of much of the existing cattle economy as well as the interior farms which were indispensable for the wintering of sheep stock. In the mid-eighteenth century the cattle trade was in a vigorous condition, much stimulated by the appetite of the English market. Between 1707 and 1760 cattle prices doubled. After a brief decline, the increase continued. By the early 1790s, prices had doubled again, reaching an average of about £4 per head. The years of the Napoleonic Wars, 1793–1815, witnessed much faster inflation and there were reports of prices greater than £18 being taken in the last years before Waterloo.[21] Yet, although the demand for cattle continued to grow in this period, it accelerated less rapidly than the demand for sheep and wool. The Highland economy possessed far greater natural production potential for sheep than for cattle. This, of course, was the reason for the sheep clearances.

Prices of sheep and wool were relatively level from the 1750s to the 1770s. Thereafter an increase began, gentle at first and with one or two setbacks, which eventually merged into the sharp and dramatic increases of the 1790s and early 1800s. When trade with Spain was interrupted by war the price of wool shot up. In 1809 it already stood at twenty-five shillings a pound, yet had been a mere four shillings only a short time before. At their peak, during the opening two decades of the nineteenth century, price levels were anything from 250 to 400 per cent more than the levels recorded back in the 1770s and the early 1780s.[22] This was the engine of growth in the Highlands, the driving force behind the Clearances. The price of 'Highland wool' rose from fifteen per stone in 1801 to thirty-one shillings in 1815, and was forty shillings in 1818. Then came the fall: in the following five-year period wool prices shrank by a quarter and continued to slump into the 1830s. The price of sheep fell even more precipitously, in quite close concurrence with the trends in cattle prices.[23] This sharpened competition in the pastoral industry, weeded out the less efficient and added the urgency for yet more efficiency and clearance.

IV. Sheep breeds

The old native Highland sheep were of no use to capitalist sheep farmers: they were diminutive and 'dog-like' and yielded far less wool and mutton than southern breeds. In the old economy it was common practice for the native stock to be literally 'housed' overnight and to be nursed through the winter for fear of their starvation. The native Highland sheep were extraordinarily unshapely and small, and the yield of wool was derisory, though it was usually very fine and soft and much prized in the Aberdeenshire stocking manufacture (a declining industry by 1815), but not at all adaptable to the demands of Yorkshire woollen manufacturers. The native sheep were overrun first by the Blackface and then, from the 1790s, by the immense success of the Cheviot flocks. The defeat of the native breeds was greatly accelerated by the 'severe outbreaks of scab and liver rot in 1807, which swept away a very large proportion of the old sheep and also of the goats'.[24] To contemporaries they were almost a different species from the new-fangled breeds brought in from the south. Eventually, by 1820,

Inverness emerged as the great centre for sheep sales, the seasonal mecca for hard-bargaining mill-owners from Yorkshire who, no doubt, met their match in the new sheep-farming élite of the Highlands.

The growing flocks of Lintons and Cheviots pushed out the cattle, and placed demands on the sweet spots of old arable lands for winter feed. They were introduced at a time when population growth was accelerating, and into a region in which the people had little alternative resort apart from potato cultivation and the kelp shores. The triumph of the alien sheep in the Highlands is suggested by a series of estimates. Thus in Argyllshire there were 278 000 sheep in 1800, 827 000 by 1855 and just over a million by 1880. In Inverness there were about 50 000 in 1800, rising to 588 000 by 1855 and 700 000 in 1880. Caithness, only marginally a sheep county, possessed 12 700 in 1800 and 72 000 in 1855, rising to 91 000 by 1880. In Sutherland, the classic locus of the clearances, there were only 15 000 sheep grazed in 1811; nine years later, there were 130 000 on the hills of Sutherland, mainly Cheviots, and their number increased to 204 000 by 1855. In 1827 150 000 animals were sold at the Inverness Wool Market and five years later it was estimated that the Highlands annually exported 200 000 sheep. The crude numbers of sheep tell only part of the story since the output of wool and meat per sheep was also increased dramatically. It was a revolution on the uplands running in exact parallel with that achieved in the factories of the south.

Local and incoming sheep-farming entrepreneurs transformed the Highlands into a productive source of cheap wool and meat for the producers and consumers of the new industrial Britain. The success of the great sheep farmers indicates also the severity of the competition which faced the resident peasantry of the Highlands. The latter could not compete with the capital-intensive, scientific, highly calculating sheep farmers, sensitive to all the economies of scale, to movements in the market prices, able to pare costs to a minimum and to call on credit and plan a cycle of production which stretched over half a decade. It was industrialised agriculture with all its benefits – and all its costs.

V. The power of the landlords

The victory of the sheep required the sanction of the landlord. He, and sometimes she, stood between the sheep farmers and the old society; the landlord faced the moral and economic dilemma ultimately controlling the resources of the Highlands. Sir John Sinclair famously described the extraordinary powers of his own class:

> In no country in Europe are the rights of proprietors so well defined, and so carefully protected, as in Scotland.

In Scotland the registration of landholdings was especially well organised and gave security to the title and conveyance of property unrivalled in the rest of Europe.

In every way, except in the collective psychology of the common people, the Highlands were ripe for development: 'To colonise at home' was Sinclair's clarion call.[25] Landlord power was demonstrated in its most naked form in the Highlands; it was something which exercised the mind of Sir Walter Scott. He recalled a childhood memory of accompanying his father, a Writer to the Signet, to a clearance in the Highlands, probably in the mid-1780s:

> It was his allotted task of enforcing the execution of a legal instrument against some MacLarens, refractory tenants of Stewart of Appin . . . An escort of a sergeant and six men was obtained from a Highland regiment lying in Stirling, and the author, then a writer's apprentice, equivalent to the honourable situation of an attorney's clerk, was invested with the superintendence of the expedition, with directions to see that the messenger discharged his duty fully, and that the gallant sergeant did not exceed his part by committing violence or plunder. And thus it happened, oddly enough, that the author first entered the romantic scenery of Loch Katrine, of which he may perhaps say he has somewhat extended the reputation, riding in all dignity of danger, with a front and rear guard, and loaded arms . . . We experienced no interruption whatever, and when we came to Invernenty, found the house deserted. We took up our quarters for the night, and used some of the victuals which we found there. The MacLarens, who probably had never thought of any serious opposition, went to America, where,

having had some slight share in removing them from their *paupera regna*, I sincerely hope they prospered.[26]

Similar scenes were re-enacted across the Highlands throughout the following half century, doubtless accompanied by similarly optimistic and sentimental hope on behalf of the displaced victims of the devastating agrarian transformation.

VI. *Rents and the turnover of ownership*

Rents rose wonderfully. On the Locheil estates in Lochaber, even without improvement investment by the landlord, rents doubled between 1755 and 1788. The Dunvegan rental on Skye also doubled between 1754 and 1769, while the rents of Skye trebled in the third quarter of the century. In North Uist the increase was from £1200 in 1703 to £1800 in 1771, and to £2100 in 1794. Torridon in Wester Ross increased tenfold from 1777 to 1805. On the Argyll estate income trebled in the first seventy years of the eighteenth century. Sometimes it appears that the rent increases were delayed until the last quarter of the century, and then accelerated very rapidly, usually in association with sheep farming.[27] In 1837 the *Inverness Courier* registered some of this inflation in rents. Since 1760 rental income in Argyllshire had increased from £20 000 to £192 000; on the Chisholm Estate since 1783 rents rose from £700 to £5000; between 1787 and 1837 the Glengarry Estate rental grew from £800 to £7000; and the Orkney Islands which yielded £19 000 in 1791 were now worth £70 000 per annum. The improved rental incomes were also reflected in capital values, and were shown by land sales. The Castlehill Estate fetched £8000 in 1799 and £80 000 in 1804. The Glenelg Estate was worth £30 000 in 1798 and £82 000 in 1824; while the Redcastle Estate sold for £25 000 in 1790 and for £135 000 in 1824.[28] Many of these increases were in advance of the sheep clearances though these eventually caused the most powerful propulsion.

One of the paradoxes of Highland landownership in the late eighteenth century and beyond was the accumulation of debt in so many families despite the rise of commodity prices and real income. Debt was a great spur to changes because clearances yielded a much higher rent. Thus the Gordon Estates in Aberdeenshire experienced very early changes, given urgency by the accumulation of family debts. By the 1770s the Gordon debts increased further as the consequence of competitive building and swelling political expenses. The Chamberlain complained in 1774: 'I do not see the possibility of raising money here to support the rate of expense that has been going on these two or three years past in buildings, politics and other articles.'[29] These kinds of strain upon landlord finances became general, and provided a powerful motive for agricultural rationalisation and for opportunistic marriages into southern wealth. Landlord obligations, in terms of consumption and the provision for large numbers of relatives, swallowed rental income and caused widespread indebtedness, even where incomes were rising. It was an age of landlord insolvency. In the county of Argyll, the 200 proprietors of the middle of the eighteenth century had dwindled to 156 by the end of it. Debts were usually connected with a more extravagant living style.[30] Yet the rewards to landlords, often with very little infusion of their own capital, were extraordinarily lucrative. Rents rose splendidly, but so did outgoings. In between were caught the small tenantry all across the Highlands.

VII. The progress of the sheep

The imperial march of the Blackfaced sheep penetrated the Highland line in mid-century. Their progression was summarised fifty years later thus:

> The change of system began in Inverness-shire about 1764 – its progress was slow – it proceeded afterwards more quickly in the Perthshire highlands and the mountainous districts overhanging the plains and glens of the Counties of Forfar, Aberdeen and Moray. The districts of Breadalbane, of Atholl, of the Gordons and of the Grants came next . . . In all these instances the demand for labour in the great towns, absorbed the population that had to look for other homes. In

Badenoch it is believed it met with some resistance. Thus further north, the facilities enjoyed in the South in disposing of the surplus population being wanting, emigration to America became the recourse. The MacDonald Clan made, it is believed, the first and most united move of the kind.

Sir George Mackenzie, a particularly robust improver amongst Ross-shire proprietors, claimed that 'the advantages of sheep farming, since it has been fairly established, have never been denied, and we have heard but a few feeble voices exclaim against the necessity of removing the former possessors, to make way for shepherds'.[31] Sir John Lockhart Ross of Balnagowan in Easter Ross, retired from the Army and threw himself into the improvement of his estate and identified the great potential of sheep farming in the northern Highlands. He became a great experimenter and advocate of the Blackfaced sheep, already at large in Perthshire to the south, where they had already proved more profitable than the resident black cattle.

As soon as the 'natives" leases ran out Ross removed the local tenantry to set up a sheep farm and hired shepherds to start the work, despite the opposition of the resident people. This experiment began, apparently, in the early 1770s, but in 1781–2 Ross gave over his sheep farms to a Mr Geddes from Tummel Bridge in Perthshire, 'a very sensible sagacious man, who understood the business thoroughly' and persevered against substantial opposition. Mackenzie claimed that 'Mr Geddes was the first sheep farmer who settled in the north of Scotland.' Soon after an Ayrshire farmer named Mitchell settled on the estate of Davidson of Tulloch on the west coast, and another trial was made by a Fort William man, Cameron, on the Culcairn estate.[32]

Ross at Balnagowan was an important local stimulant to a movement which began considerably earlier and owed most of its impetus, in the first instance, to men from Annandale in Dumfriesshire, and from the hill zones of Ayrshire, probably in the late 1750s. These were the border sheep farmers, men of enterprise and capital who, in a great northern thrust, sought cheaper lands for their sheep. They were in a literal search for new pastures and, as far as they were concerned, the Highlands were virgin territory.

Soon they could easily outbid the rents paid by local occupiers; the incomers were eager for such cheap lands; the landlords were thrilled by the higher rents.

Claims for precedence were also advanced on behalf of John Campbell of Lagwine, a native of New Cumnock in Ayrshire. Campbell had first moved north 'about the year 1747' to Dunbarton, where he introduced Blackfaced sheep in the region of Glen Matlock in the parish of Luss, on the banks of Loch Lomond.[33] Another account said that he began his career in the north as an inn-keeper, at Tyndrum, and there discovered that sheep could exist in the Highlands without being housed overnight. Campbell was described as

> a most singular, but honest character, who certainly was the first who banished cattle from the west Highland areas, and supplied their place with Blackfaced moor-sheep from his native place; and that, too, at a very considerable extent.

He had owned an estate in Ayrshire (which he subsequently sold for £30 000) and farmed sheep in the same district. A series of bad years in mid-century had ruined his sheep farming operations and he had become bankrupt. After this disaster in 1755 and 1756, he migrated to the west Highlands and leased a farm on the Ardkinlass estate at the head of Loch Fyne in Argyllshire. According to his enthusiastic advocate:

> He stocked it with stock or cast ewes from his own country; and such was the aptitude of those hills for sheep, that he said they *sprang an inch in an hour* after going there.

Thereafter Campbell leased other farms in Argyllshire, and the rents of these lands trebled over their previous levels under black cattle. Moreover the Ayrshire man spread his knowledge 'of the wonderful cheapness of lands in the Highlands when stocked with sheep'; he apparently proselytised across south-west Scotland, and initiated a flow of southern sheep farmers in quest of lucrative bargains in the Highlands. It was a trend which persuaded northern landlords to lever up their rents, which displeased Campbell, 'the father of the system', to the point at which he began to speak ill of the Highland proprietors. Campbell, a rough diamond, 'uncouth in appearance and conversation', was 'the first to demonstrate the true pastoral capabilities of the north'.[34]

Campbell had been at the vanguard of the movement of Blackfaced sheep beyond the Highland line. He was the link connecting Ayrshire with Perthshire and Argyll by way of Dunbarton. Moreover, by 1792 he was farming sheep on the borders of Ross and Sutherland; some of them were rustled during the famous insurrection of that year.[35] Southern expertise was evidently crucial and close on the heels of Campbell came a group of farmers from Annandale in Dumfries-shire who, in 1762, took leases of lands in Perthshire and Dunbartonshire, adjoining the Highlands. After that there was an increasing flow of settlers from the border areas to the north – from Clydesdale, Nithsdale and Tweeddale, and eventually from the most northerly parts of England too.[36] The minister of Kilmonwray and Kilmalie in western Inverness-shire recorded that commercial sheep farming reached his parish in 1764 and by 1796 had taken over three-quarters of the lands, exporting wool by coast to Liverpool and other English ports.[37] Meantime the value of the land had been tripled in the process.[38] The movement north seems to have been uneven: Perthshire and Inverness-shire were invaded only after 1770.

VIII. The empire of sheep extended

From the 1770s the catalogue of rural transformation lengthened and widened. At that time, in Aberfoyle, Perthshire, almost all the upper part of the parish was converted to sheep farms.[39] At the same time, at Aberarder near Loch Laggan some eighty tenants were cleared off their lands to make way for sheep farming.[40] At Blair Atholl it was claimed that the coming of the sheep had caused the reduction of the status of cottagers to the extent that some emigrated to the towns and to America.[41] At Fortingall the changes had been foreshadowed by rearrangements instituted by the Forfeited Estates Commissioners in the years after 1754 and clearances had reduced the population; at Mauchlin, the entire

Glenfernat had been denuded of its inhabitants, perhaps twenty families, to make way for the sheep.[42] In this decade a farmer named John Stewart was breeding sheep on an experimental basis near Ballachulish (Fort William); George Culley commented: 'The kind they have been recommended to are the Blackfaced or Short Sheep, a kind perhaps of all others best adapted to live upon a mountainous exposed country like this.'[43] In the parish of Morvern in Argyll sheep farming was promoted by the larger tacksmen during the 1770s. In this instance however the landlord was hesitant about the wholesale conversion to sheep and chose to delay evictions for several decades – but by 1815 the Morvern clearances had been achieved and most of the common people were engaged in working arable strips on the periphery of the new sheep farms.[44]

The rapidity of the advance varied, and large areas remained untouched, even in the southern Highlands, into the second quarter of the nineteenth century. In 1794 less than two-fifths of the arable land of Perthshire had been enclosed. The number of Blackfaced sheep had increased rapidly in that county without, according to the agricultural reporter, any reduction in cattle numbers. Yet in Perthshire, despite the capacity of its improved arable farming to absorb population, it is clear that the new pastoralism caused a substantial dislodgement of the population. The famous and successful improvements by Lord Kames on the mosslands at Blair Drummond in the far south of the county were undertaken expressly to accommodate Highlanders from the interior; the great project had begun in 1766 and continued into the 1780s. By 1811 about 400 acres of low-lying land had been recovered and 'settled by a number of families of industrious Highlanders'.[45]

It was during the 1780s that clearances occurred on a new scale, and with a suddenness which began to cause widespread public disquiet. In 1783 Thomas Gillespie, another southerner, rented a sheep farm in Glenquoich from Macdonnell of Glengarry, and two years later there were reports of the first great clearances on Glengarry's estates. These changes apparently provoked a substantial migration (perhaps 300 people) from Knoydart to Canada. At the time, it was said that:

These people, when once they settle in Canada, will encourage others, as they are now encouraged by some friends before them. They will form a chain of emigration. It is thought the country will be converted into a sheep walk. Should this grow general, and our gallant Highlanders desert us, I fear all the sheep that can be introduced and reared will form in their stead but a sorry defence against our enemies.[46]

The return of estates forfeited after Culloden to their original owners in the 1780s added to the increasing fluidity of landownership at this time. The land market was active to an unprecedented degree, which itself was a mark of the commercialism that had taken a grip on the Highlands by this time.

Although Sutherland did not enter the empire of the sheep for two more decades, there was a small experiment conducted on the estate of the Countess of Sutherland in 1787, which again involved the introduction of southern shepherds.[47] Some landlords gave thought to the idea of direct sheep farming, without the intermediary of a tenantry. In virtually every case they came to realise the actual difficulties resulting from their lack of capital, business sense and managerial ability. Most were neither willing nor able to entertain the risks involved in sheep farming. The failure of a number of landowners in the role of entrepreneur also undermines the credibility of the claim that the resident peasantry could have managed the new sheep farms on a co-operative basis.

The pressures for sheep farming were mounting in the 1780s. Some landowners came to a compromise: at Glenshiel in 1786 the landlord was offered treble the rent of a farm. This he refused, but re-let it to the current occupiers at a small increase.[48] Even where the sheep were held back, they exerted an inflationary influence on rents.

The ultimate victory of the Cheviot breed owed much to the propagandist energy of Sir John Sinclair: he convinced the world of the superior quality and higher value of Cheviot wool. By 1808 the Cheviots had made great progress. It was stated that 'Stocks of Cheviot sheep are gaining ground, because their wool is much finer, and their carcase equally large with the Linton breed'.[49] Sinclair, himself an experimenter in sheep breeding, was at the vanguard of the ovine revolution. He believed that 'under sheep, the Highlands would be six, if not ten times more valuable than under cattle if proper breeds were introduced'.[50] Nor was the improvement merely a matter of wool; he believed that under sheep the north could produce three times as much meat as under cattle.[51] Sinclair was not satisfied with these sensational increases in productivity and hoped for even further advances from the introduction of the Merino breed into the Highlands. He started three flocks on his estate in Caithness and even as late as 1821 continued to entertain extravagant expectations. He told a kinsman, 'I shall bring north with me a Flock of the finest Spanish sheep in Europe, which I hope will be the means of doubling the value of all our Estates in the lower part of Caithness.'[52] But though the Merino revolutionised output in other parts of the world, it did not succeed in the Highlands. Conditions were too wet, and lameness affected them to a severe degree. At one point Sinclair equipped his entire flock of Merinos with leather boots.[53] In the event the Cheviot was the great carrier of productivity gains in the north: the new sheep represented a technological change in no less a sense than the great mechanical changes in contemporary industry.

Within the Highlands there developed a pattern of intra-regional specialisation. In the eastern foothills, for instance, in North Angus and Kincardine, much of the land was used as grazing for wethers rather than the Cheviot ewes. In southern Aberdeenshire cattle production expanded and consequently pushed sheep into the hillier parts.[54] In Sutherland some of the south-eastern lowlands were devoted to the production of winter feed for the sheep of the interior. There were local factors which affected the progression of sheep into certain districts. Some landlords who had access to profits made in the army or in the colonies or India, sometimes ploughed their new capital into improvements which included sheep farming. Munro of Novar acquired a large fortune in the service of the East India Company and invested a great deal of it in his estate in Easter Ross, determined to reconstruct the local economy. The Macleods of Skye amassed spoils in India to the tune of £100 000 but much of this was frittered away with little advantage to the isle of Skye.[55] Others believed that the devastating famine of the year of 1782 gave a great impulse to the substitution

of sheep for black cattle, especially in Ross-shire.[56] A later commen-
tator described the general consequences of the famine in Ross-shire:

> Many emigrated to America, many placed themselves in Sutherland,
> but the kelp manufacture came to the temporary relief of the coastal
> population, though it has since fallen a sacrifice to the progress of
> modern science, aggravating greatly the sufferings of the people in the
> long run.

In Sutherland there were still sceptics among the landlords and
their agents. Some openly asserted that the social consequences
were too great to justify the change to sheep: the people would be
'extirpated' and the country de-populated and a danger to the
security of the realm. The march of the sheep continued, rarely
checked by this time. The 1790s witnessed a clear acceleration of
sheep farming, now in the shape of the Cheviot, into Ross, into the
smaller estates of Sutherland, and into Caithness on a considerable
scale. By 1792 many parts of the Highlands were being advertised
as good territory for sheep. For instance 13 000 acres in Kintyre in
southern Argyll were offered as good grazing; moreover, as the
landlord put the matter, a 'Stranger in good circumstances will
meet with encouragement'. The Monar Forest in Ross was
available, 'supposed to be able to pasture 8000 sheep', according to
its advertiser.[57] In 1792 Lord Armadale placed his tenants on the
shores of the Pentland Firth; some passed into Caithness. The hills
were stocked with sheep. In 1800 Lord Reay's country followed the
same course – some of the old tenants went to America. The
Bighouse estate did the same: 'The hills were stocked with *Cheviot*
sheep.' Soon after, the greatest of the Highland estates, that of the
Countess of Sutherland, pushed forward a series of great clearances
which were not completed until 1821. By then the sheep farmers
included men from both sides of the border with England as well as
a group of local men who transformed themselves out of the old
tacksman class into the new pastoral élite.

The sheer magnitude of operations disqualified all but men of
great capital. The two sheep farmers who pioneered sheep farming
in Sutherland, Messrs Atkinson and Marshall from Alnwick in
Northumberland, spent £20 000 on stock to inhabit their new

leases in the Highlands. Such sums were beyond the reach of most local farmers. Hugh Rose, a northern agriculturalist, remarked in 1795 that 'No mode of farming requires a greater capital to set it going properly'.[58]

IX. Local sheep farmers

The idea that the Highland revolution was exclusively the work of outside sheep farming entrepreneurs has been undermined by recent research. It is now abundantly clear that Highlanders were heavily implicated in the sheep-farming revolution and that they have been denied their proper responsibility. Tacksmen and drovers entered the sheep trade and a cadre of Gaelic speakers such as Donald Macdonald of Tulloch in Brae Lochaber in the 1780s successfully infiltrated the higher reaches of finance and trade in wool and its production. Allan Cameron of Invercaddle on the west side of Loch Linnhe was a successful sheep farmer in 1810 and worth £6000. Alexander Macdonald of Glencoe, who held great tracts of land from the Duke of Gordon, McIntosh and Glengarry, was probably the greatest Highland sheep farmer at the turn of the century. He began on his own lands and then borrowed large sums and leased land in three counties. At the time of his death in 1814 his borrowings alone amounted to £8000. Indeed many of the great new sheep farmers were Highlanders and were clearers in their own right: Glenstrathfarrar for instance was cleared by Highlanders. According to a recent analyst, much of this record was suppressed in the well-known antiquarian work of Charles Fraser-Mackintosh.[59]

One of the great flockmasters was Cameron of Corrychoillie in Lochaber, born the son of a poor crofter. He was a drover who accumulated stock and then set up independently; displaying great talent for organisation, he soon became the greatest sheep farmer in the north with 60 000 sheep and eleven farms.[60] In Sutherland, when the sheep revolution eventually triumphed, more than half of the grazing leases were held by Sutherlanders, though the most renowned were from the south. Landowners varied widely in their response to the challenge of the sheep: some of the most traditionally minded of the lairds became muscular clearers; some of them refrained; there was no covering rule.[61]

The rigour of competition for land was obvious – the repeated bursts of emigration and the growing popular agitation against sheep (leading to a climax in 1792) were unequivocal symptoms. After 1815, when wool prices slumped, the economic desirability of further expansion of the sheep economy became less obvious. In the event growth continued because the comparative advantage of sheep continued to apply despite the changed price horizons. However, in the new phase, the economics of sheep farming became interlocked with the economics of overpopulation and of sectoral decline in other parts of the regional economy. Thus, despite the precipitate decline of wool prices, the sheep maintained pressure on the landed resources (and therefore also on the human population) of the Highlands.

X. Beyond the Great Glen

The passage of the Cheviot across the Great Glen was a great symbolic moment in the history of sheep farming. Sullen disgust with the changes had occasionally broken surface in spasms of resistance in the 1780s. In 1792 resistance to the spread of sheep into the northern Highlands was brought to a head in a remarkable, concerted confrontation in Ross-shire.

During the 1790s there were many reports of evictions. J.L. Buchanan in 1793 mentioned the removal of 'several hundred souls', for the sake of sheep, in South Uist and Canna.[62] In that same year Francis Humberston Mackenzie advertised the whole parish of Uig in Lewis as a sheep farm, and in 1796 358 summonses of removal were issued by him;[63] over the period 1780–1832 he issued 2300 summonses of removal. Colonel Macleod of Macleod undertook reorganisation and removal on a similar scale also in the '90s.[64] In 1794 Alexander Macdonnell of Glengarry, whose estate had already taken a flying start into sheep farming, had no compunction about evicting any small tenants who refused to enlist for him: 'I have fully determined to warn them out, and turn them off my property, without loss of time'.[65]

At much the same time southern breeds of sheep had been introduced into central areas of Inverness-shire, notably in Kingussie and Laggan. By 1793 the sheep system was in evidence at Fodderty in Easter Ross and in Lochbroom in the extreme west of the same county. At Banff in 1794 there was already a selection of southern breeds familiar to the stock farmers.[66] Throughout the decade many landlords were contemplating plans for clearances, most notably on the great Sutherland estate: schemes were being concocted for the planned introduction of new economic structures in many places. It seems very likely that the recruitment of regiments, and the highly visible success of kelp, helped to create an atmosphere favourable to radical reorganisation. Thomas Garnett reported that many of the people displaced by sheep in the counties of Argyll, Inverness and Caithness had migrated south to the lowlands, and some had found their way to New Lanark, where they were welcomed into the arms of the managers of the celebrated milltown.[67]

The central Highlands, in the early 1790s, were passing into the rigours of wholesale rural transformation. The turmoil overwhelmed the lives of thousands of small tenantry, yet most of it occurred with only minor commentary and little audible resistance. In 1792, and quite suddenly, the community of the peasantry erupted into resistance and called for the march of the sheep to be reversed. It was the year of crisis for the ovine revolution.

Notes

1 M. Gray, 'Scottish emigration: the social impact of agrarian change in the rural Lowlands, 1775–1875', *Perspectives in American History* 7 (1973), pp. 95–174.

2 See 'Ayrshire at the time of Burns', in Ayrshire Archaeological and Natural History Society, *Collections*, no. 5 (Kilmarnock, 1959).

3 Henry Hamilton, *The Industrial Revolution in Scotland*, (Oxford, 1932), p. 41.

4 Douglas Young, *Scotland* (London, 1971), p. 172.

5 William Macgill, *Old Ross-Shire and Scotland* (2 vols., Inverness, 1909–11), vol. 1, p. 158.

6 Alexander Stewart, *A Highland Parish or the History Of Fortingall* (Glasgow, 1928), p. 179. See also Devine, *Clanship*, op. cit., pp. 35–6.

7 Walker, *Economical History*, vol. II, pp. 399, 404.

8 Robert A. Dodgshon, 'The removal of runrig in Roxburghshire and Berwickshire, 1680–1766', *SS*, vol. 16 (1974).

9 Bangor-Jones, op. cit., p. 3.

10 Walker, *Economical History*, vol. 11, p. 404.

11 *Old Statistical Account*, vol. IV, p. 281.

12 Garnett, *Tour*, p. 164.

13 Fraser-Mackintosh, *Letters*, pp. 272–6.

14 Anderson, *Hebrides*, p. 278.

15 *New Statistical Account*, vol. XV, p. 307.

16 Mackenzie, *General View Of Ross*, pp. 86–92.

17 Ibid., p. 83.

18 Ibid.

19 I.F. Grant, 'The social effects of the agricultural reforms and enclosure movement in Aberdeenshire', *Economic History*, vol. 1 (1926), pp. 89–116.

20 Watson, 'Sheep industry', pp. 5–6. See also R.M. Hartwell, 'A revolution in the character and destiny of British wool', in N.B. Harte and K.G. Ponting (eds.), *Textile History and Economic History* (Manchester, 1973).

21 A.R.B. Haldane, *The Drove Roads of Scotland* (Edinburgh, 1968), pp. 56–61, 204–7; Dairiad, *The Crofter*, p. 63; Campbell, *Scotland Since 1707*, p. 35; Cregeen, 'Tacksmen', appendix.

22 Robert A. Dodgshon, 'The economics of sheep farming in the southern uplands during the age of improvement, 1750–1833', *EHR*, vol. XXIX (1976), p. 552.

23 *Inverness Journal*, 17 February. 1809; James Bischoff, *A Comprehensive History of the Woollen and Worsted Manufactures* (2 vols., London, 1842), vol. 11, pp. 330, 406, and Tables II and VI; William Singer, 'On the introduction of sheepfarming into the highlands', *Transactions of the Royal Highland and Agricultural Society of Scotland*, 1st series, vol. II (1807); J.A. Symon, *Scottish Farming, Past and Present* (Edinburgh, 1959), p. 276; Teignmouth, *Sketches*, vol. 1, p. 129.

24 J.A.S. Watson, 'The rise and development of the sheep industry in the Highlands, *THAS* 5th. 44 (1932); see also W.J. Carlyle, 'The changing distribution of breeds of sheep in Scotland, 1795–1956', *Agricultural History Review*, vol. 27 (1979), pp. 19–23; cf. Macinnes, *Gaeldom*, p. 83.

25 Sir John Sinclair, *General Report of the Agricultural State and Political Circumstances Of Scotland* (Edinburgh, 1814), pp. 115–21.

26 J.G. Lockhart, *Memoirs of the Life of Sir Walter Scott* (7 vols. 1837), vol. 1, pp. 142–3.

27 Somerled MacMillan, *Bygone Lochaber* (Glasgow, 1971), p. 176; SRO, GD 221/54, John Macpherson to John Campbell, 24 June 1816; Leigh, 'Crofting Problem', p. 10; *The Topographical, Statistical And Historical Gazetteer of Scotland* (2 vols., Edinburgh,1844), vol. I, p. 793.

28 T. Barron, *The Northern Highlands in the Nineteenth Century* (3 vols., Inverness, 1907–13), 2 June 1837.

29 Gaffney, *Lordship of Strathavon*, p. 150.

30 See Cregeen, *Argyll Estate Instructions*, p. xi.

31 pp. 125–6.

32 Ibid.

33 David Ore, *General View of the Agriculture of the County of Dunbarton* (London, 1794), p. 63.

34 'On the sheep husbandry of the west Highlands; with some Accounts of Mr Campbell, who first introduced sheep into these districts', *Farmers' Magazine*, vol. XII (1811), pp. 25–7.

35 See Chapter 6 below.

36 Watson, 'Sheep industry', p. 8; Leigh, 'Crofting Problem', p. 138; Walker, *Economical History*, vol.1, p. 67.

37 *Old Statistical Account*, entry for parish of Kilmalie, p. 424.

38 Iain S. Macdonald, 'Alexander Macdonald Esq. of Glencoe: Insights into early highland sheep-farming,' *Review of Scottish Culture*, 10 (1996), p. 56.

39 *Old Statistical Account*, vol. VIII, p. 170.

40 Charles Fraser-Mackintosh, 'The depopulation of Aberarder in Badenoch', *Celtic Magazine*, vol. 11 (1877).

41 *Statistical Account Of Scotland*, 1791–1799 (reissue, 1977), vol. XII (North and West Perthshire), p. 8.

42 Ibid., pp. 101, 752.

43 Anne Orde (ed.), *Matthew and George Culley: Travel Journals and Letters, 1765–1798* (Oxford UP, for the British Academy, 2002), p. 140, n.99.

44 Philip Gaskell, *Morvern Transformed* (Cambridge, 1968), p. 7.

45 Garnett, *Tour*, vol. II, pp. 158–9.

46 Quoted in Fraser-Mackintosh, *Letters*, pp. 311–12; see also Macdonald, op. cit.

47 Adam, *Sutherland Estate Management*, vol. 1, p.xxix.

48 *Old Statistical Account*, vol. VI, p. 128, quoted in Leigh, 'Crofting problem', p. 7.

49 Quoted in Barron, *Northern Highlands*, vol. 1, p. xxix.

50 Sinclair, *General View Of The Northern Counties*, Appendix, p. 41.

51 Handley, *Scottish Farming*, p. 229.

52 SRO, GD 136/543, Sinclair to Col. John Sinclair, 4 June 1821. On the advantages of the different breeds, see Rosalind Mitchison, *Agricultural Sir John* (London, 1962), p. 110.

53 Watson, 'Sheep industry', p. 14.

54 James Anderson, *General View of the Agriculture of the County of Aberdeen* (Edinburgh, 1794), p. 82.

55 See Richards I, p. 149 and Mitchell, I. op. cit., pp. 265–7.

56 SCRO, D593/K/ R.S. Taylor to Loch, 23 Sept. 1850.

57 *Caledonian Mercury*, 23 August 1792.

58 Quoted in Sinclair, *General View of the Northern Counties*, p. 163.

59 Iain S. Macdonald, op. cit. Cf., Devine, *Clanship*, pp. 34–6.

60 Mitchell I, op. cit. p. 335.

61 Cf. Devine *Clanship*, op. cit. p. 43.

62 Buchanan, *Western Hebrides*, pp. 27–9.

63 Macdonald, *Lewis, A History Of The Island* (Edinburgh, 1978), p. 160.

64 SRG, GD 128/43.

65 Quoted in Fraser-Mackintosh, *Letters*, pp. 328–9.

66 James Donaldson, *General View of the Agriculture of the County of Banff* (Edinburgh, 1794), pp. 35–6.

67 Garnett, *Tour*, vol. II, p. 235.

6

The Insurrection of 1792

I. North of the Great Glen

THE SHEEP WERE ON the move from the south and from the north. In 1791 they were about to colonise the northern Highlands. Their quiet invasion seemed unstoppable. It may have been unwelcome to the people and the tacksmen wedded to the old system, but it was generally regarded as inevitable. Yet, with little warning, in late 1791, the calm march of the sheep juddered to a halt. At a spot in eastern Ross-shire, on the margins of the Highlands, the forces of change confronted those of the status quo. The improvers and their stock were challenged by the peasant mass. There was sensation in the air, and a Ross-shire gentleman captured the moment of local pandemonium when he exclaimed:

> We are at the feet of the mob, and if they should proceed to burn our houses, we are incapable of any resistance.[1]

In retrospect, the year 1792 marked the second phase in the Highland Clearances. Popular resistance dramatically erupted to form a bottleneck which now blocked further advance of the sheep farmers in their invasion of the northern Highlands, the territory beyond the Great Glen. It was a climacteric moment in Highland history and much celebrated in the oral tradition. 1792 was remembered as *Bliadhna Nan Caorach* ('The Year of the Sheep') and the powerful resistance of the people sent a shiver of fear through the Highland proprietors. It called into question, in the most public fashion, the entire future of property and progress in the Highlands. Anarchy threatened to overwhelm the civilising mission of the rationalisers of land use.

II. Borderland

Before 1792 the sheep had spread with only pinprick opposition, sporadic rumblings against the forces of change, hardly rising to the level of guerrilla resistance. It is surprising that such a society, renowned for its internecine violence and its continuing military prowess and tradition, produced so little civil conflict. Stoical passivity had been the reigning response of the people to the clearances.

Easter Ross was a borderland between Highlands and Lowlands on the north-eastern shoulder of Scotland. This region was now at the centre of the pincer-like invasion of sheep into the Highland economy. Already by 1790 the northward push had reached the Great Glen. At the same time in Caithness, the extreme north-east of the region, Sir John Sinclair had begun a southward movement of the new sheep breeds. There was also a general awareness of the threat from the south: the cattle drovers and the seasonal labourers returning from the southern harvests carried the news of the advancing sheep. Fishermen and seasonal harvesters passed through Easter Ross and carrying accounts of the changes now imminent.

The antecedents of the 1792 resistance could be found in minor symptoms of mutiny in Easter Ross in the previous few years. But now the opposition moved into a much more thorough, concerted and dangerous form of resistance. The immediate origins were in the last months of 1791 and the events reached their climax in the middle of 1792. Soon these events were talked of as an 'Insurrection'.

The episode began with the acceleration into the district of sheep farming during the previous two years. Sir George Mackenzie of Coull (an arch-improver and propagandist author himself) recorded the arrival of further new tenants into Easter Ross, including a Mr Cameron, from near Fort William, who took the Highland portions of the estate of Munro of Culcairn, in addition to part of Sir John Lockhart Ross's estate.[2] Here again were sheep graziers taking advantage of low rents and rising wool prices, and thereby pushing off the small tenants while also undercutting the old tacksmen who controlled the cattle trade. It was another episode in the eternal struggle for land, new only in its intensity. But, as was often the case, the opportunist graziers were southerners in league with Highlanders-on-the-make, probably ex-military men with a fortune to find.

By 1791, as Mackenzie of Coull put it:

> Strong symptoms of opposition to sheep farming began to appear . . . among lower orders of people, while the gentlemen were beginning to give every encouragement to sheep farmers to settle among them.

Mackenzie regarded the small tenants as the problem. They were accustomed to graze their oxen on the hills during long periods of the year. The arrival of the sheep was a direct attack upon their economy because now 'the cattle were entirely shut out from the hills'. The people of Sutherland, to the north, felt common cause, and 'when the spirit of revolution and revolt was fast gaining ground over the whole kingdom, an open insurrection broke out in Ross-shire, in the summer of 1792'.[3] This, of course, indicated that there was a widespread popular consciousness of the impending invasion of the sheep into the previously untouched northern limits of the Highlands.

The events of 1792, unlike the sporadic outbursts of petty intimidation of the earlier years of the clearances, were new in scale and co-ordination. The eruption was volcanic and there was especial alarm among the lairds that the north would become contaminated with radicalism imported from the south: the events in Easter Ross coincided with a short-lived phase of radical activity in southern Scotland.[4] The revolutionary threat from France heightened local anxiety and the timing of the insurrection naturally generated suspicions of popular conspiracy. 'Sedition' was the first word on the lips of the landlords as they strained to hear each new rumour of clandestine subversion. Minds were inflamed with the dangers of the age. The French were able to believe that 50 000 enlightened Highlanders were ready to come forward and support a French invasion of Britain. English newspapers reported that Highland regiments had recently refused to fire on United Irishmen. There was certainly opposition to the enrolment of militia in the north of Scotland. Most of all, the rights of property were thought to be at risk.[5]

III. The new sheep farm at Kildermorie

The 'Ross-shire Insurrection' started at a place called Kildermorie, immediately south of Strathrusdale. The sequence of events began on the estate of Sir Hector Munro of Novar in 1791. He had leased the greater part of his land to the two natives of Lochaber, the brothers, Captain Allan Cameron and Mr Alexander Cameron, who were, more significantly, sheep farmers. The original small tenants had been superseded but some were given grazing for their cattle on the heights of Strathrusdale at Whitsun 1791. It is likely that many of the people were evicted completely from the district to make the new sheep farm at Kildermorie. Mrs Grant of Laggan commented upon the passive response to such evictions in Ross-shire in a letter of November 1791:

> The poor people have neither language, money, nor education, to push their way anywhere else; though they often possess feelings and principles, that might rescue human nature from the reproach which false philosophy and false refinement have brought upon it. Though the poor Ross-shire people were driven to desperation, they even then acted under a sense of rectitude, touched no property, and injured no people.[6]

At Kildermorie the people had been severely dislocated but many still remained and awaited further incursions upon their land. The sense of impending eviction was in the air while their fate remained in suspense. But there had been no resistance and their passivity was admired.

In the following year it was a different story. The Cameron brothers, unsurprisingly, faced a hostile atmosphere when they brought their sheep into Strathrusdale. Cattle and sheep were like oil and water. Interminable disputes were inevitable while a co-existence was attempted. There were running disputes about the limits of the sheep farmers' grazings in relation to those of the cattle belonging to the small people who continued to use the heights. The marches of the respective grazings were imprecise or ambiguous and it is unlikely that the small tenants felt any obligation to co-operate with the new tenants, whose profits depended on a smooth return to their heavy initial capital outlays.

The Cameron brothers refused to tolerate an alleged trespass by their neighbours. They 'poinded' (that is, impounded) their cattle and demanded payments and pledges before they would release the beasts. This was the first catalyst in the dispute between the Camerons and the people. It was a predictable consequence of a partial clearance: had the entire population been evicted by the landlord, as was often the case, there would have been no friction. This, indeed, was the common argument of many sheep farmers in the Highlands, who demanded total security from the people of the hills. Wholesale removal of the old economy and its people was, they declared with increasing insistence, the condition of 'progress'.

In late June 1792 the petty dispute swelled much more dangerously.[7] Somehow all the cattle of the Strathrusdale people crossed into the Kildermorie sheep farm, where they were rounded up by the Camerons' shepherds. The Strathrusdale people, exasperated by the frequent poinding of their cattle, now resolved to pay no more fines. They also determined to release their animals by force. They sent messages to the local people of the neighbouring Ardross estate to ask for their assistance to rescue their impounded cattle. The Ardross folk, at that time busy at their peat-cutting, downed tools and joined the action, headed by Alexander Wallace, widely regarded as the champion of the district and known as 'Big Wallace'. Thus a party of fifty men was assembled.

Meanwhile, at Kildermorie, Captain Cameron made defensive preparations. He armed himself with a shotgun and a dirk a foot long. He was reported to have told the Strathrusdale people that:

he would shoot them like birds and . . . send the rest of them to Botany Bay.

This was a very early use of Australia as a deterrent to crime. But, in the event, Cameron quickly met his match in the figure of Alexander Wallace who, after some grappling, efficiently disarmed the irate sheep farmer. During the struggle, according to a later account, the barrels of Cameron's gun were twisted like a 'woodie' (a halter), and his dirk was confiscated as a trophy for Wallace's family. Cameron was roughly handled by the party; 'beaten a hundred times' according to another report. He had been deserted by his own shepherds. The cattle of the Kildermorie people were liberated and returned to Strathrusdale. There was no further poinding. It was a clear success to the people and their cattle, and an outrage against dignity, property and progress.

Cameron, humiliated by this turn of events, attempted to bring his attackers to justice and instituted a complaint upon which a precognition (a sort of coronial investigation prior to legal action) was undertaken. But on 25 July 1792 witnesses to the precognition were obstructed on their way to give evidence at Alness. The law was evidently being mocked and the people were amused.

Two days later there was a wedding at Strathrusdale. During the festivities, much aided by home-brewed ale, there were open celebrations not only of the nuptials but also the victory over the Camerons at Kildermorie. Under this inspiration the participants

> devised the bold step of collecting all the sheep in the counties of Ross and Sutherland and driving them across the Beauly river, there to wander at pleasure.

Another version of the same story was that the sheep would be collected on the border of Inverness and then driven further south. In their anger and their elation the people, according to Wallace's recollection forty years later, resolved 'To extirpate the vipers': that is, the sheep and their minders.

All this happened on Friday 27 July, and the popular plan was proclaimed on the following Sunday in the churches of Alness, Urquhart, Resolis and Kincardine, thereby implicating the church in the events. Parties were also sent into Sutherland to churches and public houses in Creich and Lairg. The grand instruction was that the people were to muster at Strathoykel (in Kincardine parish) on Tuesday 31 July in preparation for the grand expulsion of the offending sheep. The sheep would be stopped in their tracks and sent into reverse, turned south by popular action.

Associated with this plan were three specific demands made on behalf of the small tenantry of the district. They sought first a reduction of rents; they required also an increased availability of arable land so that the price of bread could be reduced for the sake of the poor; and they demanded an end to the enclosure of common pastures. It was alleged that those who refused to participate in the campaign were threatened with the 'curse of all future generations'. By any standards it was an elaborate exercise in pre-industrial popular protest and it invoked a transparent 'moral economy', an appeal to social values, often seen in food riots across Britain before modernisation.

On Tuesday 31 July an estimated 200 people gathered as planned at Brea, and there were lesser gatherings at other places. The people proceeded to collect the unwelcome sheep together, from as far away as Lairg in Sutherland. All the flocks of the parishes were brought together (with the one exception of those belonging to Donald Macleod of Geanies, Sheriff Depute of Ross, apparently out of respect and fear of him). At Amat several thousand sheep (one report said 10 000) were gathered to be driven south to Boath at Strathrusdale where, on Saturday 4 August, the Camerons' sheep were to be added to the monstrous flock. The entire operation, involving the participation of many local people, had required immense co-ordination. It had taken eight days to drive the sheep to Strathrusdale, the original source of the revolt. It was a elaborate logistical exercise.

During that time the authorities initiated several defensive moves which culminated in an action against the rebels in the early hours of Sunday 5 August. Among the local landowners there had been much nervous talk of 'insurrection' and 'sedition'; there was rumour that the people had bought £16 worth of gunpowder in Inverness; it was known that they were armed with guns, clubs, bludgeons and other weapons. The spectre of 'revolution' passed across the minds of the landowners. Local officers of the law gathered their own forces, obtained military support, and closed in upon the insurgents. They were ready to make a lightning strike on the rebels.

In the middle of the night the guards on the sheep were surprised by the landowners' attack and the entire 'Insurrection' swiftly ended in a fiasco of panic and escape. The sheep were rounded up by the soldiery, eight prisoners were taken at Boath and another four in their homes. No further resistance was offered. The entire episode fizzled out and ended with trials in Inverness in September 1792.

When the full dimension of the 'Disturbances and tumultuous associations' became apparent it was clear that the local landowning oligarchy had come together remarkably effectively to put down the revolt. A considerable body of estate owners (the 'Freeholders, Justices of the Peace and Commissioners of Supply') had met in Dingwall to consider the whole question. They included the proprietors of Fowlis, Cromartie, Novar, Allangrange, Geanies, Kindeace, Tulloch, Culrossie, Scotsburn, Culrain, Gillanders, Cadboll and Glasstullich. The local landowners, many of whom were not yet involved in sheep farming, had closed ranks impressively. Their object was to secure property, to restore order, and stamp out the suspicion of sedition in Easter Ross. Their lands were on the very fringe of the Highland territory, on the frontier of the new sheep economy.

The Ross-shire insurrection was a sensation in the northern Highlands and its reverberations reached Edinburgh soon after 'the King's Birthday riots' in the city, and created anxiety even in London. It was certainly the most alarming news from the Highlands since Culloden. The entire story entered the folk memory and remained warm in the collective psyche for several decades. But there were different perceptions of the events: the insurrection was viewed from different angles by the authorities, casual observers, the military and by the rioters too. These versions should be compared.

IV. The official story

The reserves of law and order in Easter Ross were orchestrated by Donald Macleod of Geanies, whose family had provided leadership in the district over many generations. Macleod concerted the forces at the disposal of the landowning class, and acted as their spokesman in communication with the government and newspapers in the south. At the end of July, the landlords' view of the sequence of the revolt had been relayed to Edinburgh.

The official view identified three phases in the outrage in Ross-shire. The first incident, the attack on the Camerons, was described as a violent assault by 'a great number of disorderly people' directed against a gentleman, his family and servants. It was classed as 'a very daring outrage'. The second phase was the obstruction of the subsequent legal investigation by what was described as 'an armed multitude'. This was a seditious act and ought to be 'reprobated' by all friends of 'regular government and subordination'. The third abomination comprised 'the Proclamations which were made in the name of the Populace at several Churches of this County', which was an 'absolute sedition' setting 'the laws and government of the Kingdom at defiance'. This, of course, was the great popular campaign to expel sheep from the north.

The official account therefore conceded and emphasised the popular basis of the insubordination and its seditious political intent. But the landowners also asserted that before the outrages of 1791–2, the district had been tranquil. The people had expressed no grievance against the introduction of the sheep. In any case the existing law provided ample redress to 'the injured of every rank'.

The proprietors alleged that 'the introduction of Sheep into a few farms of this Country' was simply a transparent pretext 'to cover Crimes and Outrages that are daily committed against all Law and Order'. The disturbances were unconnected with the process of sheep farming and the proprietors claimed the people from the sheep farms had made no complaint nor were they involved in the tumults. The actual participants had been deluded by their 'ignorance . . . youth or inexperience'. Their folly was leading them into misery, ruin and even loss of life. The landowners had called for military help, to protect the common people, who had refused to become involved in the outrages, and to avoid the great danger inherent in all such popular associations. In brief, the people were being contaminated by political 'associations'; there was a general level of unruliness in the population; and the rioters had behaved as a mindless mob without regard for life and property or for the consequences.[8]

Donald Macleod of Geanies, as Sheriff Depute, writing from Dingwall, had provided a running commentary on the events to the Lord Advocate in Edinburgh. Macleod gave a vivid account of the tension in the district. The people's proclamation had been read in all the parishes; it declared:

> that all the People . . . were expected to meet . . . at certain Places named, in the Highland parts of the County, where they would be joined by a very large force from Sutherland.

Macleod claimed that the rebels had rallied support by 'the most violent threats and denunciations' which were directed at 'the lukewarm' and those who failed to attend at the appointed time. He alleged a system of intimidation among the people. Thus laggards were warned that their oxen would be attacked and that the sheep would be driven over their homes if they failed to join the rebellion. Macleod, confirming the solidarity of the protest, pointed out that the constables had been unable to apprehend any of the proclaimers, and that the people had, indeed, 'kept their word'. The assemblies of people had gathered as planned, on 31 July, 'from all quarters of the County in this Extraordinary Attempt'. The plan therefore bore all the marks of widespread popular support and social solidarity.

Macleod's original idea was to intercept the rioters. But his forces were meagre and he wisely desisted:

> We were on no account to Hazard Defeat which might be attended with the most dreadful and melancholy consequences to the Troops and ourselves Judicially.

Until military reinforcements arrived from Fort George, Macleod had no alternative 'for the present [but] to permit the Deluded population to take their swing', even though it was 'an Actual Existing rebellion against the Laws'. He had no knowledge of the leadership of the revolt or its 'advisers', 'but I am hopeful that no Gentleman of this County does give them Countenance or Concurrence'. This last comment hinted at the fear of complicity among the lesser landholders, whose social and economic status was being subverted by agrarian change across the Highlands.

Macleod, exhausted by the events, indicated that without military assistance (which he had requested one week before) there could be no precognition nor capture of the rioters. In a frantic postscript he relayed a report that 'a person from Sutherland came to Inverness a few days ago and bought Gunpowder to the value of £16 Stg, and it is known that they have a good many arms among them.'[9] On the same day Munro, on whose estates much of the trouble had originated, told the Lord Advocate that the proprietors were

> at present so completely under the Heel of the Populace that should they come to Burn our houses, or destroy our Property in any way their Caprice may lead them to, we are incapable of resistance.

It was believed that the disturbances had been 'fomented in Sutherlandshire'.[10]

The Lord Advocate in Edinburgh, Robert Dundas, communicated his actions to Whitehall in response to what he called 'the alarming outrages in Ross-shire'. From the Home Office, his uncle Henry Dundas agreed to the dispatch of the 42nd Regiment to the north and authorised further support to be sent from Dundee. Dundas understood that the assault had been directed

> on the person and family of a Mr Cameron, who has lately taken in lease a Farm in the County, intending to stock it with sheep, which is a measure very unpopular in those Highland districts where sheep are not yet introduced, as it tends to remove the Inhabitants on those Estates, from their small possessions and dwelling houses.

Dundas was under no illusion about the causes of the trouble in Ross-shire. London offered every encouragement to the northern authorities to punish 'these daring offenders'. The government in both London and Edinburgh had clearly agreed in their evaluation of the gravity of the danger. They gave complete authority for the insurrection be put down 'to the last extremity', if necessary. Henry Dundas sanctioned taking 'the most vigorous and effectual measures . . . for bringing these daring offenders to punishment'. He said such action would serve to convince the lower class of people 'that they will not be suffered to continue such acts of violence with impunity'.[11]

Fraser of Lovat, another large proprietor in the disaffected district, was equally frank about the cause of the outrage. He described the rebellious people as 'Insurgents against Sheep Farming in Ross-shire'. They had either 'collected themselves from Desperation', or else been 'deluded by designing persons who proved themselves able to put up Counter Manifestos in good language to those of the Country Gentlemen'. Either way, it was not good, said Lovat, 'to permit the Lieges in Ross-shire to obtain Redress, by taking the Law in their own Hands.' He too implied that the people were supported by 'respectable' elements in the community.

Lovat described the measures taken in Inverness-shire to counter the spreading rebellion. Arms and ammunition were applied for; the authorities had issued Resolutions through the churches; the landowners 'sounded their Dependants' to be ready to face the rebels. As a consequence, Lovat claimed, the Inverness participation in the revolt had been broken. The Inverness people had not succeeded in crossing the River Beauly into Ross-shire, and various prisoners had been taken. Lovat, congratulating himself on this success, ended his report to the Lord Advocate with a plea which related to one of the most fundamental problems of the region:

> Permit me also to Entreat that in order to enable us to employ the people in Industry and Manufactures that you will use every endeavour to get Repealed or Exchanged the Coasting duty on Scots Coal.

It was a curious remark to make in the middle of the greatest threat to order in the Highlands since the Jacobite Rebellion. Lovat was alluding to the immense difficulty of generating enterprise and employment in the north – a chronic problem, obviously aggravated by the sheep clearances. Cheap coal, he thought, was essential: 'It is impossible to Inhabit or Manufacture in Northern Scotland without Fuel'. By implication the insurrection was a consequence of economic adversity and the solution was therefore to generate employment in the north.[12]

The danger from the county of Inverness diminished but in Ross-shire the rebellion had much more stamina and posed a far greater danger. Macleod of Geanies gathered his military assistance ready for action. On the eve of the confrontation with the rebels,

Macleod wrote from Dingwall to individual Inverness-shire proprietors, expressing the fear of escalation widely sensed in the district, and providing a view of the scale of the episode:

Dear Sir,

You can be no Stranger to the Tumults, Commotions, and actual Seditious Acts that are going on in this County at this time; the Flame is spreading; what is our Case today, if Matters are permitted to proceed, will be yours Tomorrow. I understand a Mob of about Four Hundred Strong are now actually employed in collecting the sheep, over all this and the Neighbouring country of Sutherland. I Intend to oppose them with what Force I can collect. The Gentlemen of the County, armed with such of their Servants and Dependants as they can confide in, [are] backed by Three Companies of the 42nd Regiment. If you suppose you can raise Volunteers hearty in the Cause, of good Order and Subordination to join us, we shall feel much obliged to you; and request, you may inform me here by Express Tomorrow, whether I may have any Reliance on your Assistance; and if so, I shall send you Notice when we wish you to move, and to what Place. I have the Lord Advocate's Orders to proceed against the Insurgents should it be necessary, to the last Extremity.[13]

The proprietors responded with great spirit. They agreed to gather their adherents 'at any Place of Rendez Vous for the purpose of giving their Assistance'. Money would be raised to defray expenses; applications would be made for extra troops and for the accommodation for prisoners. The landowners were thus mobilised.

On Sunday 5 August Macleod of Geanies wrote another breathless despatch to the Lord Advocate in the heat of the confrontation. He had received intelligence at two o'clock on the previous afternoon:

that the insurgents had drove off the sheep of Col Baillies and Charles Ross's Estate in the County of Sutherland, and were to be with them last night, at a place called Boath ten computed miles from Dingwall, that they were to leave only forty or fifty men as a Guard, and that the rest were to Proceed to collect Capt Cameron's, and to go with them by a different road and collect those belonging to Mr Mitchell, and proceed Monday and Tuesday with them by another Pass until they got the whole beyond the Bounds of the County.

In the light of this knowledge Macleod ordered three companies of the 42nd Regiment then at his command to be ready at eight o'clock on Saturday evening. He also summoned the armed assistance of the gentlemen and inhabitants in the vicinity of Dingwall: 'It does much honour to the Gentlemen of the Country, with what Alacrity the greatest part of them within reach turned up.'

This substantial force arrived at Boath at one o'clock on Sunday morning

and found from Scouts that not withstanding Every precaution we had used, they discovered our approach and fled, leaving 6000 sheep on the muirs, which they had taken from the Three Farms in Sutherland.

Macleod then decided that, the soldiers being tired, he should lead a small posse to search the woods and the locality. They were successful in that they 'Discovered about Eight of the Scoundrels either lying in the Beauly [corn?] or in the woods, and after a good deal of galloping over very bad ground, we apprehended everyone, and delivered them to the care of the military'. After this they spent the rest of the night searching the Strath and found several others who had been with the drovers but had returned home to sleep. Macleod was confident of 'bringing in all the Ringleaders of this most Unaccountable Commotion'.

Macleod's prisoners came from a wide area and included a piper and a boy of fourteen.[14] Macleod thought there was still danger that the insurgents would regroup; he was not confident enough to promise final victory. Much fatigued and still anxious about his military strength, he added another postscript to his dispatch:

I can with truth assert, that if this Business was to proceed one week more, 2000 men would not repress the Insurrection, which would ensue not only in this, but in the Counties which surround us. It may appear a little extraordinary, but the Fact I learned from some of the Prisoners, that they have not touched any of my Farms, nor did not intend to do it, unless I opposed them by force. A threat I very much despise.[15]

One week after the skirmish at Boath, Dundas was able to report that the Ross-shire disturbances were now 'completely quelled'. The ringleaders would be brought to trial in Inverness.[16]

In the intervening time great vigilance was maintained in the districts affected: the *Edinburgh Courant* reported that extra troops were required. In fact three companies were kept in Ross-shire at the request of the Sheriff, and another six remained on alert at Fort George for the entire summer.

V. Lord Adam Gordon's reaction

Macleod of Geanies represented the landowners' view of the insurrection. An outsider's reaction to the events was provided by Lord Adam Gordon, commander of forces in North Britain. Not long after the insurrection and before the trial, in August 1792, Gordon was in the north of Scotland on a tour of the military forts. Of all the official correspondence at the time of the Ross-shire insurrection Gordon's letters were the most outspoken and illuminating.

Gordon reported from Fort George on 19 August that a quietness had now descended on the district and that no more troops would be necessary. He believed the presence of troops had effectively prevented further disturbances occurring in the area. The military had stamped out the riots. Gordon then proceeded to ventilate some of his thoughts on 'this *unpleasant* business'. He wrote:

> If I was to hazard an opinion upon the matter . . . it is a decided one – that no *disloyalty* – or hint of *rebellion* – or dislike of His Majesty's [Person] or *Government* – is in the least degree [indicated] in these tumults – and that they have solely originated – in a (too well founded) apprehension – that the landed proprietors in Ross-shire, and some of the adjacent Highland Counties – were about to lett their Estates to sheep farmers – by which means – all the former tenantry would be ousted – and turned adrift – and of course obliged to emigrate – unless they could be elsewhere received – any probability of which they could not discover and it is an undoubted fact – that in several instances within the last two or three years such . . . [fears] have been realized –

and the Proprietors have by these means greatly increased their rentrolls – and diminished the number of their people – on their respective estates.

Gordon was sympathetic to the case made by the people, and his testimony reinforces the view that sheep farming had already caused substantial and unpopular dispersion of the people of this part of the Highlands.

Ruminating on the general circumstances of the Highlands, Gordon employed the mercantilist principle that 'the Strength of a Nation depends on the number of the people'. The policy which neglected this axiom, he claimed, had caused 'General alarm [which] has been spread all over the Highlands'. In those cases where proprietors had accepted 'a moderate rise of rent' and had retained and valued the population, there had been 'no disturbance . . . heard of – nor has the Duke of Gordon or Mackenzie of Seaforth lost one man on their wide extended Highland Estates'. Gordon continued:

> Everybody knows the wonderful attachment a Highlander has – to his *native spott* be it ever so bare, and ever so *mountainous* – and if these calculating Gentlemen shall by any means or from *avarice* – once dispeople their Estate and [settle?] them with sheep – and that a season or two should follow – and the sheep be thereby destroyed – I am convinced – no temptation under the sun – will be able to bring the inhabitants to Highland property – from any part of the world. If they should ever so happen I shall not hold them as objects of pity, or be of opinion the Publick (who certainly suffer) should be putt to trouble and expense – in bringing matters to their former situation.

Gordon made no secret of his personal abhorrence of sheep-farming landlords, but he acknowledged that there was no law 'to hinder [anyone] to do as he wishes with his own property'. Their actions might be against the public interest, and the ringleaders of 'the late daring mobbs . . . which are disgraceful to any civilized country' had to be brought to justice. Regardless of his own ambivalence, Gordon promised his best endeavours in the prosecution of the law. He knew also that without military intervention the insurrection would have been far greater. Even two weeks after the Boath climax he was not entirely sure of peaceability in the district. The troops had been indispensable, he said, 'The utility of which [that is, the troops], in these levelling times, appears to me, *more* than ever'. He reported that many of the rioters had been caught and others had surrendered; he commented, 'Thank God as yet – no blood has been spilt. But the law will take its course'.[17]

Adam Gordon's remarks, precisely because they came from the official side of the events, were unlikely to overestimate the popular basis of the insurrection, the cohesion of public feeling, the threat to order, or the consequences of landlord policy.

VI. The press

The clearances in Easter Ross in the early 1790s were exceptional only because they erupted into resistance. The sympathetic reaction of Gordon and some of the ministers recorded in the *Old Statistical Account* were echoed in the tone of most of the press coverage of the Ross-shire tumults. They virtually amounted to a public indictment of the landlords of Ross-shire. The *Edinburgh Evening Courant* reported the first news of the northern troubles in strong terms:

> The people there, exasperated at their being turned out of their farms, by the present prevalent custom of the landlords letting out their grounds for extensive sheep walks, and rendered desperate by poverty, had assembled in great numbers, and proceeded to several unjustifiable acts of violence, particularly in destroying the sheep, no less than 3000 of them belonging to one gentleman having been drowned. Some woods are also said to have been burnt.[18]

The press sympathy for the people was diminished by the allegation of violence, much strengthened by the report that 'all the gunpowder in Tain and Dingwall had been previously bought up by the rioters'. The *Courant* was, however, highly critical of the landowners:

> Every gentleman has doubtless a right to make the most of his property; but surely in the exercise of that right much is due to humanity – we may add justice. The lower class of people in this part of the country,

particularly in the northern parts, have hitherto been remarkable for the regularity of their deportment, and a respectful submission to the laws of their country. Some measures therefore more than commonly oppressive have, we apprehend, given rise to this outrage, and we trust it will excite the immediate attention of the Legislature. While we are commiserating and giving assistance to the distressed inhabitants of Poland [in connection with the Russian invasion and the abrogation of the constitution in May 1792], let it not be said that we suffer Oppression to stalk uncontrolled at home.[19]

These criticisms were extremely repugnant to the northern proprietors. The *Courant* and the *Caledonian Mercury* both recommended that the Ross-shire refugees from the sheep walks should be assisted to the south of Scotland 'to settle where manufactories are established, [where] they would greatly benefit the country, and the poor people would soon get into easy and affluent circumstances'.[20] This was a time when David Dale was recruiting large numbers of Highlanders into his cotton mills at New Lanark.

When the news of the collapse of the northern insurrection reached Edinburgh the newspapers took the opportunity to correct their previous reports. In particular the *Courant* now made it clear that there had been neither bloodshed nor cruelty, and this squares with the official reports:

> The insurgents themselves have behaved in a very uncommon manner; though almost starving, not a sheep had they taken for their own use, and when made sensible of their error, several troops of thirty or forty came and delivered themselves up to the Sheriff, who selected the most guilty and dismissed the rest. The civil power, it is believed, will, as it ought in such a case, be very lenient in the punishment of these unfortunate people.[21]

There was not the slightest whiff of political sedition, in any of these reports and the allegation of deliberate wanton violence was finally scotched. It was reported, 'Indeed, so far were the poor fellows from destroying the sheep, that they even carried such as were unable to walk'.[22] Hence the press reports were remarkably warm towards the people and cool to their landlords. The people had been wronged by their landlords.

VII. Punishment

The prisoners taken by the 42nd Regiment at the time of the insurrection were brought to trial in the middle of September 1792 at the Circuit Court of Justiciary at Inverness. The trial was presided over by Lord Stonefield. There were two cases. On 12 September the Court considered the charges against the eight Strathrusdale men who were alleged to have attacked the Cameron brothers one month prior to the insurrection itself. By a majority voice, they were found not guilty of the charges of 'riot, assault and battery'.

Touring Scotland in 1792, the poet and divine John Lettice, in Inverness at the time of the trials, was eyewitness to the first proceedings.[23] He reported that 'The town is full of peasants, from Ross and Sutherland, anxiously awaiting its issue'. He squeezed into the courtroom through a dense crowd. There was eloquent pleading from both sides, and the prisoners and witnesses were examined at length before the jury. In the first case the men were found not guilty: 'The cattle mentioned in the indictment, were the cows and horses of these poor men, which had been removed from their own pastures, and poinded, to make room for the sheep of the persecutor', who had not given proper legal notice. The man in question, Cameron, had met the people with guns and threatened them with violence. The jury thought the people had simply acted in self-defence.

Lettice was entirely sympathetic to the men charged at the Inverness Assizes. They were pitiable and, he thought,

> There is . . . a point of necessity, if those, who suffered, could but impartially distinguish it, beyond which no human being is obliged to bear without resistance.

The Ross-shire insurrection had arisen from 'the sudden extermination of a number of small farmers, who have been used to maintain their families by a dairy, the rearing of a few black cattle for sale, and a little tillage'. Lettice reported, on good evidence from several sources, that thirty-seven families had been evicted to make way for sheep. He thought it was a calamity which merited the attention of the government, especially in the light of the current alarming emigration. Rents had increased and the avarice of the landlords was being gratified but, he declared, 'Where individuals grow opulent by the depopulation of the country, they make more haste to grow rich, than ought to be suffered by its rulers'. The whole business, he believed, was an unusual and outrageous experiment.

Unfortunately Lettice did not attend the second trial, which dealt with the men involved in the actual 'Insurrection', the 'cottage farmers' who had opposed the sheep walks. In the second trial seven men from Rosskeen, Alness and Kincardine were charged with

> the advising, exciting, and instigating of persons riotously and feloniously to Invade, seize upon, and drive away the property of . . . our Lieges, especially by lawless and seditious proclamations made at . . . the churches or places of worship where the inhabitants are convened upon a Sunday for the purpose of attending divine ordinances.

The indictment described it as 'a preconcerted plan' and named the churches of Alness, Urquhart, Kirkmichael/Cullycudden, Amat, Creich and Lairg. The defendants were alleged to have said 'That the curse of the children not yet born, and their generation, would [be on] such as would not cheerfully go and banish the sheep out of the county'.

The indicted were alleged to have assembled more than 100 people at Brea and to have taken the sheep flocks of various farmers (including those of Campbell of Lagwine, and Mrs Margaret Geddes) amounting to 'several thousand'. They had been armed with guns, clubs and bludgeons. The case was supported by twenty-eight witnesses, mainly tenants, tacksmen, kirk officers, shepherds and sheep farmers. Some of the witnesses were illiterate, some required translation from the Gaelic ('the Erse').[24]

In the outcome the case against the men was judged proven. The Edinburgh newspapers reported that two of the prisoners were sentenced to seven years' transportation; one was fined £50 sterling and imprisoned for one month, and until the fine was paid; two were banished from Scotland for life; another was imprisoned for three months. The fate of the seventh prisoner is not known.[25] The contemporary reports were clear about the sentences, but an alternative story was alleged to have circulated to the effect that just as the accused were about to be acquitted one of the Camerons made a public demonstration in the court to the effect that 'no man's life would be safe in the country' if they were let off Scot-free. Only then were the prisoners convicted.[26] For this version no corroborative evidence survives. In any case, given the generous use of capital punishment in the north,[27] it is surprising that transportation was considered a sufficient punishment for men who had threatened the entire basis of the law in the region.

Lettice said that no one doubted the men's guilt or the justice meted out to them, but he condemned the whole business of eviction as sordid and savage. It was incredible that a landlord would 'reduce a being of his own species, happy but to earn a bare subsistence by the sweat of his brow, to such a piteous state of helplessness and despair'.[28]

Lettice did not remain in the eastern Highlands long enough to report the positively operatic sequel to the Inverness trial. On the night of 24 October, the two prisoners who were under sentence of transportation for their involvement in the Ross-shire insurrection escaped from prison at the Tolbooth of Inverness. Various versions of this episode followed. One said that popular feeling was so incensed by 'the unrighteousness of the sentence' that the prison door was opened; another said that the escape had been connived at, 'for they disappeared out of the prison no one knew how, and were never inquired after or molested'; a further account said that a fellow prisoner (allegedly insane) had employed a nail to work a hole in the prison wall.

The fugitive men were described thus:

Hugh Breck Mackenzie is about 40 years of age, 5 feet 6 inches high, black short hair, dark complexion, much pox-marked, his left eye much blemished, has a down look and walks lightly; had on when he made his escape a short, dark, dussle striped coat, a striped vest, corduroy breeches, white stockings, and a bonnet.

John Aird is about 45 years of age, 5 feet 8 inches high, broad shoulders, black eyes, a very dark complexion, straight and well-made; had on when he made his escape a black short coat, and breeches of coarse, country-made cloth, a striped vest of country-made cloth (black, red and white), with blue stockings and a bonnet.

A reward of £5 was offered for the apprehension of each of the prisoners, but they were never caught. According to local belief they were harboured by the common people until they reached the Moray Firth, and the authorities judged it best not to search for them.[29]

Notes

1 Quoted in Thomas Douglas Selkirk, *Observations on the Present State of the Highlands of Scotland* (1805).

2 See Mitchell, I. op. cit., Chapter. XXXI.

3 Ibid., p. 131.

4 See Michael Fry, *The Dundas Dynasty* (1992), pp. 167–70.

5 H. W. Meikle, *Scotland and the French Revolution* (Edinburgh, 1912), pp. 175–6.

6 Grant, *Letters*, vol. II, pp. 326–7.

7 One account dates the events as May 1792: SRO,GD127/36/Clippings from the 1890s (extracts from *North Star and Farmers' Chronicle*), 'A.M.R.', 'Ross-shire a century ago and now'. Robert Bain, *History of the Ancient Province of Ross* (Dingwall, 1899), pp. 349 et seq. See also *Ross-shire Journal*, 9, 16 and 23 March, 1951.

8 SRO, RH2/4/64, pp. 260–2, document dated 31 July 1792.

9 Ibid., pp. 262 et seq., Macleod to Lord Advocate, 31 August 1792.

10 SRO, RH2/4/Munro to Lord Advocate 31 July 1792.

11 SRO, RH/2/4/218/Dundas to Lord Advocate, 9 and 21 August 1792.

12 SRO, RH2/4/64/Lovat to Lord Advocate, 5 August 1792; Lovat to Dundas, 10 August 1792.

13 SRO, RH2/4/64, pp. 271 et seq.

14 The prisoners came from Alladale, Langwell, Letters, Drumvraich and Invernald. Other rebels were said to have come from Strathconan, Gladfield and Wester Greenyards.

15 SRO, RH/4/64 Macleod to Lord Advocate, 5 August 1792.

16 SRO, RH/4/62/Robert Dundas to Henry Dundas, 13 August 1792.

17 SRO., RH/2/4/218/Gordon to Lord Advocate, 19 August 1792.

18 *Edinburgh Evening Courant*, 4 August 1792.

19 Ibid.

20 *Caledonian Mercury,* 2 August 1792.

21 *Edinburgh Evening Courant,* 10 October 1792. See also *Scots Magazine,* August 1792, p. 412, *Caledonian Mercury,* 13 August 1792.

22 *Caledonian Mercury,* 15 August 1792.

23 J. Lettice, *Letters on a Tour Through Various Parts of Scotland in the Year 1792* (London, 1794).

24 SRO,GD127/36/*North Star and Farmers' Chronicle,* clippings, 'The indictment'.

25 Caledonian Mercury, 17 September 1792; *Scots Magazine,* September 1792, pp. 462–3.

26 SRO, GD127/36/*North Star and Farmers' Chronicle* clippings, 'The indictment'.

27 See for instance Mitchell, I, op. cit., pp. 52–3, *Edinburgh Courant* 3 November 1792.

28 Lettice, *Letters,* pp. 341–3, 363–6.

29 SRO,GD127/36/*North Star and Farmers' Chronicle* clippings. Cf. Mitchell, I, op. cit., p. 267. See also William MacKenzie, 'Bliadhna na Caorach', *Transactions of the Gaelic Society of Inverness. (TGSI)* vol. VII, p. 254. Much of the contemporary documentation is contained in SRO, JC 26/268 and I thank Peter Grant of Lyttelton in New Zealand for his assistance with this material.

7

Aftermath and the Widening Sheep Empire

I. Defeat

THE COMMON PEOPLE MAY have been defeated in the events of 1792 but the victors, the landed proprietors, emerged with tarnished reputations; they had also drawn national attention to their behaviour towards their people. In the wake of the Ross-shire events the Sheriff Depute, Donald Macleod of Geanies, attempted to straighten the record. He wrote two newspaper letters in an elaborate *apologia* for his fellow landlords. Macleod himself was widely respected and a model proprietor. He had successfully conducted large experiments for the conversion of waste muir land into arable in an arrangement with cottars who provided the heavy labour.[1] He now tried to recover the reputation of his own class.

Macleod protested that the circulating reports about the 'Ross-shire Insurrection' were inaccurate. Soon after the trial, he published a letter designed

> to obliterate from the public mind the improper and unfounded prejudices which had been industriously disseminated against the Highland proprietors of this county.

Macleod declared that in fact no sheep had been drowned and that no effort had been made to rescue the prisoners from his custody. This was a gesture towards the people. He contended that the country had been perfectly quiet until 'a few desperate men' had violently attacked the Camerons, the sheep farmers, without any 'just provocation'. One of the Camerons had been 'nearly murdered' in the incident in

Kildermorie. He said that the two Camerons (one of whom was consumptive), as well as a poor old and inoffensive woman and the three servants, had been beaten with sticks, and terrorised with the threat of arson if they attempted to bring their assailants to justice:

> This unprecedented outrage was committed by a mob of betwixt sixty and seventy persons, all armed with clubs and batons.

In their attempt to obscure their crime, these men had associated their action with the popular clamour against sheep farming. Macleod believed that the whole business had been precipitated by a particular local dispute and then converted into a wider conflict by designing agents. The verdict of the first trial in Inverness was not consistent with his judgement.

Macleod argued that 'a general spirit of disorder spread' which fed and exaggerated reports of the repugnance of the people to sheep farms. Resistance to civil power was

> preached up, and mobs of hundreds of persons did convene in a species of military array . . . [which then became] a regular plan for a general insurrection . . . The spirit of violence was carried so far as to set the civil power at defiance; the laws were trampled upon; there appeared no safety for property; and the gentlemen of the country seemed to be subjected to the power and control of an unruly and ungovernable mob.

Macleod indeed repeated each of the allegations: that a mob of up to 400 people had been mobilised; that subversion and threats were employed across the district; that nineteen churches were implicated; and that the demands of the rebels were outrageous: not only would the 'noxious animal' be banished, but an assault was promised on high rents, enclosure for pasture, and the rising price of bread. It was, he said, 'a turbulent spirit of anarchy' which affected 'the greatest number of the lower class'.

Macleod contended that the moderation and prudence of the local proprietors had prevented the rebellion spreading through thousands of local people. He insisted that, contrary to popular opinion, sheep farming had benefited everyone. It had been introduced to Ross-shire fifteen years before, and, since 'not as yet one single family [has] been obliged to emigrate on account of sheep', it was most unlikely that this was a cause of the commotions. He conceded 'that some families have been obliged to change their situations, and move from one farm to another, and from one part of the county to another'. Highlanders undoubtedly disliked being shifted in this way, but it was not 'a good reason why a proprietor should preclude himself from letting to a more enterprising and active occupant', nor why any family should remain forever at the same place.

Macleod could find no reason why Highland proprietors 'should not have the same liberty of improving or managing their properties as seems to them most conducive to their interest' – even if depopulation (which he thought unlikely, in any case) were the consequence. He affirmed that 'by introducing a source of wealth and a staple of manufacture hitherto unknown amongst them, [it would] increase their numbers and their happiness'.[2]

Macleod's vindication of the landlords of Ross-shire reflected the expansive optimism of his times, particularly the belief that new enterprise would arise and absorb the population displaced by sheep. In retrospect it is evident that he expected too much faith from the common people. The events of 1792 were the tip of the iceberg of Highland revulsion from the clearing system; nevertheless the 'Insurrection' had, in reality, little revolutionary intent. It was more a symptom of the mainly passive abhorrence with which the great change was received by the common people. Indeed even references to sheep in Gaelic poetry remained rare until the 1790s.[3]

II. Aftermath

In the aftermath of the riots there was a great deal of self-congratulation among the landed proprietors of Ross-shire. The arrangements for raising subscriptions to pay the expenses involved in the suppression were conducted without difficulty.[4] Once more sheep farming continued to extend through Ross-shire. The bottle-neck of opposition had been snapped by their solidarity and the aid of the military. The newspapers, in their advertisements, continued to chronicle the progress of the wool farmers enticed north by the low rents of under-utilised grazing land.

There remained, of course, a sensitivity among estate administrators: on the Sutherland estate in October 1792 the factor advised against the introduction of commercial sheep farming on the grounds that the sheep farmers became absentees and that 'bad neighbourhood would ensue twixt them and the poor people'.[5] Popular resistance to the sheep farmers, however, dwindled to sporadic attacks on stock and there was no further large-scale confrontation until 1812–13 in Sutherland. But thefts of sheep became a chronic irritation for the sheep farmers, and the years after 1792 were full of their complaints. Such thefts represented resistance as much as sheer hunger among the common people of the Highlands. In 1798 farmers in Inverness, Argyll, Perth and Ross set up a protection society called the Northern Association of Gentlemen and Farmers, Breeders of Sheep, 'for the purpose of discovering the Thefts already committed on their flocks and Preventing Thefts in future'.[6] It was a vigilante group defending the new sheep-farming investments in a hostile environment.

The Northern Association was the first of several efforts made in the following thirty years to curb the 'depredations' of the Highland population against the property of the sheep-farming capitalists. In a memorandum to the Lord Advocate in 1799 the 'Sheep Farmers' Association' alluded to the great advantages that had been derived by the northern Highlands from the introduction of the Tweeddale breed of sheep, and the consequent diffusion of wealth. They couched their case in the most positive way. 'Hills inaccessible to black cattle and in their former history almost useless to man have been found by experience to produce the best sheep.' The sheep, they pointed out, were left to roam over wide tracts of grazing without supervision even by shepherds. The association complained that:

> In this situation an opportunity is offered to thieves of committing depredations on the Stock with scarce a Possibility of detection. To such an extent has this malpractice been of late carried, that at one farm in the County of Ross a parcel of no less than 200 sheep had been carried away at one time, and drove [sic] openly to market.

They complained that there had been many similar cases over the previous few years. In one instance the sheep were taken at night and driven fifteen miles to market along the King's road to the low country. The sheep farmers wanted to introduce a system of certificates for sheep drovers and sought the legal advice of the Lord Advocate.[7]

The events of 1792 were set against a larger backdrop of demographic pressure, emigration and fear of radicalism. There was also a continuing hope of development in the region which, in the year of the riots, was focused mainly on the benefit to be expected from road construction. A road across the northern Highlands from Ullapool to Contin employed large numbers of Highlanders and there was optimistic talk that manufacturing development would be stimulated by better communications. Duncan Davidson of Tulloch, a substantial proprietor, rhapsodised on the revealed potential.

> Employment will be found for the numerous Inhabitants, and I trust we shall be able to keep them at home and make Emigrations unnecessary; you know the warm attachment of the Highlanders to their country and nothing but cruel oppression and necessity will drive them from their Habitations; in this quarter we are now exerting ourselves to preserve them, to employ them and make them comfortable and independent and I trust we shall succeed but without this Blessing of a Road and easy Communication all our Endeavours would have been in vain.[8]

That a landlord, such as Davidson, should testify to the 'cruel oppression' of his own class is doubly significant. It reinforces the view that clearances were implicated in the emigrations of those years and in the general dislocation of the Highland population. It also indicates that part of the proprietorship of the Highlands was actively attempting to counter or ameliorate the effects of sheep farming and population growth.

Sheep farming thus focused the social tensions which derived from a much wider mesh of agrarian and social circumstances. Demographic pressures had already created a degree of land hunger and generated more mobility in the population. The reorganisation of agriculture, especially on the arable eastern fringe of the Highlands, had disturbed the old patterns of social existence. Efforts to introduce industry, and to open up the north, had reinforced the drift of people into villages and towns such as Dingwall, Ullapool, Inverness, Fort William and Tain. Vigorous improvement schemes adopted by landlords had displaced communities. At the same time, the old fear of famine and the hardships of the years 1782–3 continued to stalk the collective mind.

III. Amelioration

In terms of the general social psychology of the region it was an alarming time for the common people, a time of communal anxiety and insecurity. Upon this mental state played all the rumours of wholesale eviction and forced emigration from other parts of the Highlands. Sheep farming undoubtedly loomed as an incoming threat to the welfare of the people; their fear was far from irrational, as the reports in the *Statistical Accounts* amply demonstrated. The contemporary reports may have exaggerated the direct responsibility of sheep farming in the dislocation of the society, but sheep farming was indubitably one of the pressures creating upheaval in the Highlands.

A decade later the government in London sanctioned and funded one of the greatest public works of the day. This would become the Caledonian Canal, connecting the east and west coasts by navigation through the Great Glen. One of its most prominent purposes was to create employment and industry in the Highlands, in part to counteract emigration associated with the increasingly negative consequences of the sheep clearances as they widened at the turn of the century. The construction of the canal certainly generated a local multiplier impact, employing relays of nearly 3000 workers for twenty years.[9]

Meanwhile the events of 1792 passed into the collective memory in two forms: as a warning to landlords, and as an inspiration to the common people. The great advocate of emigration, Lord Selkirk, invoked the Ross-shire insurrection as evidence of the mounting spirit of discontent among the Highland peasantry. Writing in 1803, he drew anxious parallels with turbulent Ireland, and referred to the long history of irritation and discontent in the north of Scotland. The riots of 1792, he said, had concerned 'poor and ignorant men, without leaders and without any intelligible plan; actuated by indignation merely against their immediate superiors', they found themselves 'committing an offence against the general government of the country'. The best safety valve for this rage, he maintained, was emigration.[10]

In opposition to Selkirk's view was that of 'Amicus' who, in 1806, retorted that the 1792 events had been purely small scale and temporary. He believed that the outside influences and the 'spirit of revolution' which prevailed in 1792, had since entirely evaporated: 'Thanks to God, these sentiments have vanished with the fever that produced them, and the peaceful disposition of the Highland peasantry is now as pure as would be their contentment, if American advisers would let them rest'.[11]

More than forty years after the original riots, several of the ministers writing for the *New Statistical Account* drew upon memories of the disturbances from their parishioners. The minister of Kiltearn gave an account completely sympathetic to the rebels. The entry for Rosskeen was equally outspoken and included reference to the events at Kildermorie and 'Big Wallace':

> An old man still living, a man then in the prime of life, and of great strength and stature . . . the principal instrument in closing instantaneously with, and disarming the shepherds, before they could use their firearms, even if so inclined.

The people had acted out of total exasperation with the system of sheep farming which was 'progressing in every corner of the North Highlands, and the people driven year after year from the fields of their fathers'. The minister finished with the observation that:

> There is one striking feature of this case, characteristic of a Highland mob, which strongly exemplifies their high moral principles, even when excited and roused by oppression to an illegal act; no sheep was injured, no lamb was hurt, by overdriving.[12]

These responses are not easily to be squared with the common verdict that the ministers of the Church lived entirely in the pockets of the landlords.

As for the original scene and cause of the 1792 insurrection, the lands of Strathrusdale were described by a gazetteer of 1844 as 'an extensive upland vale . . . disposed for the most part into a sheep walk'.[13]

The social and economic dislocation of life in Easter Ross was common to both the arable lowland and the higher pastoral lands of the district. It is significant that the riots occurred near the densely populated new village communities of lowland Easter Ross. The rapid influx of sheep focused opposition to the modernising forces which were believed to cause depopulation. Nevertheless many of the landlords genuinely believed that their changes could be introduced without any loss of people. It was naïvely supposed that manufacturing could be reproduced in the Highlands on the pattern of the Lowlands. In reality the upheaval was great, especially for the small tenants who lived at the bottom of the social scale. On this question the contemporary reports of depopulation and social dislocation are virtually unanimous. At Kildermorie the new sheep farming arrangements clearly caused the ejectment of most of the old tenantry. The residue of the old population was pushed onto the higher lands and deprived of most of their customary grazing privileges; this inevitably undermined their entire economy. It brought the people into direct confrontation with the new sheep-farming tenants; it provoked the clashes over the poinding of the cattle, and the rebellion was thereby precipitated.

Just as the Galloway disturbances of 1722–4 signified the first and last determined resistance to enclosure in southern Scotland, so the Ross-shire rebellion in 1792 provided its northern counterpart. The defeat of the resistance to sheep farming was comprehensive; co-ordinated obstruction of the sheep farmers was thoroughly broken and never again was there a chance for the old Highland society to hold back the invasion of the sheep. The last stronghold, the northern Highlands, was breached.

IV. A new century

At the turn of the nineteenth century the sheep farmers had penetrated into most accessible districts of the Highlands though they still had more colonising to accomplish. Already by 1800 sheep farming was thoroughly developed in Knoydart and there were high-pitched complaints from tenants who faced not only increased rents but a great loss of grazings. The estate of Scothouse was already laid out in sheep walks several years before sheep farmers fom the borders entered the district. In 1803 and 1804 James Hogg, the self-educated 'Ettrick Shepherd', registered the extent of the sheep empire through the eyes of a lowland tourist and farmer. The Cheviots had reached the estates of the Duke of Argyll. In Easter Ross most of the Strathconan estate had been already laid out as sheep walks, apart from a small part at the lower end which had been 'reserved for the accommodation of such of the natives as could not dispose of themselves to better advantage'. It was a sign of the tenacity of these people that, several decades later, they still occupied this remnant of their old lands and, in a later clearance, became the subject of great public outcry against their evicting landlord.[14]

At Fort William, the main town on the west coast, Hogg met Thomas Gillespie: twenty years before he had pioneered sheep farming in Glengarry, where he had been able to obtain lands on very generous terms from the landlord. Hogg described Gillespie as a rough-hewn man who was prepared to live ruggedly and to sleep in shepherds' cots whenever necessary; he had overcome great difficulties and had extended his farm whenever the opportunity arose:

He is now the greatest farmer in all that country, and possesseth a track of land extending from the banks of Loch Garey to the shores of the Western Ocean, upwards of twenty miles.

Hogg made no mention of any resultant depopulation, but he did believe that the original circumstances of many of the people had been so utterly appalling that they could not be 'worsened unless they were starved to death'.

At Strathinashalloch Hogg reported that the incoming sheep

farmers had bid up the price of land to an alarming degree. In this valley, the only inhabitants who remained were 'Mr Macintyre's shepherds', yet 'there were considerable crops of corn and potatoes left by the tenants who have removed last term'. This, of course, was the clearest evidence of the precipitate character of many of the clearances: the tenants had either chosen to disbelieve the eviction notices, or had left so hurriedly that their crops were ungathered. The sheep farmer who took over this land had obtained the lease for £200 per annum, but Hogg calculated that the current upsurge of wool prices would yield him a return of perhaps £700 per annum from his acquisition. Hogg summarised the economic and moral propositions associated with the sheep economy:

> The truth is, there are several low-country gentlemen getting into excellent bargains by their buying lands in that country ... and I cannot help having a desperate ill-will on that score. I cannot endure to hear of a Highland chieftain selling his patrimonial property, the cause of which misfortune I always attribute to the goodness of his heart, and the liberality of his sentiments; unwilling to drive off the people who have so long looked to him as their protector, yet whose system of farming cannot furnish them with the means of paying him one fourth, and in some situations not more than a tenth of the value of his land ... All things are doubled and tripled in their value, save his lands. His family – his retainers – his public burdens! These last being regulated by the old valuation, lie very hard upon him, and all must be scraped up among the poor, meagre tenants, in twos and threes of silly lambs, hens and pounds of butter.

Hogg thus defined accurately and vividly the dilemma of the landlords. Not only had most rents advanced at a sensational rate, but, under sheep, the costs and bother of managing a Highland estate were much diminished. It was well known that collecting rent from a single capitalist sheep farmer was far easier than the interminable struggles to extract payment from a numerous small tenantry. The aggressive enterprise of the sheep farmers, combined with the financial difficulties of the old landowners, helped also to increase the fluidity of land ownership in this age. Clearances changed the tenantry; the ownership of the land itself was also altering across the region.[15]

Another agriculturist toured the Highlands in 1807, reporting that there were large territories in the north which were still untested by commercial sheep farming; thus Breadalbane had hardly yet tried either the Blackface or the Cheviot. 'From the very superior value of the wool,' he wrote, 'the farmer would be enabled to pay a much higher rent; while our great staple manufacture would be much promoted.' The Cheviot, he reported, had reached into Inverness-shire at Fort Augustus, and was into Caithness and parts of Ross, and ought to be tried elsewhere. He noted that:

> One thing, at least, is certain, that this range of hills is much better adapted to the rearing of sheep than black cattle; which last practice, though formerly most prevalent, is now much on the decline.

In Wester Ross there was little sign of improvement in any form, least of all in stock, in the vicinity of Lochbroom. At Beauly a wool and sheep fair had been established to promote the industry. Cheviots were thriving from the vale of Loch Lomond to Glengarry. This author took the view that the Highlands were overpopulated and were destined for pasturage – he believed that depopulation was not only inevitable but fully necessary for the national interest. Nevertheless he entertained some qualms about the process and opposed the reduction of the population by 'any arbitrary or violent measures'.[16]

The first decade of the new century was therefore marked by a still greater extension of sheep farming, which had by then reached most places south of the Great Glen, but had only just made a start in many of the Western Isles. The debate about emigration and population growth now swelled into a considerable controversy. Lord Selkirk's defence of Highland emigration[17] was a prelude to a flood of polemical writing. Some writers sought to persuade the government to intervene in order to prevent either the outflow of migrants or the inflow of sheep, or both. Emigration was closely associated with continuing clearance in many places. In 1801 Strathglass was almost totally cleared by William Chisholm and his wife Elizabeth Macdonnell, and there followed heavy emigration from Fort William, Isle Martin and Knoydart. In 1803 four ships took 500 people from Strathglass, many of whom suffered indescribable hardships on the trans-Atlantic voyage. It was during these years that 5390 people were said to have been driven out of the west coast glens. But on one patch of Strathglass an old widow refused to budge, and remained there until her death in 1820.[18]

In the 1730s it had been easier to recruit emigrants for America in Gaelic Scotland than in the Lowlands. This was generally the case until as late as 1815 when Clydeside and the south-west of Scotland emerged as generous suppliers of people for North America.[19]

In 1802 the Highland Society received an account of the current extension of sheep farming in the north. The braes of Perth, Dunbarton and Argyll, and the entire west coast from Oban to Lochbroom as well as most of Mull, were under sheep. In Skye the change was also fast approaching the island, simultaneously with accelerated population growth, and the new sheep had entered Lewis. In Inverness the west coast was still to be claimed by the sheep, but most of the rest of the county was occupied. Ross and the north were ripe for the new pastoralism.

The reporter predicted in gloomy tones:

> I have not a doubt from what is now passing in the Seats of Great Estates – that the whole race of Highlanders will, in a very few years, be extinguished, and the sheep come down to the East, as well as West and North Coasts.

The position, he said, was much exacerbated because, though the Cheviot was enabling sheep farmers to pay initially twice the rent that had been possible under the Blackfaces it could not survive the climate 'without low Winterings, and even some hay in bad seasons. This will soon annihilate Arable except [in] Towns; and perhaps a narrow border on the Coasts'.[20]

Despite these warnings, the work of clearance continued. Fraser of Lovat issued large numbers of removal notices in the years 1807–10.[21] In 1808 Sir George Mackenzie of Coull bought a large stock of Cheviots 'for the purpose of stocking an extensive sheep walk which he has lately taken into his hands' in Ross-shire.[22] Already in 1800 there had been clearances on the southerly fringes of the county of Sutherland, at Strathoykel. The plans for the utter transformation of the Sutherland estate (which comprised the lion's share of the entire county) began to take effect in 1807 when seventy families were removed from the parishes of Farr and Lairg. In neighbouring Reay country the conversion to Cheviots occurred first in the hands of Dunlop at Balnakill in 1800, and the process was completed by Major Forbes at Melness sixteen years later.[23] In the first decade of the century clearances were instituted in Kintail by the Seaforth factor, Duncan Mor Macrae and his father, 'who used the land to add to their own sheep farms'. These events, known as the Glenelchaig evictions, were followed by further evictions in the Letterfearn district, where fifty families were reputed to have been turned off their lands.[24] Between 1798 and 1808 the number of sheep in the county of Inverness had doubled.

On the estates of the Locheils in Lochaber the first clearances were those of Donald Cameron of Clunes – he pounced when leases expired in 1801. According to one account, Cameron's 'poor tenants were forced to spend the first night with their wives and children in the old graveyard above Clunes after being evicted, where they watched their humble dwellings being consigned to the flames'. These people moved, in the first instance, to Fort William. Fear of clearance was widespread among the people and may have persuaded them to emigrate in the exodus of 1802 and 1803. By July 1803 the estate was advertising lands in Lochaber in the newspapers. A letter of the time spoke of much 'spurring and hauling' which gave the local tenantry little realistic chance to compete in the rents asked. The letter writer suggested:

> I believe that the highest bidder of rent, whether from Moffat or Lochaber will be preferred . . . [The] proprietor encourages extensive grazing, which is greatly against the poor tenants who would incline to go to America, but the Government has fallen upon a plan to stop their career, as they will not be able to pay freight, as each passenger young or old must take up two tons of the ship, with every other allowance of provision, surgeons, attendance.

In March 1804 Duncan Cameron of Fassiefern remarked to Archibald MacMillan that Locheil's lands were being reset, and 'the present possessors are certain to be turned out'. The incoming pastoralists were offering double the current rent for the land. In another letter, dated December 1804, the full implications were spelled out:

> Everything is turned upside down since you left Lochaber, and the remainder of the unfortunate people you see emigrating, or at least as many of them as have the means in their power. Families who had not been disturbed for 4 or 500 years are turned out of house and their possessions given to the highest bidders. So much for Highland attachment between Chief and clans. But my own opinion is that the great gentlemen alluded to are doing a general good without any intention of doing so, by driving those people to desperation and forcing them to quit their country.

It was this Highland paradox of eviction and liberation that weighed on the mind of Archibald MacMillan in the following year when he wrote in similar terms:

> We cannot help looking to our native spot with sympathy and feeling which cannot be described, yet I have no hesitation in saying that considering the arrangements that daily take place and the total extinction of the tyes betwixt chief and clan, we are surely better off to be out of the reach of such unnatural tyranny.[25]

V. Land Leviathans

In the first decade of the new century, therefore, large tracts of the Highlands, even beyond the Great Glen, had been turned over to sheep and many of the inland communities dispersed or resettled on the coasts. Shepherds' cottages were now dotted about the mountains, inhabited by 'the servants of the opulent tenants'. But there were still many districts untouched by clearance, like the Isle of Kerrera where there existed seven hamlets composed of miserable huts, and to each a herd of about thirty cattle and a few patches of oats and barley, with some potatoes and flax. The island of Mull was not yet much affected by the improvement movement, unlike the Glencoe district where clearances had benefited the sheep farmers and landlords and both reaped excellent returns, and the wool produced was of splendid quality, though it was pointed out that 'twelve or sixteen families are thrown out of their usual line of employment . . . the greatest number of them are obliged to emigrate'. In the county of Inverness, Thomas Garnett saw that the coming of the sheep was 'wearing down the population', but he thought that those 'thus driven from their farms' found employment in the manufacturing towns. At Kenmore, Garnett discovered that even a relatively indulgent landlord found that his people were deserting him by emigrating to America: this was the Glenorchy estate which, far from clearing its inhabitants, had acted as a resettlement refuge for people evicted from other estates to the north.[26] It was a telling example which suggests a corrective to the notion that clearance was the exclusive cause of dislocation, land hunger and emigration in the Highlands during this period.

By 1810 the sheep had made prodigious progress across the Great Glen. There were other incursions around the main flank: a movement around the east coast establishing separate beach-heads in the Moray Firth and Caithness, and up the west coast slightly in advance of the mainland thrust. During the 1810s there was faster expansion in several districts. In North Uist, minor and unsung clearances were executed during this decade (and continued sporadically until 1850).[27] In February 1813 further sheep farms in Glengarry were advertised.[28] In Glenorchy the Marquis of Breadalbane was engaged in major clearances through the period 1806–31 and caused substantial depopulation. In many parts of Ross-shire people were being shifted to make way for the Cheviots. These changes went unrecorded for the most part, except in the anonymous statistics of estate rentals where groups of tenants disappear in favour of one large new tenant paying a much higher rent. It was as though the inhabitants had been erased by a stroke of a pen. Much of the history of the clearances was of this silent character.

In 1810 Walter Thom reported from Easter Ross a relatively small episode near Tain where a new tenant farmer had just turned eighteen families off their land. There was no manufacturing employment in the district and the people who had been evicted were 'too proud to serve on a property, where they have been masters'. The abhorrence of a perceived reduction of status from peasant to proletarian was a recurrent theme throughout the clearances, an essential aspect of the psychology of popular response to agrarian change. The Tain people emigrated to America where, thought Thom, their evident attachment to feudal notions would usefully serve as a counterpoise to the restless democratic spirit of that country.

Typical of the experience of small tenants living on estates on the fringes of the Highland land mass was that of Kiltearn, also in Rossshire. Here the population clearly declined in the decade after 1811 and the local clergyman had no hesitation in blaming the landowners for the loss of his human flock:

> During this period, numbers of small tenants were ejected in order to make way for farmers from the south, possessed of some capital, who, by their superior management, were able to afford higher rents. The more elevated districts of the parish, which were altogether unsuitable for cultivation, were converted into sheep walks; and numbers were thus deprived of all means of subsistence, and driven to seek in a foreign land for the shelter and protection which were denied them in their own. The right of landlords, however, to manage their properties according to their own pleasure, no one will pretend to doubt.[29]

Robert Southey, the poet laureate, visited the Highlands in 1819 and was shocked at the demolition of the old society, though he made no bones about the squalor of the traditional settlements in the hills. He was appalled at the tyranny of the clearing landlords. He described avaricious behaviour of landlords whereby an adviser would be employed simply to recommend a doubling, even a quadrupling of rents, which were then demanded of the people. The collapse of cattle and other prices after the French Wars placed the tenantry in extreme difficulty, and some of these rackrenting lairds seized the goods of their defaulting tenants. Southey called it the action of 'grasping and griping' landlords. One of these men had raised his rents from £500 to £7000 per year; his estranged wife took £3000, and his accumulated debt left him only £600 a year upon which he lived in London, 'kept needy by his debauched course of life . . . eking out this pittance by cutting down his woods. The roads at this time are almost destroyed by the carriage of his timber'. It was indeed the classic tale of landlord prodigality, of rapacious relatives, and of the suffering of a hapless tenantry. Southey recognised the sheer arbitrary power invested in such men, in contrast to the 'sober, moral, well disposed people, who if they were treated with common kindness, or even common justice, would be ready to lay down their lives in his service'.

The fifty 'Land Leviathans' who effectively possessed all the land in the Highlands were, according to Robert Southey, 'fools at heart', seeking only increased rents, and entirely careless of the human costs involved in their hedonistic pursuit of their own priorities. Southey believed that the Highlanders, given ordinary encouragement and goodwill, could exist as well as the English: the more so if they converted completely to potatoes as their staff of life.[30] It was a heroic assumption, but given no credibility by the events of the following quarter of a century.

Notes

1 *Old Statistical Account*, vol. VI (Tarbat).
2 *Edinburgh Evening Courant*, 18 October 1792.
3 See Leah Leneman, *Living in Atholl, 1685–1785* (Edinburgh, 1986) p. 67.
4 *Caledonian Mercury*, 15 October 1792.
5 Adam, *Sutherland Estate Management*, vol. I, p. xxix, n3.
6 SRO, GD 28/36/Fraser-Mackintosh Collection. For a later version of this type of vigilante association see Bangor-Jones, *The Assynt Clearances*, op. cit., p. 26.
7 SRO, GD128/47/4/Copy of 'Memorial and queries for the Sheep Farmers' Association, 1799'. See also the 'Petition of Donald Macleod of Geanies and others, 1798', GD128/36/8.
8 SRO, RH/2/4/64/Davidson to Mackenzie, 19 August 1792.
9 See Mitchell, op. cit., I, pp. 14, 334.
10 Selkirk, *Observations*, pp. 122–3.
11 'Amicus', *Eight Letters on the Subject of The Earl of Selkirk's Pamphlet on Highland Emigration as they Later Appeared Under the Signature of Amicus in Some of the Edinburgh Newspapers* (Edinburgh, 1803).
12 *Old Statistical Account*, entry for parish of Rosskeen, p. 266 n.
13 *Gazetteer of Scotland*, vol. II, p. 607.

14 See above, Chapter 2.

15 Hogg, *Tour*, pp. 27, 37–8, 49, 89–90.

16 Quoted in Richards, *Clearances*, op. cit., I, pp. 211–2.

17 Thomas Douglas, Earl of Selkirk, *Observations on the Present State of the Highlands of Scotland* (London, 1805), pp. 122–3.

18 Mackenzie, *Highland Clearances*, p. 187; Day, *Public Administration*, p. 84.

19 See for example, Anthony W. Parker, *Scottish Highlanders in Colonial America* (Athens, Georgia, 1997) and the unpublished work of Lucille H. Campey.

20 SRO, GD 51/5/28–52 (Questionnaire).

21 SRO, GD 128/32, Fraser-Mackintosh Collection, Evictions 1807–10.

22 *Inverness Journal*, 22 April 1809.

23 SCRG, D593/K/Horsburgh to Loch, 27 September 1850.

24 Mackenzie, *Highland Clearances*, p. 143.

25 MacMillan, *Bygone Lochaber*, pp. 181–3.

26 Ibid., pp. 13, 88, 235–6.

27 Iain Crawford, 'Contribution to the history of domestic settlement in north Uist', *SS*, vol. 9 (1965), pp. 35 et seq.

28 *Inverness Journal*, 12 February 1813.

29 *New Statistical Account*, vol. XIV, Ross and Cromarty, Kiltearn, p. 322.

30 Southey, *Journal*, pp. 40–1, 67, 137–8, 149, 158–60.

8

Clearing Sutherland: Lairg, Assynt and Kildonan 1807–13

I. The statue

IN 1994 A GROUP of people in the north-east Highlands mounted a public agitation to demolish, preferably by dynamite, the 100-foot statue of the first Duke of Sutherland which sits atop Ben Bragghie overlooking Dunrobin Castle and Golspie on the east coast of Sutherland. It was erected by the grateful estate tenantry in 1834, a year after the Duke's death. The idea in 1994 was to take retrospective retribution on the man regarded as responsible for the Sutherland clearances which had taken place almost two centuries before. It would be a grand symbolic action which James Hunter, prominent historian and spokesman for the modern crofter, likened to the public destruction of the icons of Stalinism which followed the collapse of the Iron Curtain in 1989.[1] Other historians have drawn powerful parallels between the events in Sutherland at the start of the nineteenth century and the extirpation of the Jews under the Nazis in the Second World War. Phrases such as 'final solution', 'genocide' and 'ethnic cleansing' repeatedly spring into the vocabularies of the condemners. As a spokesman said:

> The Gentleman on top of this pillar is perhaps one of the most evil men there ever was. Like Stalin and Hitler, he destroyed people's homes without cause. He was guilty of enormous cruelty. He has no honour in Scotland, and he is despised in the Highlands.

The Duke was 'symbolic of everything that is evil in Scottish history', said another.[2] It was the language of vilification and hatred; Websites, with cosmic anonymity, now continue the work, so that the communal memory shall never forget the crimes committed by the Sutherland aristocracy upon the common people of the northern Highlands.

All this sustained and barely diminished anger derives from the period 1807–21, a time of intensive removal and reorganisation on the great Sutherland estate which occupied most of the county of that name. Thousands of people were cleared from the inland straths and replaced by great sheep farms occupied by capitalist graziers who revolutionised land use and productivity on the estate. It was all done at a velocity and on a scale which were breathtaking even by the standards of the day. It was movement *en masse*; most of the change was telescoped into a single decade. The dislocation for the people was great and the psychic wounds inflicted did not heal; a sense of wrong was carried from generation to generation. Hence the Sutherland clearances were the most dramatic and sensational of all the removals and they occupy centre stage in all accounts of the Highland Clearances. They were also very well recorded because they were planned by an estate bureaucracy which prized planning and rationality above most other considerations.

In reality the first Duke of Sutherland was not the main force behind the Sutherland clearances; he merely provided the money that was lavished on the estate during the dislocations. This expenditure was mainly designed to mitigate the adverse consequences of the transformation. Lord Stafford (1758–1833, created first Duke of Sutherland in the year of his death) was an English millionaire who channelled extraordinary amounts of money taken from his English estates and English canals and (later) railways to subsidise the less remunerative Highland property of his wife, who was the principal source of energy and intellect behind the Sutherland clearances. She was Elizabeth Gordon (1765–1839), Countess of Sutherland, Marchioness of Stafford and finally Duchess/Countess of Sutherland. She was a talented, intelligent, attractive woman who had married extremely well – connecting a poor Highland dynasty with the richest family in the country. She was also ambitious and clear-minded in her resolution to turn her northern empire into an efficient paying property. This required modernisation – 'improvement' in the contemporary terminology – and this was the common obligation of any landowner. The challenge in Sutherland was greater than in most other places and the dislocation so much the harsher. It was a classic example of means and ends. The verdict of posterity has been kinder to the Countess than to her statued husband.

Lord Acton, who more famously remarked on the corrupting tendencies of power, declared that: 'We have attached political influence to property so closely that rich old women like the Duchess/Countess [of Sutherland] or Lady Londonderry, are dreadful powers in the land'.[3] The sacred rights of landownership were preserved by the political system and the law and the Duchess/Countess represented wealth and power in its most conspicuous form. That she used that power to clear her people from the glens seemed like the ultimate crime of the aristocracy over the loyal clansmen. It has never lost its capacity to anger each passing generation.

Not surprisingly, given the scale and rigour of the events in Sutherland, there was also considerable turbulence. Riots broke out on several occasions and these eruptions were given greater publicity than even the 'Insurrection' of 1792 in Ross-shire. The people who were actually cleared made themselves heard (indirectly but often eloquently) through the medium of popular protest.

II. The perfect plan

The events in Sutherland were the more cataclysmic because they were delayed by conditions which limited the scope of estate management and reorganisation until after the turn of the new century. Then they accelerated at a pace designed to catch up with the lost opportunities of the previous two decades. These opportunities were those beckoning all Highland proprietors and they sprang from the great inflation of the prices of wool and mutton.

Until 1803 the Countess of Sutherland was too poor to undertake a great rationalisation of her territorial empire: but in 1803 her husband became Marquess of Stafford and inherited the richest fortune in the kingdom – only then did clearances and reorganisation become practicable. His brilliant wife persuaded him to pour a very large part of this extraordinary fortune into her Highland territories in the belief that this would bring great improvements to the people and to the proprietor alike. It would be an intelligent investment, the more sensible because the opportunities were so ripe. In retrospect the Sutherland estate seems like a sump into which some of the richest profits of English industrialisation were lost in Highland bogs. Eventually the loss to the nation at large was appalling and rarely accounted in the balance sheet of the clearances.

There were two further problems in Sutherland. Most of the land was locked up in the hands of tenants and wadsetters[4] until their leases either expired or were bought out by the landlord. The Countess did not gain full control of her estate until after the turn of the century. Her other problem was the disposition of the people who occupied the inland of the estate and remained wedded to the old cattle and meal economy. Their numbers were increasing and they were resolutely 'unimproved'. No improver could be satisfied with the squalor and poverty of these people: they and their living conditions were anachronisms. But any change, radical by necessity, would require their succour and co-operation. The managers in Sutherland were acutely conscious of the unhappy reputation of improving landlords across the Highlands. They would not make the same mistake.

Two ideas loomed large in the thinking of the Sutherland estate when a great new plan eventually emerged at the turn of the century. The first was the growing conviction that the estate, which was close to a million acres in extent, was capable of spectacular economic advance. The propaganda of advanced thinkers such as George Dempster and Sir John Sinclair entered the minds of the Countess and her advisers: they knew that sheep farmers were prepared to pay vastly enhanced rents for the mountains and glens of the interior. The conversion of large territories to sheep could be allied, without great difficulty, to a parallel advance of fishing and manufacturing industry in designated places along the coast of the estate. There was a flush of confidence which eventually persuaded the estate owners and entrepreneurs that a literal replication of the industrial success of Lancashire and Lanarkshire was practicable in far away Sutherland and the west Highlands.

The second pillar of thinking in the Sutherland plans was about the poverty of the common people of the estate. They fell victims to recurrent famine which haunted the old Highlands in a way by then long forgotten in most of the rest of the British Isles. The people lived in precarious conditions and they were periodically dependent on the landlord for large outlays of famine relief. Unless the people were to live in permanent or worsening misery, a fundamental rearrangement of the foundations of their lives was imperative. This was the message of improvement transmitted across western Europe.

Thus, the diagnosis was clear and blazoned forth in the doctrines of Improvement. With or without sheep farming, the condition of the people had to be transformed. Better still, the plans for sheep farms and the solution for the problem of poverty could be connected by balanced progress. Sheep could be introduced; the landlord's income would be greatly augmented; her ability to succour her people would be enhanced; and the people could be removed from the shadow of famine and established on new and more secure economic foundations. Clearance and social advance were, under this formula, perfectly compatible.

III. Famine and progress

The realities behind these assumptions are less secure. It is true that the condition of the people was periodically awful.[5] Sutherland was remote, and poor in arable resources; in the several decades before the clearances there was unambiguous evidence of poverty and strain among the common people. Emigration was heavy in 1763 and 1771–2 and there were vivid contemporary descriptions of the agony of the refugees from famine *en route* for North America. The rigour of the famine in 1771 was attested by the attempt of the tenantry of Assynt to throw up their leases, and by the landlord's extraordinary action to alleviate their difficulties.[6] Near-famine conditions recurred in every decade to the 1870s and always required external relief. Between times, however, economic conditions were often generous enough to maintain the population in reasonable comfort. It was a perennial Highland paradox. The recurrent meanness of nature was not the only cause of these privations: the pressure of the tacksmen and the growing rent demands of the landlord cannot be discounted. Population growth compounded the difficulties of an impoverished peasantry, especially on the west coast of Sutherland. In Assynt the number of people increased by 44 per cent in the forty years after 1774, although some Sutherland parishes appear to have registered a decline in the same years. The increase of population was probably contingent more upon the recession of disease than on improvements in the general conditions of life. In 1803, on the eve of the clearances, famine struck Strathnaver, a relatively favoured and populous area in the north of the estate.[7] It became estate policy to clear all such people out of the interior glens.

These ideas brewed with increasing urgency in the years following the marriage of the Countess in 1785. In the eighteen years before her husband came into his mammoth inheritance the Highland estate remained typically impoverished. The Countess was unable to live within the income of her Highland property. Her consumption and expenditure exceeded her income and she accumulated debts. She and her husband were able to spare nothing for the capital improvement and until the great inheritance in 1803 they drained the local economy of its surplus. Until then they were typical unimproved Highland proprietors.[8]

Other parts of the county had already begun to introduce sheep, which helps to explain the involvement of Sutherland people in the Ross-shire Insurrection in 1792. In 1790 the Balnagowan estate of Sir Charles Ross, which overlapped into the northern county, was converted to sheep farming. Some of the people evicted in the process settled on the Sutherland estate as squatters and sub-tenants.

From 1792 to 1794 a group of southern sheep farmers entered the far northern estate of Lord Armadale but in this case the people ousted were resettled on the north coast at Portskerra and Armadale, where they were encouraged 'to improve and be industrious seamen'.[9] Other local landowners followed a similar pattern: that is, people generally were cleared to new settlements along the coasts while the landowners counted the great increase of their rental from the sheep farmers. These crofting settlements were usually less than two acres per lot, and the expectation was that the people would devote their energies to fishing. There were variations: at Eddrachillis, for instance, there were reports of fifty families being cleared without any provision for resettlement.[10] Such people were added to the swelling problem of squatting and overcrowding in the uncleared districts of the Highlands.

On the estate of Rosehall (in Creich) the lands had been arranged traditionally into five farms until 1788 when the owner, General William Baillie, consolidated them into a single large sheep farm, let to a sheep farmer named Campbell – 'the former tenants being driven away'.[11] The large estate of Reay was cleared mainly in the years 1810–15; its people were encouraged to settle on the north coast. Some resettled in Orkney. Even before this, many families had already been forced to emigrate to Orkney from Strathnaver, where 'their farms had been converted into sheep pastures'. According to the minister they had been 'comfortably situated in their former residences, as they all brought with them, to this place, a very considerable stock in horses, cows, sheep, and goats and also in grain'. In common with many other Highland emigrants they appear to have been relatively prosperous, yet they were evidently unable to avoid expatriation in the face of the incoming sheep masters and their flocks.[12]

The estate of the Countess had considered the introduction of sheep farming as early as 1767 but was held back by lack of capital, by inertia and by an unease about the social consequences.[13] A sheep-farming expert, Andrew Ker, visited Sutherland in 1791. He reported that the estate was contemplating the new system. Ker spoke to Fraser, the agent of the Countess, who was

> pretty certain a great many, if not the whole of the tenants on that coast would give up in a great measure, their black cattle, and take to sheep, provided that they had an example shown them. But as they know nothing about sheep, or the management of them, they do not chuse to run any risk.[14]

When sheep farming came to Sutherland, as to the rest of the Highlands, it was not so much the ignorance of the small tenantry, as the level of capital (in very large amounts), which appears to have disqualified them from even the slightest involvement in the new sheep-farming economy.

The attempt by the Sutherland estate management to farm sheep on its own account also proved signally uneconomic. But the first approaches from professional sheep farmers from Ross-shire in 1792, for leases at Wester Lairg, were not well received. The Sutherland factor was sceptical of the whole idea of large-scale sheep farming. He believed that it would create bad feelings between the various grades of the tenantry. He probably also feared that the disturbances which had rocked Ross-shire only a few months before would spread northwards.[15] The factors, trained in the old ways, positively resisted the new disruptive ideas of Improvement and Clearance. Eventually the Countess found it necessary to sack the old managers.[16] Meanwhile, however, indigenous tacksmen were taking part of the process into their own hands and were clearing out their own sub-tenants in advance of their landlord.[17]

IV. Impatience

Although held back by the timidity of her advisers, the Countess began thinking seriously about sheep farming and resettlement zones as early as 1791. In 1799 she was planning 'thinning' the population of the western districts and thinking about ways of accommodating the people thus cleared into coastal villages.[18] She knew, however, that the revolution would have to wait upon the expiration of leases in 1807.[19]

Meanwhile estate life continued in the old ways but in the context of the great war with France. Sutherland was a supplier of men to the regiments and this was still an assumed obligation of both landlord and people, a traditional reciprocation. Even as she planned to dispense with the relics of feudalism on her estate the Countess of Sutherland reasserted her claim on the military service of the common people. The ironies of the situation began to multiply. In July 1799, for example, she became angry about her people's evident reluctance to accept wartime recruitment into her regiment. She wrote that they 'need no longer be considered as a credit to Sutherland, or an advantage *over sheep* or any useful animal'.[20] Some tenants were placed under notice of eviction because they had joined the wrong regiment;[21] and such people were actively discriminated against in the subsequent removals in Kildonan in 1806–7, when they were refused resettlement on the estate.[22]

If recruits were not delivered by these communities the common people could evidently expect no special favours or indulgences, 'or be permitted to remain on the Sutherland estate any more than the Countess's own immediate tenants who are in the same predicament'.[23] This was evidently the voice of change from above.

The estate management effectively acknowledged that military service was related to the occupation of the land and that 'loyalty and regard to the character of the country' continued to operate as obligations. Though there may have been 'a relaxation more or less of the Ancient Spirit of Clanship and Vassalage' in some parts, there remained a set of accepted reciprocities in landlord–tenant relations. Hence the common people could expect landlord assistance 'when a year of scarcity or any particular accidental distress reduced them to temporary difficulties'.[24] In time of war the Countess was prepared to invoke the old loyalty in a direct way, thereby implicitly renewing the traditional 'contract'. The young Glengarry had made the same determination in Knoydart in 1794.[25]

In 1802, when the Countess and her husband visited the northern estates, the plans were in an advanced state of readiness. Offers, often at very high rents, were already being gathered from prospective sheep farmers in advance of any announced plan for clearance. But the estate factors continued to express hesitation and disquiet about the anticipated effects of sheep farming on the common people. The old generation of factors could see no easy solution to the problem of the co-existence of sheep and people. In June 1803 the factor remarked that

> When so great a range is thrown into one farm, and the system of
> management is changed from Black Cattle to sheep, there ought to be a
> rise beyond double rent.

Sheep farming would raise rents very rapidly. In 1806, when the rental of the estate had stood at £5859, the estate factor predicted that a figure in excess of £20 000 could be achieved.

In March and October 1803 the husband of the Countess of Sutherland inherited the fabulous fortunes of his uncle the Duke of Bridgewater and his father the Marquis of Stafford. The restraints on capital investment were now relaxed, even though many leases in Sutherland did not expire until 1807 or later. By August 1805 the broad lines of the plan for Sutherland had been specified in terms of both sheep walks and village development. The current factor predicted that the 'New Arrangements . . . will be beneficial to the Estate and the Country at large . . . I am persuaded the country never will be improved or civilised till totally New Systems are introduced'. He added, with emphasis:

> Our constituents are always tender of the people and will not be less so
> now but it will be a blessing to a great proportion of them to be taught
> a new and improved application of their industry and labour.[26]

V. Tender clearances

'Tenderness' was to be the mark of the new arrangements, but the Countess herself told her husband in 1805 that 'a proper degree of firmness' would be essential. Social control and improvement travelled in tandem. The people would be resettled without leases so that they could be easily shifted in cases of bad conduct, or be 'ready to settle in another part of the country where we conceive fisheries will speedily increase'. She believed that the success of the new fisheries and other public works would confound the pessimism of Lord Selkirk (who advocated wholesale emigration). 'In a few years,' she told her husband, 'this country will be benefited by preserving its people to a reasonable degree.'[27]

The Countess was buoyed with optimism at this time: she spoke of one fishing village which 'will employ numbers of people, establish them, and bring riches and industry into the Country'.[28] Moreover the Countess believed that the creation of fishing villages would attract the common people out of the hills voluntarily, somewhat in advance of the new sheep farms. This was a measure of how little she understood the inertia and psychology of the inland people; there was no anticipation of the social dislocation and turmoil which eventually enveloped the estate plans. From the beginning the consistently reiterated theme in the clearance programme was that the retention of the population was vital. All their pronouncements were couched in the language of retention.

The financial prospects for the Sutherland programme were assumed to be highly favourable for the investment of English capital. The factor remarked however that

> This is evidently impossible without sweeping away what *at present* is a *superfluous* population but which when our roads, villages, and harbour are made, and a little time allowed for enabling example to operate, will become the means of enhancing the value far even above £20 000 a year.[29]

With the elimination of the middlemen, rents for the common people could be reduced and the estate might even be able to accommodate more people than before, and they would be 'happy and contented'.[30]

Some of the estate managers recognised the severity of the transformation about to be set in motion. The Countess was told about the likely problems in unequivocal terms:

> A great proportion of . . . your population is totally ignorant of the means of gaining Subsistence in a Village and this ignorance if construed into Contumacy would be punished by leaving them only an option between Starving and Emigration, which last if adopted from voluntary choice I would certainly not restrain but can never Consider it as otherwise than impolitic as well as cruel if forced upon the people prematurely requiring of them to change suddenly all the habits of their lives. In my humble opinion the end in View will be obtained by patient and steady Measure *gradually* brought to maturity, while any

attempt at an instantaneous change would fail and only involve the bulk of the people in misery and Ruin.[31]

These sentiments were reiterated frequently throughout the painful years of the clearances although there was always a gulf between the conception and the execution of the plans. It was a recipe for conflict.

VI. The new beginning

The Sutherland plan moved into gear in 1806 with the advice of Thomas Gillespie of the Glengarry district, an established grazier who had been among the first generation of commercial sheep farmers in the Highlands. The new sheep farms were advertised, and at Whitsun 1807 the first big sheep farm began operations at Lairg at a rent thrice its previous level. The settlement of the displaced small tenantry, even at the outset, proved to be the fundamental weakness of the experiment. The people concerned were placed, very unhappily, on the northern banks of Loch Naver. It was the first of a long succession of problems which derived from the poor synchronisation of clearances and resettlement facilities along the northern and eastern coasts of the estate. As R.J. Adam observed, the practical difficulties were consistently underestimated. The numbers involved in the Lairg clearance were at least 300. Progress in the development of the new coastal villages was slow. The flow of English capital into Sutherland was still limited and the conditions for expansion were further dislocated by the famine that marched through the northern Highlands in 1807–8; it was the worst harvest since the ill-famed years of 1782–3.[32]

The negative reaction of the small tenants to the clearances of 1806–7 was a matter of disappointment to the Countess and her advisers, and reflected a general repugnance for resettlement schemes among the people affected. Many of the families removed from Strathnaver spurned the offer of other accommodation along the north coast. They emigrated instead to North America in a ship which was lost with all hands off the coast of Newfoundland.[33]

These first clearances undoubtedly created turmoil in the minds of the people, even among those not directly affected by the current changes. Emigration accelerated. The factor, Cosmo Falconer, reported that a group of Sutherlanders had taken

> a *freak* in their heads to leave the country because they foresaw that they had no chance of possession did they remain, and there was a sort of discontent among them, and also a stirring up by some disaffected persons which led to the embarkation.[34]

The people who remained on the estate and resettled on the north coast faced inadequate and congested conditions and many were forced to seek work on an itinerant or seasonal basis.

The Countess of Sutherland was much abused locally for her clearances of 1806–7 and her factor testified to 'the Commotion occasioned by the formation of the large sheep tenement'.[35] There had been an alarming lack of co-operation from the people in the first round of clearances, and the reception arrangements were, on the admission of the management itself, insufficient. A pilot scheme to resettle people on improvable moors at Achavandra on the east coast proved equally unattractive to the people.

The surly resistance of the people can be sensed in the exasperation of the factors, and in the reactive pattern of emigration. As for the proprietors, they felt that the material state of the people could be improved only by change, and that their old mode of living was deplorable, indeed scarcely human. The Countess's son, Lord Gower, expressed this attitude when, in August 1805, he described some of the people of Assynt 'as a dirty set, and no very prepossessing specimens of the Lords of Creation'. Falconer was hardly less contemptuous when he justified expenditure on resettlement facilities for the people, essentially on grounds that it 'would shut their mouths against the clamours and prevent a plea of hardship'.[36]

VII. The second round

The first round of the Sutherland clearances had produced a local explosion of rancour and difficulty. The Countess lost confidence in her managers. She now sought stronger guidance, more enthusiastic energy and new initiatives for her Highland empire. In 1809 these qualities were supplied by two dynamic Morayshire agricultural entrepreneurs, William Young and Patrick Sellar. The old factor was sacked and the management of the Sutherland estate fell into the hands of the two Moraymen who did not regard themselves as Highlanders.[37]

Young and Sellar gave new direction, as well as ambitious solutions, to the problems of the estate. Their ideas were essentially an extension of those of the Countess, but they accelerated and expanded the plans into a great exercise in social and economic planning.[38] They powerfully reinforced her idea that the estate economy could be radically reshaped by the introduction of capital and enterprise. Sheep farming was inevitable and the interior population should be resettled in villages built for fishing and industrial employment. Young and Sellar were convinced that the two processes were complementary. The Sutherland estate was extraordinarily backward, primarily because the poverty of the people was occasioned by the misapplication of their labour and the mismanagement of the soil.

There was a glorious opportunity to develop the natural and human resources of the estate. In common with the Countess, Young and Sellar rejected all suggestion of overpopulation: the people were poverty stricken only because their energies were dormant or misapplied. The notion that there were actually too many people, they reasoned:

> must be a mistake . . . for England, although less fruitful and more populous, is richer than Spain; and it is so, *only because* it is more populous, and because every nation pays tribute to the well directed industry of its people.[39]

Sellar and Young were full of Adam Smith's doctrines, extolling the virtues of the division of labour at all times. With boundless enthusiasm they painted fantasies of progress which amounted to the industrialisation of the population of Sutherland. They talked expansively of quadrupling (and even more) the rental income of the land in the estate. It was a plan of forced economic advance which included specific plans for coastal development, involving tanning, cotton, flax, salt, brick and lime manufacturing, coal-mining, fishing and 'muir' improvement. These plans were meant to be entirely complementary to the ongoing plans for clearances from the interior. The justification of the changes rested squarely on the premise that the peasantry of the inland glens lived in conditions intolerable both to themselves and to the landlord. The near famine of 1807–8 gave particular point to this assumption.[40]

The first stage in the new sequence of agrarian revolution was to be the clearance of Assynt, the extreme north-west of the estate, under the direction of William Young. In a report on Assynt written in August 1811, Young recommended that most of that large parish be converted to Cheviot sheep, while 'reserving accommodation for kelp makers, fisheries, lime burners, and other labourers'. Such resettlement provisions were vital because he knew that 'Lord and Lady Stafford will in this and other districts rather sacrifice their interest than that the people should be entirely dispossessed'. He had therefore proposed extensive village development on the west coast, centred upon Lochinver which would become, he predicted, 'the *Metropolis* of Assynt'. He recommended that settlers on the coast be given potato land but he insisted that they would have to be shaken from their current 'sloth and idleness'. Most of the interior parts of Assynt were tied up in tacks until Whitsunday 1812.[41]

Euphoria warmed the estate discussions in 1810–11. There was now a feeling that no inherent contradiction existed between the interests of the landlord and those of the common people. The clearances would be benevolent. The Sutherland system promised a mode of absorbing the people displaced by the sheep walks: it reconciled the issue of rent increases with the welfare of the people. As one relatively independent observer (and a critic of the clearances) wrote in 1811, the Sutherland plan was unprecedented in its scale and expenditure. Sheep farming was to be introduced without any reduction of the population. The plan would

tend most effectively to increase the number as well as the comfort and happiness of the population of this country.

Sutherland would become the model for all other Highland proprietors. It would moreover put an end to emigration.[42]

VIII. Calm clearances in Assynt, 1812

Assynt was the first test of the new management. In Assynt great new sheep farms were carved out of the old tacks and the small tenantry were extruded to the coasts. The arrangement was executed in 1812 and, though brimming with confidence and self-belief, Young and Sellar half expected trouble and resistance to erupt. The local harvest had been very poor again. Nevertheless the sheep farms had been accepted by the new farmers, drawn not from the south but from the local tacksmen who had, somewhat desperately, outbid all other competition.[43]

At Whitsunday 1812 Patrick Sellar, Young's right hand man and implementer, carried out the clearances in Assynt and the events passed relatively quietly. Sellar attributed this surprising peacability to the fact that the new sheep-farming tenants included Assynt tacksmen, who exercised a calming and controlling influence over the people, so that 'little or no interference of mine was necessary'. The people of the west were commended as sober, industrious and uncorrupted by illicit distilling. But even in Assynt it is clear that some of the common people 'would not listen to a seaside settlement' and remained in the hills. Lady Stafford told her son, Gower, that 'the People of the lower class in general appear so unwilling to come to any plan for bettering the general condition'. It was, therefore, reasonable to encourage the unco-operative elements to emigrate.[44]

At a critical time in these removals in 1813, it became clear that the resettlement schemes were unpopular to many of the people. Lord Selkirk discussed the whole problem with Lady Stafford. He said that the arrangements made by William Young were 'more liberal', but 'in the state of mind of these people, many would not accept'. Selkirk offered to take many of the married men to Canada to serve in a regiment, their families to follow at the end of the war. Lady Stafford vetoed this idea as 'totally inadvisable', which left the problem unsolved.[45]

IX. *Turmoil in Kildonan and Clyne, 1812*

Assynt was, in the outcome, a misleading dawn. Nor did the peaceful character of the clearances 'mean that they were not traumatic'.[46] The people of the rest of Sutherland had become thoroughly alerted to the impending spread of the removal movement. Next on the list were the wider valleys and deep straths of Kildonan and Clyne. Here open conflict erupted at the end of 1812. Soon the district looked as dangerous in potential for popular resistance as Ross-shire twenty years before.

In Kildonan and Clyne, Young and Sellar had made the 'sett' of several large sheep farms and the dispossessed tenantry were offered allotments on the northern and eastern coasts. Several hundred people were involved in the clearance and transplantation, many of them, according to Young, smugglers who would do better for the estate as fishermen. Events came to a rapid crisis in the first week of 1813. A group of factors, shepherds and valuers who were surveying prospective sheep farms near Suisgill were confronted by a large body of people bent on ejecting them and their sheep out of their lands. Young exclaimed, 'The natives rose in a body and chased the valuers off the ground and now threaten the lives of every man who dares to dispossess them'. The tenacity of the recalcitrant Kildonan people was attributed to their whisky smuggling, which they would undoubtedly lose if resettled on the coasts. The elimination of the tacksmen was another potent cause of disaffection.

The subsequent precognition of these events left little doubt that, in Kildonan, a plan had been 'concerted to oppose the introduction of sheep into the parish'.[47] The surveying party had been threatened by a group of men armed with bludgeons, and told 'that if sheep were put upon that Ground there should be blood . . . and not little of it'.

It was, so far, intimidation and threat rather than violence. The antagonism was directed in part at the inflation of rents and prices caused by 'those English Devils who had come into the country'. One of the assailants, it was reported, 'swore that it was sheep farming which had made the Boll [of meal] so dear, that formerly they would have got the Boll for twenty shillings whereas it now cost them two pounds'. It was also alleged that threats had been made to the effect that 'every shepherd's house in the Country should be set on fire . . . and burned down to the bare walls', and that there would be a general rising of the people of Kildonan (aided by those of Reay and Caithness) to 'drive the Sheeps [sic] out of the country'.[48] It was an accurate echo of the sounds of 1792.

In a petition from 'the tenants of Kildonan' it was asserted that they were prepared to pay as much rent as offered by the sheep farmers; they denied allegations of intimidation, but refused to sign a bond to keep the peace 'until they had received satisfaction in the conflict'.[49] They had clearly adopted an uncompromising attitude towards the landlord. The law was flouted: it proved impossible to capture the miscreants or to continue the precognition; the entire investigation was stymied by collective resistance.

A law officer thought that the people could muster '1000 men, a great proportion of whom have been in the army'. There was talk of 'a general rising'.[50] It was another 1792 nightmare in the making, and now more serious still since the country was at war. The people said that they had furnished sons as recruits to the 93rd Regiment and that this 'entitled them to their own land' and that they would hold it at least until their sons were returned. This was the voice of an obstinate, aroused and indignant peasantry. William Young was now thoroughly embittered:

> Everything I do is in a manner at the point of the sword. Both rich and poor (with very few exceptions) are hostile to every plan of improvement. They are absolutely a century behind and what is worse a great many want common honesty.

He described the common people as a set of savages, worse than American Indians; they were 'banditti' threatening the entire course of progress in Sutherland. He alleged that they were supported by the dispossessed tacksmen, and that 'the whole country are on the watch to see how the *war will end* and so act accordingly'. If the rebels were not quelled, he warned, 'we may bid adieu to all improvement.'[51] It was, palpably, a collision between the forces of change, of improvement, and those of tradition and the past.

The agrarian resistance in Kildonan was formidable by any standard and it continued for more than six weeks. It was therefore more sustained than the resistance in Ross-shire in the so-called 'Year of the Sheep'. In mid-February 1813 William Young told Lady Stafford:

> The matter is now come to such a point that either Lord Stafford or your Ladyship are to renounce every title to dispose your property as you see proper, or an Armed force is to support the Laws of the Country . . . it is impossible to proceed with any business in the present State of the Country.

The management of the estate was conspicuously unable to recruit the moral support of the 'Gentlemen of the Country', moreover 'the whole Population feel desirous of success to the Rioters, knowing that they have common interest in the Expulsion of the Strangers'.

The point of confrontation had now been reached. Lady Stafford, the prime mover in the events, recognised the diametrical opposition of the inevitable collision:

> In short, I do not see anything more that can be done by us, our efforts being rejected, and as the people resist by force, no one can complain if they are brought to reason by the same means.

With cold precision she saw the logic of improvement following its inevitable course, regardless of the accompanying conflict.[52]

The resistance was clearly based on broad popular support. It persisted into March 1813 and negotiations repeatedly broke down. Petitions were sent to the Stafford family and to the Prince Regent. The Sheriff Depute, Cranstoun, who considered the riots as 'a very extensive and well organised combination among the tenantry', ordered troops into Kildonan. At the same time the management offered various concessions to the people, particularly a provision for the purchase of the people's cattle at generous prices, and arrangements that 'the Crofters will be allowed to continue in their houses until their new ones are ready for them'. Six months' notice was given for the removal. Undoubtedly, despite dire warnings from Patrick Sellar, the estate adopted a conciliatory attitude and the commotion simmered down in the latter part of March. Two other factors may have assisted the diminution of tension: a number of neighbouring lairds in Caithness offered the people accommodation on their estates, and Lord Selkirk also offered to assist the migration to Canada of Sutherland Highlanders. Astonishingly, 580 people from Kildonan had accepted the opportunity by the middle of April, though fewer ever fulfilled the engagement.[53]

The Kildonan riots represented a critical moment in the evolution of the Sutherland clearances. It is evident that the people's co-operation in the social and economic change had not been engaged. The entire programme of clearance and redevelopment had come to depend on compulsion. The people remained at all times either sullen or actively hostile. The Countess of Sutherland and her advisers were genuinely astonished at this response to plans which they regarded as wise and benevolent. They believed the common people were ungrateful and foolish. 'The annals of History', claimed William Young, 'do not afford proof of any proprietor of a Highland Estate having done so much for a tenantry.'[54] But the Countess acknowledged the hostility among the people: when the question arose of giving estate encouragement to the people to emigrate to America, she remarked that they 'would suspect that they had not fair play and that it would defeat its own purpose'.[55]

The people of the Highlands, the record indicates, were not easily inflamed into riot and resistance to their lairds, and the behaviour of the Sutherlanders at this time is therefore powerful testimony to their moral outrage, their fear and their tenacity in clinging to their allegedly ancient rights and possessions.

There was a significant sequel to the anti-clearance activity in July 1813. In this case the trouble arose not from evictions but from the induction of a new minister unacceptable to the people of the parish of Assynt. William Young had previously commended the Assynt folk for their industrious, sober and uncorrupted demeanour. In July 1813 he accompanied the Revd Duncan Macgillivray, a native of Nairn, to Assynt. The people believed that they should determine the ministerial succession and now made their feelings abundantly clear. Young and Macgillivray were assaulted by a group of 'Mountain savages . . . and it was ten to one that lives were not lost'. They had been driven out of the parish and had narrowly escaped being handcuffed and pushed out to sea in an open boat. It was, Young advised, a complete threat to all public order in the district. He added that 'The Kildonan riots were a mere nothing [compared] to this and [in Kildonan] the people had some shadow of excuse'.[56] The Sheriff Depute, Cranstoun, began an investigation and arranged for military assistance. A 'King's Cutter' with 160 men of the West Norfolk Militia arrived at Lochinver but the disturbances had already subsided.[57]

In his subsequent discussion of the riot in Assynt, Patrick Sellar claimed that the disturbances indicated a pattern of general popular resistance to the Sutherland family in the county. It was part of a widespread conspiracy among the common people who were harassing every shepherd in the north. They had pledged themselves to drive all the south country people out of the Highlands.[58] Indeed all the evidence about these events suggests that the Assynt riot was an expression of anti-landlord feeling of a type with the popular disorder in Kildonan. The mood of the people, and their reaction to the clearances, was transparent. Religion was now mixed up with clearances, and the people were equally inflamed on both issues.[59]

The common denominator was resistance to landlord authority. The Sutherland clearances, designed as a scientific exercise of improvement planning, had run into the bogs of communal opposition. And the planners had hardly yet tackled the best parts of the estate, including the still densely populated parts of the great strath of Naver, the subject of 1814 and a critical moment in the long history of the Highland Clearances.

Notes

1 See Rob Gibson, *Toppling the Duke – Outrage at Ben Bragghie?* (Evanston, 1996).

2 Quoted in Charles W.J. Withers, 'Place, memory, monument: memorialising the past in contemporary highland Scotland', *Ecumene* vol. 3 (1996), pp. 325–44.

3 Lord Acton, quoted in Bernard Falk, *The Bridgewater Millions* (1942), p. 132.

4 Wadset: the conveyance of land in satisfaction of, or as security for, a debt, the debtor having the right to recover the lands on payment of the debt. Much of the background to the Sutherland clearances is treated expertly in M. Bangor-Jones, *The Assynt Clearances* (Dundee, 1998).

5 See Richards, *Leviathan*, pp. 160–8.

6 Fraser, *The Sutherland Book*, vol. I, pp. 482–3.

7 On the 1803 famine, see *Inverness Courier*, 16 July 1845; and David Forbes, *The Sutherland Clearances* 1806–1820 (Ayr, 1976), pp. 12–14.

8 See Richards, *Leviathan*, Chapter XII.

9 SCRO, D593/K1/38/Loch to Anderson, September 1850.

10 Richards, *Leviathan*, p. 169.

11 Rosehall Memorandum Book, Reading University Library.

12 OSA XIX (Orkney) p. 205, quoted in *Parish Life in Eighteenth Century Scotland.* (1995), p. 133.

13 Adam, *Sutherland Estate Management*, I, p. xxix.

14 Ker, *Report to Sir John Sinclair*, pp. 22–3.

15 Adam, *Sutherland Estate Management*, vol. 1, p. xxix, n3. See Bangor-Jones, op. cit., pp. 4–5.

16 Eric Richards, 'The prospect of economic growth in Sutherland at the time of the Clearances, 1809–1813', *SHR*, vol. 49 (1970), pp. 154–72.

17 See Bangor-Jones, op. cit., pp. 4–5.

18 Richards, *Leviathan*, pp. 169–70; Adam, *Sutherland Estate Management*, vol. I, p. xxix, n.3.

19 See Fraser, *The Sutherland Book*, vol. I, pp. 483–4.

20 Adam, *Sutherland Estate Management*, vol. 1, p. xxix, n4.

21 Ibid., vol. I, p. 3.

22 Ibid., vol. I, p. 9.

23 Ibid., vol. II, pp. 3–4

24 Ibid., vol. II, pp. 6–l0.

25 First Report from the Select Committee on Emigration, Scotland (1841). Irish University Press series: Emigration, vol. 3, p. 9.

26 Ibid., vol. II, p. 24.

27 Ibid., vol. II, pp. 39–43, 45–6.

28 Ibid., vol. II, p. 43.

29 Ibid., vol. II, pp. 59–60.

30 Ibid., vol. II, pp. 40–41.

31 Ibid., vol. II, p. 60.

32 Ibid., vol. II, p. 62; vol. I, pp. xxxiv–xxxv.

33 Henderson, *General View Of Sutherland*, p. 26; Richards, 'Prospect', pp. 155–6.

34 Richards, 'Prospect', p. 160.

35 Adam, *Sutherland Estate Management*, vol. II, p. 126.

36 Richards, 'Prospect', p. 161.

37 See Richards, *Patrick Sellar and the Highland Clearances*, Chapter 6.

38 Adam, Sutherland Estate Management., vol. 1, pp. xl et seq.; Richards, 'Prospect', passim.

39 Richards, 'Prospect', p. 159.

40 Richards, 'Structural Change'.

41 Adam, *Sutherland Estate Management*, vol. I, pp. xix, 127.

42 Henderson, *General View of Sutherland*, Additional Report, p. 158.

43 On rent increases see Bangor-Jones, op. cit., pp. 19–20.

44 Adam, *Sutherland Estate Management*, vol. II, pp. 90, 167.

45 GD268/216 Lady Stafford to Loch (undated 1815).

46 Bangor-Jones, op. cit., p. 44; cf. Neeson, op. cit., passim.

47 SRO AD/14/13/9/Documents relating to the Kildonan Riots 1813.

48 Ibid.

49 SRO, ADl4/13/9.

50 Ibid., Cranstoun to Lord Advocate, n.d.

51 Richards, *Leviathan*, pp. 179–83.

52 GD268/216 Lady Stafford to Loch, undated [1813], p. 166.

53 SCRO, D593/K/Mackenzie to Loch, 21 February 1813.

54 Adam, *Sutherland Estate Management*, vol. II, p. 190.

55 Ibid., vol. II, p. 144.

56 Ibid., vol. II, p. 194.

57 Richards, *Leviathan*, p. 183.

58 Adam, *Sutherland Estate Management*, vol. II, pp. 180 et seq., 281–4.

59 On the impact of religious zealotry on the response to the clearances, see Devine, *Clanship*, op. cit., pp. 103–8.

9

Sensation in Strathnaver 1814-16

I. *The factor-cum-sheep farmer*

THE CLEARING OF SUTHERLAND occurred in several stages which stretched from 1807 to 1821. These dramatic dislocations were executed under the central authority of the Countess of Sutherland. In each of the great phases of removal hundreds of people were ousted from their inland homes, usually to be resettled in new reception zones along the coast. The turmoil was alarming at each site of clearance: there was indignation, resignation, anger, protest and passivity. The broader drama was always dominated by the particular events surrounding the name of Patrick Sellar (1780–1851), especially during the Strathnaver eviction of Whitsunday 1814. Sellar, the sub-factor from Elgin, attracted all the hatred and vilification that the idea of the clearances generated at that time and ever thereafter.

Sellar had been employed in the Assynt and Kildonan arrangements: he was responsible for some of the most disagreeable work on the estate – collecting rents, serving writs of removal and debt, distributing relief supplies and extracting repayment, evicting debtors and prosecuting poachers and illegal distillers. Sellar brought a missionary zeal to his work. He believed he was introducing progress and civilisation to the benighted people of the remote Highlands. They were barely civilised, were exploited by their tacksmen and leaders, and were corrupted by alcohol. He was a man of precision, a legalistic mind among people used to customary ways; he was finicky and pedantic. He was also extraordinarily combative and clumsy with all about him and made enemies at every turn. During the Assynt riots he became known as a hard and unfriendly agent. His pursuit of poachers was especially resented by every level of the community, which regarded game as customary sport in one degree or another. Sellar knew no discretion in his adherence to the law. His most courageous and dangerous act was to catch the main law agent in Sutherland, Robert Mackid, in the very act of poaching. This caused immense embarrassment to all parties and Sellar inevitably became a marked man. His accumulating enemies were ready to do him injury.

Sellar had been under-factor to the Stafford family since 1810. He had entered the service of the estate as partner to the older and more esteemed agricultural improver William Young, also from Moray. Sellar's ambition caused him to transcend his role as agent and to establish himself among the great capitalist sheep farmers. At a critical moment in December 1813, when William Young auctioned off the great territories of Strathnaver to competing tenants, Sellar suddenly entered the fray and outbid the assembled company in the Golspie Inn. This was less spontaneous than it may have seemed because Sellar had already come to this arrangement with Young and the Countess. Sellar would become lord of Strathnaver, the people would be removed and he would remain as Young's right-hand man in the management.

II. *The Strathnaver clearances 1814–15*

The first clearance of communities in Strathnaver occurred at Whitsunday 1814, six months after Sellar had arranged to convert the territories into a grand new sheep farm. Sellar was punctilious in his arrangements and gave elaborate notice to the people involved, but eventually the whole episode turned into a nightmare for the factor/sheep farmer. These particular events, which essentially involved only twenty-eight families, generated the most spectacular and controversial outcry in the entire history of the Highland Clearances.

There were, inevitably, complicating factors in the events. For instance, though Sellar had clear legal access to the lands he was persuaded by humanitarian arguments to delay and stagger the removals. He came to an arrangement with the various people of the strath for some of them to remove in mid-1814 and for others to remain until the next phase of the change. Virtually all the people were offered the option of resettlement on the north coast where lots were being prepared. These arrangements created ambiguities and uncertainties in the mind of the communities affected, and the reception lots were not readied sufficiently in advance of the flittings. The entire community, and Sellar himself (now committed to vast capital outlays on stock and greatly swollen rent payments), were restless and in a state of anxiety. Some of the people simply delayed and prevaricated month after month; some of them did not believe that the Countess of Sutherland would force this obnoxious dislocation upon them; and some were too poor and sick for the move. It was an unhappy time and Sellar was irritated with the muddle and confusion that impeded his own progress.

In the winter of 1813–14 Sellar organised himself and perambulated his new lands, serving notices and designating which people would move first. All this he combined with the collection of rents. He had to display resoluteness to the people; they could not be allowed to misunderstand his determination. As he journeyed between the inland townships he sensed the simmering resistance and the danger of tumult, but he displayed no fear. He believed that they were behaving in a bloody-minded fashion which had to be outfaced. In March 1814 he reported his activities of the previous three months in connection with rent collecting and removal arrangements. In characteristically vainglorious prose he recounted:

> I know that the people would not meet me, but I also knew that, if I was not found at my post, it would stand then as a good apology for not paying at all, and so necessary in the proper arrangement of the Estate, it needs *much* vigilance to prevent them from carrying with them their last rent, piously 'borrowing from the Egyptians' all that is possible. After several weeks perambulation in this manner: in the Course of which one of my guides was nearly lost and has actually lost several of his Toes by the frost and returned home; have been receiving the rents, in *Retail* daily, since . . . I am now in the middle of my notices for

> Removal, which in this county is carried on by Suit before the Sheriff, and my number of Suits are forty-nine, of dependents, better than 700.

He expected the removals (which eventually led to his indictment on charges of culpable homicide) to be completed by the second week of April 1814.[1]

William Young was also aware of the truculence of the people of the inland townships who, he believed, literally did not know what was good for them. Nevertheless he remained confident of the general removal plan of which Sellar's new sheep farm was merely a portion. At the beginning of March 1814, immediately before the removals, Young said that he would reshape the people of the hills into 'labour and independence' even though 'they prefer idleness and grovelling'. Two months later Young described the frenetic turmoil amid the clearances:

> Our present hurry is beyond what any person who is not on the spot can have an idea of and I shall for the next 14 days be altogether in Strathnaver and Brora where we have at least 430 *families* to arrange in different allotments, to double their present rents, and put them in a more industrious way of life.

The average per family was probably in excess of five. Thus Young's task involved, in all likelihood, about 2000 people and his account demonstrated the huge scale of the removal operations.

The people themselves were in poor circumstances. They were at all times stretched hard to provide even their rents. Young explained what it was like for a small tenant about to be removed:

> Before a poor Sutherland man can pay [rent] he must often sell his cow, his wife and daughters must spin and his son go to the roads or some distant quarter to gain it by his labour.

Young divided the people into two categories. First were 'the idlers and the blackguards'. They ought to be 'rooted out of the estate'. Second were the 'industrious and diligent' who certainly 'deserved careful nurture'. The latter were like children: 'Give them a thorough knowledge of right and wrong, show them that they must earn their bread by the sweat of their brow, hunt down all vagabonds, and the thing will come round'.[2] These were the thoughts of the man responsible for the Strathnaver removals in 1814–5 and were uttered immediately before the great Sellar controversy erupted.

III. *Trouble with the people*

The clearances in Strathnaver were eventually forced through at a frantic pace. The actual timetable of the events began at the auction of leases in December 1813 at the inn in Golspie. In January 1814 Sellar arranged to meet the people and, with the help and mediation of the Gaelic-speaking minister, the Revd David Mackenzie, he explained the arrangements. In the middle of exceptionally severe weather, Sellar had travelled about the countryside giving the people notice to quit at the following Whitsun. William Young had intended to have the coastal allotments ready by early spring 1814 but the surveying was delayed until the last moment. Nevertheless many of the people in the inland townships moved ahead of the legal deadline. There were temporary buildings available near their lots and they gathered their possessions and building timbers and made the shift within the terms dictated by Sellar and the Sutherland estate.

Others among the inland people, however, remained until the last moment. Some were undoubtedly old and sick and very difficult to move. There were some who thought they could stay on if they prevaricated enough. Some had no right to be on the lands at all – they were the unofficial people, cottars, or sub-tenants or tinkers and their families.[3] Sellar could not tolerate disorder and foot dragging. In any case, virtually all removals required some intercession of the law to complete the process. After a sequence of delays, at the start of June, Sellar eventually instructed the law-officers and their bailiffs to execute his legal right to possession of the land. Sellar himself accompanied the posse on some occasions as it passed from village to village in the upper ranges of Strathnaver.

It was during these removals that Patrick Sellar was alleged to have set fire to houses and barns, and caused the deaths of several people, including a nonagenarian woman called Chisholm.⁴ These sensational allegations, especially those of murder, did not emerge until a considerable time after the events, and it was twelve months before the charges were investigated by the law, and a further nine months before Sellar was brought to trial in Inverness. Bringing Sellar to trial was a saga in its own way and made all the more melodramatic by the fact that the case against him was almost certainly led by his known enemy, Robert Mackid, the Sheriff Substitute of Sutherland – the very man Sellar had caught red-handed in the act of poaching the Countess's deer before the Strathnaver clearances. The truth became varnished in these events and, towards the end, Sellar seemed to welcome the trial which, in reality, could have destroyed him in every sense.⁵

IV. Common elements

Some of the circumstances behind the sensation became manifest in the trial which, despite the diametric opposition of claims about Sellar's behaviour, contained accounts which had considerable overlap. The removal party had consisted of about twelve men and they moved from township to township, armed with writs and the implements of eviction for those of the houses and outbuildings which had not been adequately vacated. Their purpose was perfectly clear. Their task was to render the lands immediately accessible to the new tenant, Sellar, and to ensure that the buildings would not be reoccupied as soon as the party went out of the district. This necessitated a degree of demolition and destruction, all of which was governed by the law, by the custom of the county, and by the instructions of Sellar himself. There were conventions which allowed the outgoing tenantry to take with them certain timbers and they were allowed facilities by which to gather in their final crops even if they were still growing in the fields. The subsequent controversy which led to Sellar's arrest a year later related to the degree to which the evictions overstepped the legal, customary and moral requirements of the episodes.

Sellar himself accompanied the removal party; he was on his way south to his arable farm at Morvich but could not spare the time to attend the party for all their proceedings and once he was satisfied that the work was being done he left the scene. The removal party moved from village to village, destroying buildings and ensuring that the people would not return. The officers later claimed that Sellar had insisted that they take extreme care to remain within the law and avoid all damage and cruelty. This, of course, was in a context in which, by definition, people were being evicted from their houses and their houses deliberately rendered uninhabitable. Axes, hatchets, hammers and the torch were, as usual, the instruments of eviction.

At Badinloskin the party arrived on a Monday morning, probably mid-morning. They were particularly instructed to evict William Chisholm, a tinker and allegedly a bigamist, and a man unpopular with his neighbours, who wanted his comprehensive ejection. Sellar had seen him the previous day and told him that he would be evicted and must make ready. The eviction party arrived to find that the Chisholm ménage had not removed; the inhabitants included the mother-in-law of Chisholm who was aged and sick. It is not clear whether Chisholm had already begun to unroof his house or whether the old woman had been shifted to another part of the house or to an outbuilding. Sellar himself did not arrive till about midday; eventually, despite being told that the woman should not be moved for grave fear of her life, she was placed in an outhouse in particularly squalid conditions. Her daughter tended her and meanwhile a fire had been set to the main buildings. Sellar had been present and had said that the removal would have to proceed. He then left the scene.

The episode in Badinloskin produced the subsequent allegation of culpable homicide against Sellar but there were other events which also generated complaint. These were eventually the subject of petitions to the landlord and eventually to the law officers and culminated first in a precognition conducted by his enemy Mackid in May 1815, then the arrest of Sellar and his incarceration for several days, and his subsequent bailing. A second precognition was eventually ordered and, in April 1816, Sellar was brought to trial.

V. *The indictment*

The indictment of Patrick Sellar covered eight pages of detailed accusations. There were numerous charges that Sellar had repeatedly set fire to heath and pasture which were used by the people of eight inland townships. These acts of burning had been done with malice and wickedness and had reduced the people to great distress and poverty. Sellar had also destroyed the mills and barns of the people before they had been able to secure their crops and grain – all of which was against the practice of the county. In a sense these charges were all technical questions relating to property offences. Added to them, however, were allegations that the people had also lost other property when their houses were dismantled, destroyed or burned. There were charges that furniture and roof timbers and money were lost in the process and had been uncompensated. Such charges were not uncommon in any removals under duress, but they added to the scale of Sellar's offences.

Beyond the destruction of property were the much more serious and sensational allegations that Sellar had acted brutally during the removals and had indeed caused deaths and injuries. These charges involved several episodes and a bewildering number of individuals, echoing the testimonies taken in Mackid's precognition. All these charges related to the violence and inhumanity with which Sellar and his men had behaved during the removals. The general charge was that Sellar pulled down, set fire or demolished houses, barns, kilns, and mills 'whereby the people and lawful occupiers . . . were turned out, without cover or shelter'. The list of individual cases was thus:

1. Donald McKay of Rhiloisk, about eighty years old, had been turned out of his house. Unable to travel to shelter, he was forced to lie in the nearby woods for several nights 'to his great distress and to the danger of his life'.[6]

2. Barbara McKay of Ravigall, pregnant and confined to bed after a serious fall, was compelled by Sellar to get out of her house or else it would have been pulled down about her. Her husband,

with the help of a local woman, carried her a mile across country 'to the imminent danger of her life'.[7]

3. Donald Monro, a young lad who lay sick in his bed at Garvault, was summarily forced out of his house by Sellar and thereby also endangered his health.

4. Donald McBeath, of Rhimsdale, was 'culpably killed' by Sellar. Sellar had pulled down his house while McBeath lay on his sick bed within. Sellar left only 'a small space of roof' over the sick man (no more than five or six yards in extent and in 'a cold and comfortless situation') McBeath was therefore exposed to the weather, never spoke again, and died about eight days later from the consequences. Sellar had ignored the entreaties of McBeath's neighbours and had, in a rage, exclaimed: 'The devil a man of them, sick or well, shall be permitted to remain'.[8]

5. Margaret McKay, ninety years of age, was lying in the house of her son-in-law William Chisholm of Badinloskin who lawfully occupied the house. Sellar was told that Mrs McKay could not be moved without endangering her life. Sellar set fire to and demolished the building. Margaret McKay, 'the flames approaching the bed on which she lay, shrieked in Gaelic "O the fire"'. Her daughter carried her out, her blankets burnt in several places. She never uttered another word, remained insensible and died five days later 'in consequence of the fright and alarm' and from the cold and uncomfortable place in which she was placed. She had, therefore, been 'culpably killed' by Sellar. [In the destruction of Chisholm's house it was alleged that £3 in bank notes was lost as well as furniture and crops.][9]

There were, therefore, two particular deaths enumerated in the indictment, together with three other cases of severe injury to which was added a great catalogue of losses and of injustices. Counsel for the Crown, Henry Drummond, concluded the indictment by saying that Sellar '*ought* to be punished with the pains of law, to deter others from committing the like crimes in all times coming'.[10]

The trial began at 10 a.m. on 23 April 1816 before the Circuit Court of Justiciary in Inverness. Sellar was tried by jury before

Judge Lord Pitmilly. There were fifteen jurymen (none of them from Sutherland for fear of local contamination) and a large number of witnesses for both sides of the case many of whom, for both prosecution and defence, were not actually called during the trial. Sellar was represented by J. Gordon and supported by Henry Cockburn and Patrick Robertson; he was accompanied by 'a friend' throughout the proceedings but he did not submit to cross-examination. Sellar sat silent through the fourteen hours while, about him, his fate was determined.

Sellar's own counsel, Gordon, challenged the prosecution to provide any proof of the allegations. All Sellar's ejectments had been not only lawful but executed with 'great indulgence'. There was no question of cruelty or oppression. Sellar had committed no homicide and had, in reality, been himself the victim of 'the most unfounded local prejudices' which produced the defamations he now faced. The intention of the allegations was, in truth, to undermine 'the whole system of improvements' on the Sutherland estate. Sellar rejoiced in the opportunity to demonstrate his complete innocence before a dispassionate British jury. Sellar had been selected as the 'victim' by which a 'stab' was made against the improvements of Lady Sutherland. As a consequence he had been 'branded with the name of a tyrant, oppressor and murderer'.[11]

VI. Prejudice

The Crown case against Sellar depended on evidence which would prove the allegations which flowed from the original precognition. To this purpose the prosecution assembled a large number of witnesses from Strathnaver. But first the central figure in the drama was called, namely Robert Mackid. His appearance brought immediate objection from the defence counsel on the grounds of his 'malice and partial counsel' against the defendant. The objection was based on his imprisonment of Sellar 'without a complainant', without legal warrant, his refusal of bail, and the evidence that Mackid had exposed his prejudice against Sellar in an inflammatory letter to Lord Stafford. Mackid had also advised

Young to 'have as little to do with Mr Sellar as possible'. Mackid had said that if Sellar 'is not hanged, he will certainly go to Botany Bay'.

In the outcome Judge Pitmilly ruled that most of Mackid's evidence was indeed inadmissible and this was a large hole in the Crown case. Nevertheless there were numerous eyewitnesses to call. These included first William Chisholm the tinker, whose mother-in-law had died after the eviction at Badinloskin. In his long testimony Chisholm repeated the story and claimed directly that Sellar had been involved in the atrocity. Sellar had been warned about the old woman's condition; she had been in the house when it was afire; she had been removed in singed blankets to a turf-covered sheep cot. Three pounds in bank notes had been consumed in the fire. Chisholm's wife gave evidence which generally followed that of her husband but also exposed serious inconsistencies about the time and precise sequence of events. For instance, she said that her mother had not been in the building when it was fired; she knew nothing of the three pounds. It was unclear whether the woman was or was not sick at the time. But another witness confirmed that Sellar, ignoring warnings about the old woman's condition, had insisted that she moved and that she had been very alarmed at the action.

Other witnesses testified to Sellar's harsh treatment of people and to the burning of pastures and the destruction of buildings. In reality none of them claimed that houses had been demolished with people still inside; the main gravamen was that Sellar had insisted on the removal of people who were in no condition to remove without danger to their lives and health. Sellar would not be reasoned with, and had been cruel. There were claims that the resettlement zones were not prepared until a few days before the clearance. This last claim was confirmed by the Revd David Mackenzie and by William Young, both called by the Crown.

The second half of the trial concerned evidence about Sellar and his action. It began with evidence about the interrogation of Sellar conducted by Mackid at the time of Sellar's arrest in mid-1815. The transcript was read in which Sellar defended himself with vigour and precision. He had acted absolutely within the law, he claimed. He had given the people special concessions to help in their relocation. Chisholm was a vagrant, a bigamist and a thief. Sellar had ensured that all timbers were made over to the people: he had been the perfect humanitarian. At Badinloskin he had been present only after the process had begun; when he arrived the furniture had been removed and the house was unroofed; Sellar had told the people to leave the Strath but they said the old woman was too unwell; she had already been removed to a small house and was being cared for by her daughter. Sellar had tried to ensure that the houses would not be reoccupied. Sellar left but Chisholm had indeed returned and rebuilt huts and he was still *in situ*. The legal proceeding had been concocted by 'artful and designing men to complain of oppression.' Barns had been destroyed only where absolutely necessary: he had preserved enough to guarantee the crops for the season.

In defence of Sellar several respectable references were exhibited to demonstrate his remarkable character for humanity and upright behaviour; Sellar was simply a 'person of the strictest integrity and humanity, incapable of being even accessory to any cruel or oppressive action'. Then witnesses to the evictions were called who described the events which differed from the Crown only in terms of the alleged cruelty of Sellar. The old woman at Badinloskin had certainly been present, she had been taken out to the byre by Chisholm; she was well clear before the house was destroyed by fire. Chisholm had already partially demolished the house; he had dropped burning divots near her bed. Sellar had certainly rejected requests to preserve the house. There had been no complaint about compensation at the time. Sellar had been 60–100 yards from the scene. He had given explicit instructions that there should be no harsh treatment of the people. At the end of the evidence it was decided to dispense with many other defence witness on the grounds that they were superfluous to the needs of the case.

In the face of this defence, and the revealed weaknesses in its own case, the Crown immediately gave up most of the charges against Sellar but nevertheless persisted with the most serious allegation, concerning homicide and the destruction of mills.

The outcome was reached swiftly. The jury unanimously found

Sellar not guilty. He burst into tears and the judge consoled him for his ordeal. Pitmilly told Sellar directly that he should feel great satisfaction with the outcome. His feelings must have been agitated, but he would not regret the trial since it would have due effect on the country which had been so improperly agitated.

The outcome of this trial was a rout of the people of Strathnaver and a triumph for all that Sellar had come to symbolise. It was greatly reinforced in the following months by the dismissal of Mackid from the legal position he held in Sutherland. He was also forced, under threat of total financial ruin, to write an abject confession and apology to Sellar. Sellar was always able to produce this as ultimate evidence of his innocence; yet, in the long run, posterity was never persuaded. Sellar instead came to epitomise all the inhumanity of the clearances.

The acquittal of Patrick Sellar at the Inverness Court in 1816 was greeted with great relief by the Countess of Sutherland and her family. The verdict appeared to disperse the obloquy which had descended upon their plans for improvement in the Highlands. In effect, it meant that the programme for the rest of the clearances in Sutherland had been given a green light. The law had absolved Sellar from the charge of murder. The legal proceedings also demonstrated that the landlord was entitled to clear the people, resettle them, and destroy their houses and barns, so long as proper compensation was paid. Thus, while the estate management became much more sensitive to public opinion, the effect of the trial was to confirm the legality of its radical policies.[12]

VII. Relief

There was a collective sigh of relief in the Sutherland management when the news of Sellar's exculpation was received. In reality the Countess of Sutherland and her closest advisers had been opening some distance between themselves and Sellar. Soon Sellar and Young were both eased out of the management and replaced by new men who would complete the work with less sensation and more financial control. In the interim the old team continued.

Remarkably enough, the mood of confidence evident in 1814 survived until 1817, despite the appallingly unpleasant publicity of the Sellar affair, despite the patent inadequacy of the resettlement zones, and despite the downturn in the prices of the basic commodities of the northern economy. The main infrastructure of the new economy had been established, notably at Helmsdale, and there was no thought of abandoning the original intention to resettle large numbers of people cleared from the interior.

In October 1815, James Loch, the Lowland lawyer who was taking over central control, expressed great pleasure in the progress at Helmsdale, and a belief that more Kildonan people should be sent there. Their continuance in the hills was not possible: 'in the middle of sheep farmers they will always be sheep stealers and whisky smugglers,' he said. But he urged that the people be thoroughly prepared for the changes, both psychologically and in terms of their physical wellbeing. Loch, extremely anxious about the dangers inherent in precipitate and unpopular removals, told Lord Stafford of his apprehensions: 'I do not think a removal of the whole people at Whitsunday without their own consent, would be just to them'.

This was a novel concept. The idea of gaining the concurrence and co-operation of the people was never brought to reality; it was indeed the prime weakness in the planning procedures associated with practically all the clearances across the Highlands. Loch continued:

> In the next place I am very sure that if any fracas should take place, either from real or pretended grievances upon occasion, that it would make a very serious impression upon many most respectable persons, who now entertain the opinion that in executing these changes he [Young] has shewn too little attention to the people's prejudices by not giving them time enough.

Loch added: 'Besides these reasons for not doing the thing too hastily there is another powerful one, which is that the people will take much more readily to their new occupations if they come down in good humour than otherwise.' He suggested a timetable which prepared the resettlement zones several months ahead of the evacuation of the people, with generous rent-free terms in the interim, which 'would give them every proper indulgence and the loss of rent would be no object'.[13] Loch's anxiety was centred on the question of the public opprobrium attaching itself to the Stafford family, and on the practical problems of the removals. It is not hard to imagine that the feelings of the people themselves were vastly more agitated.

VIII. *End of a phase*

The sensation over Sellar's trial was a crisis for the Sutherland plans. But the outcome was a welcome signal to proceed with the rest of the programme of clearance, only half of which had yet been executed. A great deal of Strathnaver and Kildonan had still to be cleared, some of it to complete the undertaking made to Sellar on his entry to his sheep-farming operations.

Immediately following the trial of Sellar there were further clearances to the east coast of Sutherland. Young's optimism redoubled and he predicted that the coastal enterprises would soon rival the fishing ports of Wick and Pultneytown in Caithness. In May 1816 he reported that all the Helmsdale lots had been taken up by new settlers, that some of the lots had been reduced to one acre only, and that the incoming sheep farmer who had taken over the land in the interior had entered a lease very favourable to Lord Stafford. Young remarked that all the coastal lands suitable for lotters had been occupied, and no further resettlement could be considered until 1818, when more lotting land would become available to 'accommodate a great many from the interior'. A rash of sheep thefts and mutilations following Sellar's trial persuaded Young that further clearances were indispensable.[14]

The immense difficulties of the planners associated with the clearance and resettlement of large numbers of people from the interior glens of Sutherland were paralleled by problems with estate finances. The Sutherland clearances occurred in a context in which the landlord lavished unprecedented and (for a while) uncontrolled expenditures on the improvement of the estate. The bulk of the money was used specifically to create facilities for the reception and employment of the people removed from the inland. It was expected to yield an economic return, but only in the long run. From 1802 to 1811 the estate expended an aggregate sum of £70 867; between 1812 and 1817 the expenditure was £140 488. These outlays, which depended upon capital inflows from the Stafford family's English properties, greatly exceeded the current revenue of the Sutherland estate, even though this rose from £9984 to £22 212, between 1812 and 1817.[15]

In later years these expenditures were invariably quoted when the Sutherland estate was attacked for its alleged inhumanity to its tenantry. It was always said in defence that the landlord had subsidised the estate, and provided for the welfare of the people, to a degree unrivalled in the Highland experience. Estate expenditure continued to exceed revenues for several decades; moreover, between 1800 and 1833 the Sutherland family spent £554 149 on buying up almost all the rest of the county.[16] Nothing spoke more clearly of the boundless reserves of the Stafford fortune than this conspicuous blaze of buying in the north of Scotland. Its wisdom, in retrospect, looks highly questionable. Here was a great English aristocrat drawing the profits of industry and trade in the new southern economy and pouring them into bottomless sinks in the northern Highlands.

The financial outcome of these great changes was certainly not lucrative in the short run. The runaway expenditure was partly the product of William Young's financial ineptitude. In R.J. Adam's words, this was a phase of 'Large plans, eager beginnings, defective controls, soaring expenditure, disappointing returns: the catalogue is formidable'.[17] The entire business of costing was neglected and Lord Stafford's financial resources were in large measure wasted in the grandiose plans over which William Young presided until he was sacked in favour of Francis Suther and James Loch in 1816. The great investments made by the Stafford family in the coastal economy yielded poor results, caused in part by the poor design, and the worse accounting, of the various projects that were set going. It was also in part because the programme was overtaken by adverse conditions which could not have been predicted. The years

1813–21 were very hazardous for all industrial development on the fringe of the national economy. In the long run there were secular trends in the British economy which operated against industrial development in peripheral regions.

Many of the enterprises associated with the Stafford investments in Sutherland simply withered away in the face of these circumstances after Waterloo. Some of the fishing survived as a permanent addition to the economic structure, but most of the rest failed. Moreover many of the older sources of income in the region (kelp, linen and especially cattle) declined very rapidly during these years. Even the sheep farmers felt the pinch of falling prices. The result was tragic in the sense that the new economy was no more reliable than the structure of subsistence inherited from the pre-clearance days. The fact that the population continued to grow until 1831 (or 1841 in several parishes) compounded the resultant problems. The most that may be said in positive terms is that the actual expenditures on capital projects generated substantial temporary employment in this marginal economy. But it was a short-term benefit, and the outlays did not yield long-term growth. The developmental effects of the investments were slight.[18]

IX. Pause

The clearances in Sutherland between 1813 and 1816 caused the sudden shifting of several thousand people. The accommodation on the coast was mean and depressing; many places provided were already congested by 1814. In terms of human engineering the resettlement zones were inadequate and inhospitable, regardless of the original intentions of the planners and the landlord.

In May 1816 James Loch ordered a pause in the removal programme:

All the Coast Side Lands suitable for lotting out are now *brimful* and I can think of nothing before the year [1818] when Kintradwell will be open unless a bargain could be made with Leith of Kilgower which would accommodate a great many from the interior. There is no other way to dispose of the present Inhabitants of Badenloch etc, unless the

Marquis and Lady Stafford depart from their present wise system not to turn out a single inhabitant against whom crimes have not been proved until a situation on the coast side is pointed out.[19]

Inadequate planning and managerial incompetence further contributed to the weakness of the coastal arrangements for the reception of the people dislodged by the sheep clearances. Loch recognised the problem when he contemplated the antagonism of the common people at the time of the clearances.

They had been shifted from lands they had held for generations, and had been forced out of their ancient habits. It was natural, said Loch, that they should feel a sense of inconvenience and loss:

This state of things must have tended to keep alive that feeling of regret and disquietude which their sudden and not well digested removal from the hills in the first instance produced.[20]

This was an interior voice from the management plainly admitting the essential miscalculation of the policy.

The plan for resettlement, the sincerity of which was not open to doubt, had been botched. The lots were not ready in time to receive the people and they were given too little time to prepare their crops. A senior adviser to the Countess reported in August 1816 that:

The disturbances in Strathnaver appear to have had their origin in neglecting to have the allotments intended for the dispossessed tenants divided and pointed out to them in proper time.[21]

By 1816, the year of the trial of Sellar, a rethinking of the resettlement provisions had become imperative. Future clearances would be much better prepared and there would be no further sensation. Sellar, specifically, would play no further direct part in the process.

Notes

1 SCRO, D593/K/Sellar to Loch, 3 March 1814.

2 SCRO, D593/K/Young to Loch, 24 May 1814.

3 On the invisible unofficial population see Bangor-Jones, op. cit., pp. 9, 45–56.

4 Thomas Sellar, *The Sutherland Evictions of 1814* (London, 1883), p. 31.

5 See Richards, *Patrick Sellar and the Highland Clearances* (Edinburgh, 1999), Chapter 6.

6 Robertson, *Trial Report*.

7 Ibid., p. 8.

8 Ibid., p. 11.

9 Ibid., p. 13.

10 Ibid., p. 14.

11 Ibid., passim.

12 See Eric Richards, *Patrick Sellar and the Highland Clearances* (Edinburgh, 1999).

13 SCRO, D593/K/Loch to Lord Stafford, 30 Nov. 1815.

14 SCRO, D593/K/Young to Loch, 26 May 1816.

15 Adam, vol. I, p. lxxxiii, and Appendix A.

16 SCRO, D593/N/4/1/la/Report to the Marquis of Stafford, pp. 1–2; see Richards, *Leviathan*, op. cit., Part 3.

17 Adam, *Sutherland Estate Management*, vol. I, p. 1x.

18 See Richards, 'Structural change', and *History of Highland Clearances*, vol 2.

19 Richards, *Leviathan*, p. 198.

20 Richards, *History*, vol. I, p. 192.

21 Ibid., vol. I, p. 210.

10

The Greatest Clearances: Strathnaver and Kildonan in 1818-19

FOR DECADES, LONG AFTER the events, the descendants of Patrick Sellar as well as those of the Dukes of Sutherland were repeatedly outraged by the continuing vituperation poured upon their families by the crofters and their supporters. In 1885, for instance, Lord Ronald Gower, a younger son of the current Duke, was unable to contain his anger:

> I allude to the stories and reports stating that cruel and arbitrary evictions had been practised on the people of Sutherland. These stories and reports, although they have been repeatedly proved false, are even now brought up again by a Press that should be ashamed of repeating such stale inventions. There are those, however, who, like the scriptural dog, love to return to their vomit.[1]

Gower was writing at a time when the crofters across the Highlands had captured political attention and publicised the chronicle of dispossession and inhumanity that they had suffered at the hands of landlords over the past three generations.

While Gower and Patrick Sellar's sons denied the 'stories and reports' about the original events, much of the truth of the matter continued to slumber in the records preserved efficiently in the estate offices of Gower's own family. They were especially full of the detail of the last phase of the great Sutherland clearances in the second half of the 1810s.

I. Preparations, 1816

By 1816 James Loch, the Commissioner to Lord Stafford, had taken over the reins of the great northern policies of Lord and Lady Stafford. Loch, like Sellar, was a lawyer trained at Edinburgh University during its golden age at the end of the century. There he had studied under Dugald Stewart and learned the precepts of classical political economy which informed his ideas of estate management. He had been in the employment of the Stafford family for four years when he took command of the Highland estates from Messrs Sellar and Young. He brought to the task a more stringent attitude to cost accounting; he was altogether more efficient and intelligent than his predecessors, and more sensitive to the political consequences of change in the north. He was more sophisticated, and better connected than the Morayshire improvers.

In 1816–17 the pressure for clearance in Sutherland was yet again reinforced by the descent of new famine conditions in which 'mildew' destroyed much of the potato and oat crops of the people in the inland glens.[2] The 'spirit of emigration' was also again roused and the Sutherland management instituted large plans for the relief of the hungry, but now on the most rigorous terms. The destitution of 1816–17 gave added credence to the fundamental assumption that the clearance of the people out of the interior was the only feasible solution to the problem of poverty in Sutherland.

Patrick Sellar expressed his view in his usual forthright fashion. He told James Loch in December 1816:

> You really will not find this Estate pleasant or profitable until by assisting Emigration or by drawing [the people] to your coastside you have got the mildewed districts cleared.[3]

Relief measures continued throughout 1817. James Loch felt that the people were often treated too charitably for their own long-term good, as the policy 'tended to increase their numbers, their idleness and their attachment to their mountain spots'.[4] The estate administrators now believed that overpopulation was a serious problem in the north and that clearance should properly be considered in conjunction with emigration. The estate was, however, reluctant to give overt encouragement to emigration, and Loch told a shipping agent in November 1817:

> It is not Lord Stafford's wish to promote any emigration from the estate of Sutherland, as he provides lots for all he removes from the hills upon the sea coast, but he at the same time does not wish to stand in the way of such a disposition upon the part of any who wish to go to the Colonies.[5]

This was the repeated protestation: the Sutherland policy was designed to resettle, not to evict, the common people.

By the autumn of 1817 James Loch (who then controlled the estate) was organising the plans for the second great round of clearances, which were scheduled mainly for Whitsunday in 1819 and 1820. Every precaution against the possibility of inhumanity and homelessness was to be taken: Loch was extremely anxious to avoid all public notice and criticism of the coming events. He feared that any further public excitation would attract parliamentary inquiry into landlord policy in the north.

In part, the pressure for the new round of clearances came directly from the sheep farmers. One of them, Patrick Sellar, who held large leases of land in Strathnaver, made bitter demands for immediate removals. He suffered from sheep thefts, which aggravated his native impatience. Loch explained that:

> The land [in Strathnaver] is to be added to Mr Sellar's farm. It is part of the Bargain with him that these lands should be converted into a sheep walk before now and [this] was postponed but the enormous losses which he had experienced during the last summer call for the only effective remedy the case admits of, the complete removal of the people from the vicinity of this and every other sheep farm.[6]

Sellar was angrily agitated about the delay which forced him to kick his heels and lose capital on his lease. Nevertheless, under Loch's regime, Sellar was allowed no role in the actual business of clearing the people. The policy was explicitly quarantined from Sellar's influence. The work was placed in the hands of Loch's protégé, Francis Suther, a Lowland Scot who had considerable experience of estate management in England. He was brought into Sutherland to reform the estate office and to complete the last of the great clearances and the resettlement plans. He was a man of mild temper, efficient and intelligent, with none of the deficiencies of personality of either Sellar or William Young.

II. 1818

The revamped clearance programme was set in motion in 1818 and over the following three summers the great bulk of the clearing work was completed. These were to be the most sweeping removals ever seen in the Highlands and possibly one of the largest single coerced relocations of rural populations achieved in modern British history to that time.

Under Loch's ukase the highest priority was now given to the synchronised availability of reception allotments. One estate agent recognised that the previous settlers on the north coast had possessed neither the means nor the inclination to take to the sea as fishermen. Loch was emphatic that rents for the resettlement lots should be set low enough to avoid forcing any dependence on the profits of illicit distillation. Moreover, he wrote:

> I am particularly anxious that their lots should be so small as to prevent their massing any considerable part of their rent by selling a beast, their rent must not depend on that. In short I wish them to become fishers only, but if you give them any extent of land or of Commonality they will never embark heartily in that pursuit. To induce them to exertion they must pay more than a nominal rent and yet not so much as to oppress them.[7]

This, then, was the carefully calibrated scheme which was designed to persuade the ousted inland people to take up their new coastal livings.

Loch, therefore, was as fully committed to the clearance and resettlement system as his employers and his predecessors. His greatest fear, however, was another publicity fiasco. He lectured Suther heavily on the dangers. He wrote:

> Let me beseech you don't do it in too great a hurry, but give them time

and not only let them know their new lots as soon as possible but their new rents also which make as moderate as your duty to the proprietor and the real interest of the tenant will permit . . . When you find any obstinacy in those who are to be moved and who owe money you can manage by shewing them if they go quietly they may both get a cheaper lot and be excused their arrears.[8]

Rising arrears among the small tenantry gave the estate another lever and this could be used to expedite clearance.

We can see the mechanism of a typical Highland clearance. The sequence began with a formal summons. Each small tenant to be cleared from the interior received a standard and much-feared 'Notice of Removal'. It read:

Parish of_____

The Marquis and Marchioness of Stafford having determined to lay the following places under stock, viz. [. . .] Intimation to the Tenants herein is hereby made that allotments on the Coast will be prepared for them by the end of January next when such Person will be informed of the Allotment marked off for him in order that he may prepare to enter it at the Term of Whitsunday first if he so inclines. Intimation Is also made that each of the Tenants who behaves himself to the satisfaction of the Proprietors and their Factors shall have permission to occupy their present holdings as pasturage rent free from Whitsunday 1818 to Whitsunday 1819 and they shall also possess their New Allotments rent free for that year in order that the Tenantry who conduct themselves as aforesaid may have full time to remove their property from the Grounds and erect their Houses on their new allotments and in order that they may have every advantage in removing.[9]

No stone would remain unturned in ensuring the smooth passage of the policy. The response of the people to these plans was not directly recorded, but in March 1818 the Revd David Mackenzie in Kildonan wrote to Loch, effectively on their behalf, a letter which boldly challenged all the assumptions of the Sutherland clearances. Mackenzie was asked by the landlord to explain the essential humanity and wisdom of the coming removals to the people who were about to be uprooted. He was to tell them that the policy would benefit everyone involved. Mackenzie, a respected figure at Dunrobin Castle and smiled upon by the Countess, found himself unable to lend his pulpit to this purpose. He explained to Loch that he had told the people about Lord Stafford's generosity and about his plans:

> But [I] beg leave to be excused from giving any observations to the people of the change being so much to their advantage, as you anticipate after it takes place. I take it as I infer from your letter, it is the wish of Lord and Lady Stafford, that the population of the Parish should remain undiminished.

He noted that in his parish alone some 220 families were to be removed, probably well in excess of a thousand people. Mackenzie bluntly refused to believe that they would be any less subject to famine on the coast than in Strathnaver.

Mackenzie (making an exception of Strathy) pointed out that all the waste lands on the coast were already 'thoroughly inhabited'. And, he insisted to Loch, 'Let me assure you as a positive fact, that the calamities of last year were as general and as severely felt among the Inhabitants of the Sea Coast, as many of the upper parts'. Indigence was as great on the coast among the settlers as it was in the interior; moreover, he

> could not conceive how the great addition to be made to their numbers [on the coast] can live without being more than ever indebted to the Bounty of the Landlord. The lands on the coast are not very extensive, neither are they in some places, calculated to give good returns; the surface of the ground is extremely rugged, and incapable of improvement to a great extent.

There was virtually no limestone, marl or seaweed for manure and few good landing places for boats; there was no industry or opportunity for day labour; it was all highly inhospitable. He went on:

> From what I have heard and seen of the quality of land which can be given them according to the new arrangements, it will not produce of Corn what will support their families for half a year; and being totally ignorant of sea faring their supplies from the Ocean must be scanty and precarious during the storms of winter and spring.

They would have great difficulty establishing houses and building boats, and many of the people were too young or too old for either. Mackenzie concluded from these observations:

> I candidly submit to you, with all deference, I am persuaded that the great population to be removed at Whitsunday 1819 from the upper parts, to the sea coast of the Parish, cannot, if left to depend for subsistence on the production of their new Stances, have a comfortable living, and from this persuasion, I cannot attempt to convince the people that the change will be for their advantage.[10]

Mackenzie's intervention was the most comprehensive rejection of the foundations of the Sutherland policy uttered during these years. It voiced the sceptical and incredulous state of mind of the people about to be removed from Strathnaver to make way for Sellar's sheep. If Mackenzie resisted the basis of the removals it is certain that the people were totally unconvinced and therefore deeply resentful of the coming dislocation of their lives. If Mackenzie was sceptical, it requires no great leap to imagine the fear and loathing in the minds of the people.

James Loch was unshaken. He adamantly denied the implications of Mackenzie's letter. The removals, he insisted, were not to be undertaken 'in the mere wantonness of power' but for the benefit of the people and landlord alike. Loch accepted personal responsibility for the entire consequences. He pointed out that, in logic and in practice, it was immaterial whether the landlord supported the people in charity on the coast or in the hills; in the former case it would at least leave the interior free for much more profitable sheep farming. But in reality, he asserted, the people would be far better off on the coast. He felt compassion for the people, but spoke with renewed determination for their removal and resettlement. He ended his response to Mackenzie with these words:

> I hope you will assure the people not to deceive themselves by thinking that the plan can or will be changed and that therefore they must make use best of the ensuing summer.[11]

From the sheer scale of the operations, the practical details of removal presented greater difficulties than Loch was prepared to admit. Only five days after Loch's assurances to the Revd

Mackenzie, the local factor in the Strathnaver district told the Sutherland commissioner that many of the Strathy people, who were settlers from earlier clearances, had chosen to relinquish their coastal lots because their lands were to be reduced in size in order to accommodate the new removees from Strathnaver. The ground officer remarked that:

> Mr Suther and myself are fully persuaded that the more of them that quit the estate the better, as besides the great increase of population within the last few years, there would be a deficiency of lots were all the people to remain and the generous and humane conduct of the Noble Proprietors in relieving them from their arrears will be ultimately for the benefit of the estate.[12]

The same official vouched for the fact that very few of the lots were 'capable of being made anything of and few would be acceptable to the people'.[13] This, like Mackenzie's intervention, demonstrated that the people of the interior were unlikely to benefit significantly from the change about to revolutionise their lives.

Patrick Sellar had no doubts about the necessity of the removals. In typically excited prose, he reported that the public notification of the estate's determination to press on with the removals had caused 'a most astonishing effect on the minds of the aboriginals. Several – I believe most of these half pay captains – are meditating or have already planned their flight' and his own sheep losses (from theft) had already begun to decline.[14] Suther also reported that many of the people, on the prospect of clearance, had shown signs of emigrating to Caithness, the Cape of Good Hope, North America or elsewhere; he facilitated the exodus by absolving the emigrants from their accumulated rent arrears. He arranged for them to sign the following tendentious statement:

> We the undersigned tenants voluntarily refuse to take possession of the lot of land pointed out to us on the Estate of Sutherland and freely relinquish all claim to any holding thereon and we farther feel most grateful to the very liberal conduct of the noble proprietors in relieving us from all arrears due by us to the Noble Proprietors.

Dislocation was inevitable in the removals: this was indeed the literal purpose of the policy. The extreme reluctance of the people to co-operate with the Sutherland estate administrators was beyond doubt. Many could not comprehend that the clearances would actually occur. They retained a naïve and pathetic faith in their landlord. As Suther reported:

> Many of the people believe that when Lady Stafford comes to the Country their entreaties will induce her Ladyship to permit them to remain – this idea is by no means general but several expect it.

But Suther also testified to the acquiescent demeanour of the people:

> I found them inoffensive and timidly pliant rather than otherwise on all occasions. I do not recollect of an instance of any of them refusing to do what I desired. The Ministers appear to look upon the changes quite coolly – they see plainly and I have convinced them all of it, that the thing is determined on and will be carried through.[15]

The plans for the clearances directed the people thereby removed to four widely separate locations: Strathy on the north coast, Lochinver and Culkein in the west, Brora and Helmsdale in the east and Dornoch in the south-east. The Dornoch reception lots were mainly 'improvable' muir-lands, for which prospective removees had special aversion. It would be a travesty to suggest that the business of clearance was greeted with anything less than incomprehension and repugnance by the people involved.

In 1818 all the sheep farms had been let satisfactorily, in advance of the evacuation of the people: Sellar would occupy territory in the Upper Naver and at Morvich; Paterson of Sandside had land on the east side of the lower Naver; James Hall had land at Strathbrora, and Messrs Matheson and Gilchrist would farm their sheep at Shinness. In 1818 stock losses persuaded sheep farmers, factors and landlords to establish a new alliance, 'The United Association of the Noblemen, Gentlemen in Sutherland and Caithness for the Protection of Property'.[16] Indeed the sheep farmers were in the best of spirits. Marshall and Atkinson, the pioneer sheep farmers in the country, had rented their lands at £200 a year and already had stock worth £20 000 on it. Patrick Sellar, it was said, was 'universally understood to have an amazing bargain of his new farm, and he has made most advantageous purchases of stock to lay upon it'. Economic conditions were temporarily auspicious, even for the common people, in the sense that high cattle prices allowed them to depart their old economy without heavy loss.

The sale of their cattle – assisted by arrangements made by the landlord with itinerant drovers – was the moment when the traditional economy ceased and the people converted to the new crofting existence. The rule adopted by the estate management placed a high premium on peaceability:

> Those who go to their lots quietly or who prefer leaving the country under the regulations established by Government, are all excused all arrears and have their land to Whitsunday 1819 for nothing.[17]

James Loch instructed Suther repeatedly, and with insistent emphasis, that the managers must use great kindness in the forth-coming clearances. The idea of a kind and humane clearance he did not regard as oxymoronic.

III. The summers of 1818 and 1819

In June 1818 the new round of Sutherland removals was in full swing. Some of the people displaced fled into Caithness and others joined an emigration scheme to the Cape of Good Hope. Emigration was popular at this time but, in 1818, there was no sense of active resistance to the clearances.

Francis Suther, despite the scale of the programme, did not expect trouble. He was preoccupied with the settlers, who were not only reluctant but also painstakingly selective in accepting lots offered to them. A good fishing season and the relatively buoyant market for cattle and sheep caused James Loch to exude confidence. To Lady Stafford in the south he reported glowingly with news of the progress of the east-coast settlements, especially of the fishing at Helmsdale. In August 1818 he described the scene:

> The going out of the boats was one of the most cheering sights I ever saw – the manner they dispersed themselves along the coast having the most picturesque effect. I got up the following morning to see them

come in at four o'clock; upon the coast it was mild, but the moment I turned round from Portgower into Helmsdale, I was like to have perished with the cold coming down the valley, shewing how unfit the hills and valleys among them are for growth of the corn. The boats coming in and the women pouring in from the Hills on all sides gave the whole so different an appearance of what this place had been when I knew it as to strike me very forcibly.

The Sutherland estate managers battled against the distrust and antipathy of the people, who would not believe any promise made by the landlord, such as the offer of a prize for the best boat constructed by the fishermen.[18] This was a measure of the psychological havoc created by the clumsy behaviour of Patrick Sellar in the early years of the clearances and by the continuing suspicion of the estate management. Nevertheless, in the event, the 1818 removals passed off without resistance and without adverse publicity. An even larger series was planned for the following year.

The plans for Whitsunday 1819 required the shifting of about 425 families (probably about 2000 people), and a further 475 families one year later (a figure subsequently revised to 522 families). Loch was anxious to complete the clearances because

there never was a better season for letting the sheep farms and never so good a time for the people selling their cattle to the best advantage – indeed it would be doing them a favour to force them to sell between this and Whitsunday.[19]

These were concentrated clearances on the greatest possible scale, matched only by the ambitious plans which were designed to reaccommodate the people. The year 1819 therefore was an even larger test of the skill of the planners as well as the amenability of the people. In the planning for these events Suther, in November 1818, assured Loch:

You must not be in the least afraid that I am in the least unprepared for the worst – I am ready to meet any one or all of them [that is, the people to be removed] now and I will be so every day till Whitsunday.

Whitsunday was the season of removal.[20]

At the beginning of 1819 Loch reported that some of the Strathnaver people on notice to be removed at Whitsunday had accepted small farms in Caithness. Some Caithness landowners actively encouraged settlers from Sutherland, and they made good rentals by very close settlement of such people on their arable land.[21] This was a further manifestation of greater pressure on land resources caused by the new sheep economy.

Reluctant or otherwise, most of the Strathnaver people took up their assigned allotments on the north coast. Similarly the Kildonan people were moving to Helmsdale. The people of Strathbrora and Abercross were slower, and some went into Ross-shire. Nevertheless Suther was constantly urging all the people to settle on the allocated reception zones on the Sutherland estate. These were resettlement plans and much more than a mere token of landlord benevolence. They were clearances, not evictions in the sense of summary ejections from the entire estate.

The determining principle was that fishing and cultivation could not be combined successfully. The settlers should be either fishermen or farmers, but never both. It was a principle which, in the long run, proved unworkable. Eventually the lotters became typical crofters who divided their time among several different activities, in violation of Loch's original thinking. But in 1819 the principle stood intact.

Little is known about conditions on the lots at the time of the great 'flittings' except that in August 1819 there was a plaintive report that some of the old widows from Kildonan had experienced difficulty in building houses on their new allotments. The estate provided some basic assistance with the construction materials but mostly the settlers bore the costs of rehabilitating themselves. This was the usual expectation of a small tenant at the end of a tenancy.[22]

There was no resistance in the 1819 clearances but a critical error by Suther attracted public opprobrium. Unknown to Loch, he authorised the clearing parties to use fire during the removals. In 1819, as before, the constables who accompanied the clearing parties set fire to the houses after the people had been ejected. It prevented their repossession by the former inhabitants, who were normally paid compensation for their particular effects. It was not an unusual practice in Highland removals and had been employed extensively in the period 1811–14. But it was an extremely unpopular and emotive issue which had been at the centre of the accusations against Patrick Sellar in 1816. To Loch this was a terrible blunder. It produced an automatic denunciation from all people who heard of it. Loch was aghast that Suther had sanctioned this inflammatory method once more. The unsavoury news travelled rapidly and the Lord Advocate commented adversely that 'it was a matter of great regret that the Engine of fire had ever been resorted to – to pull down the houses was nothing'.

Loch told Lady Stafford that the renewed burnings had 'created a good deal of observation and reflection; it is very provoking that a measure which had been conducted with temper and moderation should be liable to the misrepresentations which such a circumstance may give rise to'.[23] There had been a great deal of clamour and bad publicity about the firing of the people's houses. In a confidential note to Suther, Loch chastised him in the strongest terms and also warned him about the consequences of any cruelty during the removals:

> Depend upon it . . . no one shall ever hear of this but yourself, and even you never again. I trust no acts of cruelty have been committed, they cannot be passed over if they have, and the punishment of them will be a triumph to the Highlanders, and make the next year's movings more difficult.[24]

In his own defence Suther pointed out that the sheep farmers, especially Gabriel Reid, had experienced great annoyance from the recalcitrant people of the Heights of Kildonan who had rapidly rebuilt their huts from their old timber. Reid said that they simply drove their cattle out of sight when the clearing parties approached and later returned to their old pastures when the constables departed.[25] These were the realities of Highland clearings. Loch conceded part of this argument but absolutely forbade Suther to employ fire on any future occasion.

In later years one of the clearing officers made a remarkable and highly unusual statement about the events during this time. In almost confessional tones J. Campbell of Lairg recollected his involvement in the clearances at Abercross in Strathfleet. Three crofters, he recollected, resided near the Mound Wood. 'The wife of one of the them, named Macdonald, was about to give birth to a child.' The factor, along with half a dozen servants, went to burn down the houses:

> They burned the rest of them; and this crofter's was the last. He pleaded hard to be left in the house till his wife was well. The factor did not heed him, but ordered the house to be burned over him. The crofter was in the house, determined not to quit until the fire compelled him. The factor told us the plan we were to take – namely, to cut the rafters and then set fire to the thatch. This we did, but I shall never forget the sight. The man, seeing it was now no use to persist, wrapt his wife in the blankets and brought her out. For two nights did that woman sleep in a sheep cot, and on the third she gave birth to a son. That son, I believe, still lives, and is in America. That is only one instance. I could give many more did space permit.[26]

Ten years after the clearances Beriah Botfield, a literary tourist, came across some of the burnt-out remains of the old houses and wrote that 'all was silent and dead; no token of its once peaceful and happy inhabitants remained, save the blackened ruins of their humble dwellings'.[27] In later years, the stories of burning houses in Sutherland were the subject of much scepticism, but the contemporary evidence is indisputable. Burned-out houses provided the most palpable proof of the act of eviction and it never failed to stir the emotions of the enemies of the Highland landlords.

In the western clearances in 1819 there were reports that the people had actively co-operated in their own removal: 'most of them assisted the Ground Officer when he was going through the ceremony or putting out their fires, and such as go to Rhue Stoir are now busied in building houses on their lots'. The minister, Mackenzie, had accompanied the removal parties 'to the several towns and used all [his] influence and arguments with the people to submit with cheerfulness to the proprietors'. The people were, however, generally hostile to the idea of taking up a career of fishing on the coast.[28] Opposition, for the moment, remained mute or dormant; some of the people left the inland without word, others hung on sullenly to the last moment, until the arrival of the removal posses. Reports from the land agents on the clearances in 1819 were unanimous. One wrote:

It is gratifying to me having to report that my poor countrymen have acted in submission to the Laws and defference [sic] to the rights of their superiors. Many are going to America – as many to Caithness, and several to Glasgow.

Suther explained the general reaction among the people: they were highly reluctant to relinquish their houses and usually stayed until the very last moment; in Strathbrora, for instance, 'had I not sent a party with Brander . . . [to] eject them and pull down their houses they would not have budged of themselves. On Saturday the party had cleared all that were to be removed on the Strathbrora'.

It was close to Brora that 'a spirit of determined resistance was evidenced'. About forty people had assembled close to Colonel Sutherland's house, intent 'resolutely on stopping the progress of the party'. Removals and demolition work had proceeded, and when Suther confronted the resisters he, by his own account, 'scolded and threatened them heartily – they all of course denied all mention of opposing us and promised to behave as they ought to do when the party came'.[29] This, indeed, was a case in which incipient resistance to clearances had begun to form, but which failed to erupt into action. The clearances of 1819 in Kildonan, Strathnaver and Assynt were accomplished essentially without violence from the people.

Many of the people cleared from the hills, disdaining the coastal lots set aside for their resettlement, simply left the estate altogether. The estate managers, their efforts to retain them spurned, admitted partial defeat. The destination of the removees who left the estate was the subject of careful investigation. There were three main destinations: America, the heights of Ross-shire, and lowland Caithness. In Caithness the people spread themselves very widely, but the parish of Latheron received most and Sir John Sinclair's estate in particular. Several estates proved hospitable and provided the Sutherland refugees with small arable plots for oats and potatoes, with the addition of pasture lands in the higher parts. This, of course, was an approximation to their circumstances in Sutherland before the clearances. According to Suther, the people paid higher rents in Caithness and were given no security of tenure.

He remarked: 'It appears to me that the chief and only cause of the people's going to Caithness in preference to taking lots on the Coast here is the matter of Hill ground and an extent of pasture'. Such land, he pointed out, would enable them to keep at least four milch cows:

> by which they can live without working which they mortally hate – indeed I have lately found out that the people in the Hills all considered themselves *farmers* and took it as a degradation to be compared to Labourers and Fishermen.

Suther's observation penetrated to the heart of the matter, to the loss of status and the loss of the basic framework of the traditional life, both inevitable consequences of the removals. The people could not bear the idea of proletarianisation. Hill pasture was the foundation of life as they saw it. Suther wrote: 'I am now convinced if there is an opening for them any where in the Hills, they will prefer it, though worse than being on the Coast'.[30]

At the end of May 1819 Suther summarised the numbers of families who had just been cleared, and those who were to move in 1820. They were accounted in 'families':

	1819	1820
Assynt	50	86
Farr	236	–
Kildonan	123	50
Clyne	42	50
Rogart	59	133
Golspie	78	–
Dornoch	49	15
Loth	67	–
Lairg	–	30
Total	**704**	**364**

In two years 1068 families would be cleared of a population of perhaps 5400.[31] In the space of twelve months more than a quarter of the entire population of the county was cleared. It was a social reorganisation of staggering proportions in such a society. James Loch, who presided over the policy and channelled all responsibility and criticism to himself, was highly conscious of the gravity of the operation. He emphatically denied that it was a 'rash and ill considered system, it was too serious a matter and the happiness of so many of my fellow creatures was not to be so trifled with'.[32] The scale of the clearances had been much greater than Loch had originally contemplated.

Notes

1 Lord Ronald Gower, *My Reminiscences* (1885).

2 SCRO, D593/K/Sellar to Loch, 30 September 1816; Mackenzie to Loch, 14 November 1816.

3 SCRO, D593/K/Sellar to Loch, 11 December 1816.

4 SCRO, D593/K/Loch to Lady Stafford, 21 June 1816.

5 SCRO, D593/K/Loch to Mackay, 27 September 1817; Loch to Allan of Leith, 22 November 1817.

6 SCRO, D593/K/Loch to Mackay, 27 September 1817.

7 SCRO, D593/K/Loch to Mackay and Gunn, 9 February 1818.

8 SCRO, D593/K/Loch to Suther, 7 February 1810.

9 SCRO, D593/K/Suther to Loch, 6 December 1817.

10 SCRO, D593/K/Revd David Mackenzie to Loch, 19 March 1818.

11 SCRO, D593/K/Loch to Revd Mackenzie, 20 March 1818.

12 SCRO, D593/K/Capt. Mackay to Loch, 25 April 1818.

13 SCRO, D593/K/Capt. Mackay to Loch, 4 June 1818.

14 SCRO, D593/K/Sellar to Loch, 13 April 1818.

15 SCRO, D593/K/Suther to Loch, 17 May 1818.

16 Bangor-Jones, op. cit., p. 26.

17 SCRO, D593/K/Grant to Loch, 14 July 1818.

18 SCRO, D593/K/Suther to Loch, October 1818.

19 SCRO, D593/K/Loch to Suther, 13 November 1818; Loch to Suther, 8 May 1819.

20 SCRO, D593/K/Suther to Loch, 26 November 1818.

21 SCRO, D593/K/Loch to Suther, 25 February 1819.

22 SCRO, D593/K/Mackay to Loch, 17 August 1819.

23 SCRO, D593/K/Mackenzie to Loch, 30 September 1819; Loch to Lady Stafford, May 1819.

24 SCRO, D593/K/Loch to Suther, 18 July 1819.

25 SCRO, D593/K/Suther to Loch, 5 June 1819.

26 Joseph Mitchell *Reminiscences*, II, p. 91, quoting a letter from Mr J. Campbell of Lairg to the *Inverness Courier*.

27 Botfield, *Journal of a Tour*, p. 152.

28 SCRO, D593/K/Gunn to Loch, 2 June 1819. See Bangor-Jones, op. cit., passim.

29 SCRO, D593/K/Suther to Loch,12, 26 May 1819.

30 SCRO, D593/K/Suther to Loch, 29 May, 26 June 1819.

31 SCRO, D593/K/Loch to Suther, 8 June 1819.

32 SCRO, D593/K/Loch to Mackay, 8 June 1819.

11

The Last of the Sutherland Clearances

I. Mounting tension

THERE WAS NO VIOLENT resistance in the great Sutherland clearances of 1819. But there were distinct rumblings of dissatisfaction. Emigration was good evidence of a rejection of estate plans. Within and beyond the county of Sutherland there was rising public criticism of the Stafford family. The *Scotsman* was critical throughout the summer of 1819. This alarmed James Loch and his employers, who believed it could easily provoke a parliamentary inquiry, their greatest fear. The estate resolved to suspend all clearances after 1820. But meanwhile the estate was committed to the last great round of clearances in Sutherland, scheduled for Whitsunday 1820.

There was a second negative reaction to the 1819 removals, unusual in form and, potentially, equally dangerous to the landlords. A popular co-operative movement sprang up among the evicted people to organise emigration to North America. They formed a friendly society called 'The Transatlantic Emigration Society', which was regarded by the landlords of the country as a mask for activity of a much more subversive and dangerous character. The society became a vehicle for opposition to the estate polices and to evicting landlords in general.

The formation of the 'Transatlantic Emigration Society' added a new tension to the final round of comprehensive clearances planned for 1820. Its meetings, on the borders of Sutherland and Ross, some involving several hundred people, revived memories of the troubles of 1792 in the same area, and created intense alarm in the minds of the estate managers. Sir John Sinclair told Loch that he much regretted that some means are not taken to put an end to the clamour that has been excited, respecting the management of the Sutherland Estate. It is to be lamented that such a circumstance should take place in the North of Scotland, at the same time that popular commotions are so prevalent in England.[1]

The Transatlantic Emigration Society organised large meetings, collected subscriptions from the people and conducted lengthy correspondence in the newspapers about the plight of the people cleared on the Sutherland estate. It became the mouthpiece for the swelling criticisms of the Sutherland regime.

Loch and his agents were excruciatingly embarrassed at the publicity that flooded forth. Their great fear was that the organisation of the Transatlantic Emigration Society would incite active resistance, especially if it became linked with southern radicalism. The main organiser and spokesman of the popular agitation, the secretary of the society, was Thomas Dudgeon.[2] He conducted much of the controversy through the correspondence columns of the *Scotsman*, which also reported the meetings. Dudgeon wrote that Suther was 'not a bad man', but the truth was that hundreds of houses had been burned, that the 'appreciators' had been the appointees of the estate, and that the churches had been forbidden to give shelter to the evicted. It was true that the Sutherland estate had promised to pay £5 for every acre the new settlers brought into cultivation at Dornoch Muirs but, asserted Dudgeon, it was virtually impossible to trench the muirs at that rate. The tenants could not possibly gain by the arrangement: they would spend two years in poverty and hard labour primarily for the benefit of Lady Stafford. A petition from the people stated that no people in the whole of Europe could cultivate that ground, and that

> to offer such places is no more than a gentle excuse or rather a shew of humanity, where the greatest cruelty and barbarity is intended, which will undoubtedly bring its accepters to ruin and beggary.

Loch countered this allegation by saying that there were people already farming the Dornoch Muirs who were 'living well by their industry without any of the advantages which are offered to the new Lotters'.[3]

The furore in the aftermath of the 1819 clearances continued through the autumn and as Whitsunday 1820 approached, there emerged more serious allegations of 'cruelty' and 'severe distress' caused to evictees during the recent removals by the estate factors. Once more there emerged detail of the actual trauma inevitable in mass removal. For instance, it was alleged in the newspapers that the pregnant wife of a William Matheson had died in 'consequence of being prematurely delivered, his house having been set fire to'. It was another echo of the type of allegations made five years earlier against Patrick Sellar.

It is impossible to judge the truth of these charges and exculpations. The only firm inference is that most of the people left their old homes in the hills ahead of the removal party; that a few stayed behind because of illness or in the hope of a last-minute reprieve; that the party of constables burned off the old timbers to prevent re-entry; and that at least one death occurred during the 1819 clearances. Whether the death was attributable to the evictions is uncertain.

James Loch regarded the renewed public outcry as profoundly depressing, but he took great comfort in the palpable advance in the villages of the east coast. At Helmsdale the new village was a miracle of change:

> so full of life and increasing wealth and industrious exertion, about 2000 people hard at work tumbling over each other like ants, living in dozens of houses half finished and without roof [which] put me in mind of the erection and progress of an American town.

To Loch it was evidently a kind of colonisation of the Highlands. Meanwhile in the interior, he claimed, the physical appearance of the hills had also improved: 'They are getting so much greener, especially those under sheep, in fifty years [heathing?] hills and the Gaelic tongue will be rarities in Sutherland.'[4]

II. Whitsun 1819–Whitsun 1820

In October 1819 some of the sub-factors of the Sutherland estate reported a growing hostility, and some petty intimidation, among the people. They detected generalised threats against 'all law and order' and specific threats to resist removal. They heard also that people had 'determined to have blood for blood in the struggle for keeping possession'. Anonymous threatening letters were sent to the Stafford family in residence in London which referred to Lady Stafford as 'a damned old Cat', and her husband as a 'Butcher' and a 'Hyena' and a 'monster'. One such letter said that the day was 'coming when she will tremble'.[5] Suspicion of radical connections added considerably to the alarm. Extensive publicity for emigration was circulated by the Transatlantic Society and expectations were raised that 400 families might leave. In the last three months of the year the country was in ferment.

Lady Stafford and her ailing, elderly husband could not understand why her family was singled out as the target of public condemnation. In her perplexity she asked James Loch to discover how other landowners in the district treated the people that they removed from the sheep walks. In a small exercise in 'Comparative Clearances', Loch reported that, in Ross-shire, Lord Moray bought the cattle from the people where necessary, but made no other provision for them: they were evicted, they received no other type of compensation and they were not offered resettlement places. On the estate of Munro of Novar the people were simply evicted without any provision, and Loch said that the people had to emigrate. Significantly, it was on the Novar estate that some of the most violent anti-clearance riots developed later in 1820 (see below).

By the end of 1819 some of the people from the removal zones on the Sutherland estate were shifting to their new lots on the coast in the approved manner. From inland Kildonan they were placed at Gartymore and Morvich where, according to Suther, they were satisfied with the facilities: they 'will not only give no trouble but, before the removing time they will actually have their houses up and be settled in them'. In Strathfleet, another group of interior people designated for removal were discovered to possess a lease (drawn up in William Young's time) which protected them until 1828.[6] They had become 'riveted' to the land and their exception reduced the scale of the forthcoming clearances by half. It was another unambiguous sign that resettlement was the last preference of the people of Sutherland.[7]

For the remaining removals Loch ordered that special care be taken by the clearing parties. He told the sub-agents that 'meliorations' and building materials should be supplied to the people with generosity. 'Don't be rigid', he ordered, 'it is a vast arrangement which is in the course of being accomplished and which can never happen twice and therefore lead to no bad precedents, giving a little more to make all smooth'.[8] In the west, in Assynt, the estate organised a fête with dancing, which it was thought might generate a better feeling towards the landlord. It would help to break the hold of the radicals upon the minds of the people.[9]

Loch's rational philosophy intruded most fiercely when he sought to clamp 'marriage rules' upon the common people. In January 1820 he declared that 'only one son of each Tenant should after he marries be permitted to remain in his father's place'.[10] This, perhaps the most notorious aspect of Loch's clearances, was a quasi-Malthusian rule concocted to check population growth by preventing the sub-division of holdings which, he believed, threatened to swamp all the benefits of estate planning. The principle was invoked recurrently in the following decades and became known as the 'Loch policy'. It was regarded widely as a particularly loathsome form of social control. To all the world it seemed as though Loch was prohibiting marriage among the ordinary folk of Sutherland. It was, to most people, an unnatural and a disgusting abuse of landlord power.

III. *The 1820 clearances*

The 1820 clearances were scheduled for Whitsunday. In February and March, on the very borders of the Sutherland estate, there was an explosion of anti-clearance rioting at Culrain on the estate of Munro of Novar in Ross. Here the clearances had been forced through without any resettlement provisions for the 600 people involved. The resistance was violent and troops were called in to crush a popular revolt. Many feared that the Culrain revolt would cohere into a comprehensive northern rebellion against the landlords. It threw the Sutherland managers into a panic regarding their own forthcoming removals. 'In these times,' wrote commissioner Loch to his man in the north, 'depend upon it every motion is watched and if you do anything at all which will occasion public observation it will be brought before the house of C[ommons].' The tense atmosphere on the Sutherland estate was heightened by the knowledge that Sutherland people had participated in the Culrain events.[11]

Suther, for all the turmoil about him, somehow managed to retain his optimistic equanimity. 'Our people are all quiet and will I think go peaceably off,' he reported in mid-March. Loch ordered him to 'avoid using fire in any way whatever' in the coming clearances.[12]

At the end of April 1820 all reports from the sub-agents about the clearances on the estate spoke of the peaceability of the people and the diminution of radical influences in the county. At the end of May Suther told Lady Stafford: 'The Removals are now completed and they have all been effected in the most peaceable and easy manner. The people have behaved most excellently.'[13] From Assynt the agent, George Gunn, was able to say 'That the removals in this parish are completed, and that with the utmost order and without a murmur of discontent.'[14] About eighty people emigrated to America from the estate during the month of June.

The Sutherland clearances of 1819 and 1820 had involved several thousand people yet provoked no violent physical resistance. This is not to say that the people cleared were anything other than sullenly acquiescent, but the contrast with adjoining estates was marked and, in June 1820, there was further sensational resistance on the estate borders at Gruids in Ross-shire.[15] It is surprising that the disaffection did not spill over on to the Sutherland estate which, at that moment, was in the throes of its last great removals. It is not improbable that Sutherland remained immune from riot in these years because it had arranged elaborate provision for the resettlement of the people. In this sense the Sutherland estate was, despite its reputation, in strong and positive contrast to most other clearing proprietors.

A large part of the 1820 clearance programme had taken place in the western and heavily populated part of the estate. Many of the people, apparently, had committed themselves to emigration during Dudgeon's campaign with the Transatlantic Emigration Society. According to the local factor, many of them changed their minds at the last moment, 'but it was too late – the Master of the vessel insisted on their going or standing a prosecution for breach of contract'. Others in Assynt, also discouraged by poor accounts sent home from emigrants who went to America in 1819, decided to go instead to Caithness which was more attractive than the coastal lots because there was more land on offer.[16]

Two sets of figures relating to the 1819 clearances were gathered by the Sutherland estate (see Chapter 10). The first referred to rent-paying tenants removed at Whitsunday and indicated that 68 per cent of the people shifted were resettled on the estate, 7 per cent went to neighbouring estates, 21 per cent went to adjoining counties, and 2 per cent emigrated. Two per cent were unaccounted for.

The second group of figures referred to 'sub-tenants and persons paying no rent', mainly squatters. Of these people removed 73 per cent were resettled on the Sutherland coast, 7 per cent went to neighbouring estates, 13 per cent entered neighbouring counties, 5 per cent emigrated, and the estate managers were unable to discover the destination of the remaining 2 per cent. These were the most marginal people of the Highlands, the lowest stratum, with the least claim on the land. The apparent low rate of departure from the estate did not, of course, preclude subsequent migration and it is likely that removals operated as the first step on the long road to ultimate emigration.[17]

The statistical comparison suggests that the Sutherland estate did not actively discriminate against squatters and sub-tenants when granting resettlement lots. It also indicates that the shifting of the people caused a loss of at least a quarter of the previous population. Surprisingly, the estate retained more of the sub-tenants and squatters than of its direct tenants. Unfortunately, there are no equivalent figures for the 1820 removals. It is also clear that, though there was hostility to the removals in Assynt, there was no evidence of 'burnings' during their implementation.[18]

The population of Assynt, despite clearances and emigration, increased from 2479 to 2803 between 1811 and 1821. Some of the settlers were engaged in the doomed kelp industry, but more switched into fishing. A description by the western factor, George Gunn, hints at the severity of the economic and social change that had overcome these communities as a result of the clearances:

> The new lotters in Rhue Stoer appear contented and reconciled to their change – the young men who were never at sea before Whitsunday 1819 are now constantly engaged in fishing, and some of them are preparing to go to Caithness – this I think is a proof that their habits of idleness are not unconquerable and that we may look forward to the time when their services will be useful to themselves and others.[19]

Further indirect evidence of the people's attitudes to the change in tenure came in another report from Gunn concerning the Rhue Stoer people. They had previously held their land by runrig, but the removals provided them with separate and individual lots with 'each person permanently settled in possession during his lease'. Gunn, undoubtedly understating the case, reported that

> Many of them are at present rather averse to this change for they are equally so to any arrangement which interferes with their former habits, but a very short time will be sufficient to convince them of the advantage of it, and then, I hope they will evince some spirit of competition, for the improvement of their lots.

But Gunn was generally optimistic; the lotters had no complaints, and he believed that in a few years they would make as much clamour about removals if they were ordered back into the interior Highlands.[20] It was, of course, an idle speculation.

The summer of 1820 saw the end of the great displacement of population on the Sutherland estate. Loch believed that arrangements on such an extensive scale had never been 'effected with so little individual misery . . . and to do so has cost Mr Suther many a sleepless and anxious night'.[21] There was relief that the change had been engineered without further catastrophe for the public reputation of the Stafford family. A legal adviser to the family, responding to Loch's recently published *Account* of the policies, summed up the position:

The whole scheme is now effected and no circumstances whatever can ever throw back the people of that country to their former state now that the communications are so perfect and so much actively employed in every department.[22]

But Loch's book was not universally applauded and at least one respondent continued to raise the question of 'particular acts of hardship alleged against the managers of the Sutherland clearances'.[23]

IV. Smaller removals

The main body of Sutherland clearances was accomplished during the years 1819–20; but there were a number of much smaller removals in the following years, and ejectments occurred on this scale in smaller numbers for decades. They were relatively minor adjustments to the grand plan. But even small clearances were liable to generate as much disturbance as the larger events.

In March and April 1821 the Sutherland estate conducted a number of ejectments at Achness and Mudale and in both cases the people's hostility was entirely disproportionate to the scale of the removals. The turmoil was influenced by further anti-clearance violence in contiguous Ross-shire, notably at Gruids again, where troops were called in to quell the riotous populace. At Mudale, the local factor faced a defiant community of about thirty families when he attempted to execute his warrants of ejectment. He reported:

I intend to send a party to eject them and to demolish their houses, by cutting the timbers. I am not aware that there will be any resistance offered, but if there should be . . . I will myself with a second party effect the business completely.[24]

At Achness and Ascoilmore, however, the physical obstruction of the clearance in 1821 was far greater than anything witnessed on the estate in the previous two years of mass clearance. Loch described the events in the north at this time as 'a regular and organised system of resistance to civil power'. It required the intervention of fusiliers to bring the Achness people to heel.[25] Once again the local evidence gives the lie to the idea that the clearances were unresisted and that the people were stoically acquiescent.

The 1821 clearances in Sutherland, though small in scale, were executed at the point of the sword. By the end of May 1821 Suther expressed great relief that the work had been done: 'We are extremely busy just now with our Removings which God be praised will be completed eventually and without a whisper on Wednesday.' The people went to their lots on the coast, or further afield. And while Suther congratulated his employers on the eventual passivity of the people involved, a number of ugly and damaging accusations of wanton cruelty and negligence were again voiced against the estate. An internal investigation of the events absolved Suther and his men from wrongdoing, but it is highly improbable that the great evictions had been accomplished without suffering among the population at large.

At the end of 1821 Loch gave Suther instructions which marked the termination of both the clearances and the development of the coastal economy. No further expansion at Helmsdale and the other coastal centres was to occur. Henceforth the people would have to do everything for themselves. They had been spoiled by Lord Stafford's benevolence and they would now have to 'swim for themselves'. All the turmoil of the removals, the arrangement of leases and the rest of the development had been, said Loch, a great burden on the management. That had now finished and he told Suther: 'You must do what Lord Stafford sent you to Sutherland to do – to economise, methodise.' The Stafford family believed they had created the basic structure for future progress on the northern estates. Lord Stafford wrote to say that he expected thenceforth a clear income of £12 000 per annum from Sutherland.[26] This would be the return on his investment and the upheaval of the people. Estate retrenchment was added to the other depressive elements in the local economy.

V. Consequences

In the Sutherland clearances the common people were removed from their old places in the interior and they lost the traditional bases of their lives. This was the simple meaning of the clearances. The net effects are extremely difficult to gauge, partly because the experience in the east was in substantial contrast to that of the west, both economically and demographically. Population growth in Sutherland was varied. The population of the parish of Eddrachillis in the far north-west grew by 60 per cent in the 1820s, and strong increases were registered in most of the other parishes in the early decades. Indeed all the parish populations continued to rise until 1841, and several through to 1871, which was relatively late by the standards of rural Britain.

The consequences of the Sutherland clearances were complicated, perhaps beyond untangling, because there were manifold influences simultaneously at work – such as the departure of the herring from the Sutherland coasts, and the concomitant collapse of commodity prices. There is no measurable way of determining the fate of the people had they stayed in the hills. Contemporary opinion was certainly divided. The problem of population growth and increasing vulnerability to the weather and to the externally determined prices had certainly not been solved in the old economy as many parts of the region testified in the following decades. And the situation in Sutherland was complicated by the landlord's undoubted effort to reconstitute the small tenants' existence on a new footing.

In 1825 Alexander Sutherland visited some of the eviction sites in Sutherland as well as the reception centres for the resettled people from the interior. In Strathbrora he came across a recently cleared township:

> All was silence and desolation. Blackened and roofless huts, still enveloped in smoke – articles of furniture cast away, as of no value to the houseless – and a few domestic fowls, scraping for food among hills of ashes, were the only objects that told us of man. A few days had sufficed to change a countryside, teeming with the cheeriest sounds of rural life, into a desert.

Sutherland spoke to some of the people leaving this place and reported:

> They argued that they had a presumptive claim to the soil: that they did

their 'lady' [i.e. Lady Stafford] justice, if they farmed it as their fathers
had done; and that, chieftainess though she were, she had no better title
to eject them from their humble tenements, than they had to drive her
from her castle.

In any country, save the Highlands, arguments of this sort would
not be listened to. Here, owing to the peculiar structure of society,
they were not merely heard with indulgence, but warmly
advocated.

Sutherland then proceeded to one of the main fishing villages
which had been created for the future life of the people. He
described the prospect:

> Port Gower is a modern village, and, as its name imports, indebted to
> the Stafford family for its existence. The inhabitants are chiefly
> fishermen, to which life it has all along been her ladyship's desire to
> direct the attention of her superfluous tenantry. We have seldom seen a
> neater fishing village than Port Gower; and everything considered, one
> would think it no difficult matter to allure inhabitants thither from the
> solitary glens of the interior: but it is no easy task to teach men,
> habituated from infancy to tend herds on the hillside, to drag for
> subsistence in the deep sea.[27]

The careers of the people who chose not to settle in places such as
Port Gower are more difficult to follow. Within Scotland they
dispersed south into Ross-shire and probably drifted towards
Inverness, Glasgow and Edinburgh. Some went north, even to
Orkney,[28] but mostly into neighbouring Caithness. There are two
reports on a group of people who fled to Caithness in 1821 which
demonstrate the dependent state of all the common people living
on Highland property, and the amazing disregard that characterised
much landlord policy. In 1823 George Gunn, a Sutherland factor,
reported the unfortunate plight of some of these migrants:

> The poor creatures who were enticed to Mr Traill's property in
> Caithness two years ago, have met with nothing but misery and distress
> – they were no judges of the value of land, and consequently offered
> any rent he thought proper to ask – he took care however to bind them
> all for each other, and as might be expected, they have fallen in arrears,
> he swept away every article a few days ago and left them destitute and

houseless. I have had doleful petitions from them, begging permission to return, were they only to occupy huts without land, but now they are away, it is certainly better to keep free of them as they would just become so many paupers and burdens on the Parish. Mr Traill has deprived them of their effects, and I think it is only fair that he should now be allowed to take charge of them.[29]

Some of the same people were still on Traill's property twenty years later, but most had departed. Traill's own factor made a candid statement to the Poor Law Commission in 1843 which spoke eloquently of their problems:

Mr Traill took a fancy to give them crofts on part of his property. Several hundreds of them were thus provided in crofts, and planted very densely. In the course of a few years the experiment proved to be a failure. The Highlandmen, had never been accustomed to the laborious life which their new situation required of them. They soon fell into arrears of rent; and, when this happened, they generally ran away. The proprietor was well pleased when he heard of their flight. They were, in point of character, respectable and decent men, but really wholly useless as regards active and laborious exertions.[30]

The Poor Law Inquiry gave the ministers of Sutherland and others the opportunity to look back over the twenty years that had elapsed since the clearances, and to report the consequences for the common people. In the absence of any quantitative measure of the economic and social (much less the psychic) benefits and costs of the clearances, such evidence is indispensable even though it could not claim to be entirely representative.

The ministers were at variance in their judgements but the Revd David Mackenzie, who lived through the entire upheaval and was later vilified for his alleged complicity in the clearances, judged that 'the people have been decidedly losers by the change'. In food, clothing and bedding they used to be better off, but their habitations were improved. The Revd George Mackay of Clyne observed that the decline (through the 1820s) of coal and salt workings on the coast had produced poverty among some of the settlers. The surgeon at Brora believed the people were in better health than ever before. The Revd Hugh Mackay of Tongue, who had known the Reay country since 1806, had absolutely no doubt that the condition of the people had 'been very much deteriorated by the change' and that distress was more recurrent than previously . The Revd W. Findlater of Durness recollected that

> While the population were settled in the Interior, though they were no doubt more liable to be affected by unfavourable seasons than they now are, yet from the number of cattle and sheep which they kept, they could generally, by the disposal of part of their stock, purchase the meal requisite for their families.

The most interesting testimony came from George Macleod, who had been a small farmer in Kildonan for eighteen years until his land was taken from him and converted into a sheep farm. He was resettled at Helmsdale in company with many other people at the time of the Clearances and no longer had land for stock. Macleod, therefore, was the classic victim of the Sutherland clearances and his account is doubly valuable. He described the change that he had experienced as a consequence of the removals:

> There is no place for sheep [in Helmsdale], but I have now about seven acres of arable land. When I came to it it was a heathy bare moor. When I came I got a 14 year lease of it for a shilling an acre, and I was to receive a premium of £5 for every acre which I made arable in the first seven years. I made them all arable and received the five premiums. Mr Gunn paid me honestly. In Kildonan I had about 5 acres of arable land. The land was as good as at Helmsdale if it was a good season. There were not many bad years in my time there, but there have been many bad years since I left it, and I was told there had been many bad years previously. There was only one bad year while I was at Kildonan among the cattle, which was owing to 'the black disease' which got among them. I am as well off where I am as I was in Kildonan. There is more work going on at Helmsdale, especially during the fishing season, and I can get more employment at day's wages. At Kildonan there was not employment for the generality at day's wages.[31]

One contented resettled crofter did not, of course, make or break the argument. In truth the contemporary evidence is contradictory. Lord Teignmouth's account of a journey through the Highlands in the early 1830s contained high praise for the Sutherland arrangements,[32] but favourable judgements such as his are easily counterbalanced by equally adverse reports.

Even the estate factors were sometimes critical or equivocal. Thus George Gunn was prepared to state publicly in the *New Statistical Account* that 'the peasantry cannot procure the same quantity of animal food, and of the produce of the dairy, as when they lived in the interior and occupied a greater extent of land'. But Gunn believed that they obtained a more regular supply of food than before the clearances.[33]

In the long run the Sutherland experiment evidently did not fulfil the extravagant expectations of the planners of the years 1806–10. The coastal economy did not develop enough non-agricultural income to counterbalance the consequences of the disengagement of the people from the soil. Most of the resettled tenantry became crofters dependent on a mixture of activities – keeping a few cows, some cultivation, some labouring, some fishing and some seasonal work in the south or at Wick. This was the antithesis of Loch's prescription – he had wanted to create an independent population which would reap the benefits of a proper division of labour. Moreover, it is likely, as Malcolm Bangor-Jones estimates, that 'the amount of arable land per household was much less in the coastal townships as compared with the inland townships.'[34]

This is not to say that there were no positive results, but the long-term consequences of the resettlement were, at best, the relocation of congestion from the interior to the coast. Sixty years later, one of the advisers to the fourth Duke of Sutherland expressed the point in the starkest terms. Reflecting on the current furore over the crofting question in Sutherland in 1882, he declared that it was

> the result of a great many crofters being huddled together on small pieces of land, entirely inadequate for their employment, and consequently unequal to that support. To extend the area of these small holdings is impossible, and to remove the half of the people to make room for the other half, at one stroke to reform, would be a social change, calculated to cause a civil revolution.[35]

As for the results of the clearances and the local living standards, it is salutary to bear in mind that the northern Highlands were the least favoured region in Britain and one which did not receive clear benefits from industrialisation. Indeed industrialisation in the south probably created de-industrialising effects in the Highlands. Yet even in the most progressive regions in Britain, at the very centre of the most dynamic economy the world had ever seen, the benefits accruing to 'people' were still in 1850 no better than equivocal in any measurable sense. The considered verdict, from the most informed modern opinion, should be set beside the condition of the average Highlander in the age of the clearances:

> Most British workers and their families did not experience an actual deterioration in their standard of living during and after the Industrial Revolution. But neither did they enjoy the rapid progress which the super-optimists have discerned. For the majority of the working class the historical reality was that they had to endure almost a century of hard toil with little or no advantage from a low base before they really began to share in any of the benefits of the economic transformation they had helped to create.[36]

VI. Rare voices

The dispossessed in the Highland clearances did not speak clearly into the record except during the occasional eruptions of physical resistance. The oral tradition of the Highlands, always a slippery source to interpret, carries most of the burden of the story. Much of it was sustained by symbol. There was, for instance, a story told by the Revd David Mackenzie, the Free Church minister of Farr, who had witnessed the greatest of the clearances in Strathnaver as well as the aftermath. His story concerned one of the people who had been shifted, probably in 1819:

> An old woman who was in the habit, as many others were, of paying an occasional visit to the scenery of her youth, was asked on her return by one who was himself ejected, what did she see? She was sad and silent for some time. At last she said, 'I saw a raven's nest in the chimney of your own ruined house, and I saw the minister's study turned into a kennel for dogs.'[37]

A more direct voice of the people may be heard occasionally in the stilted phrases of petitions sent by the people to the Sutherland family. Often they expressed the assumptions and perceptions of the common people, but always between the lines of obligatory deference. In 1831, for instance, the Sutherland estate decided to execute a small clearance of a community of people at Gorval in Strath Halladale, to create a sheep farm. The people were a problem because their cattle repeatedly damaged the embankments on the River Halladale.

The Halladale people were offered lots on the north coast at Melvich where the young people would be able to fish, and the elderly could graze a few beasts. Their furniture would be carried without cost, they would be given timber for their new houses, and they would be exempt from rent for two years. By 1831, however, the landlord had become cautious, even inhibited, and clearances were executed with greater stealth. Loch told the northern factor who was sceptical of the adequacy of the Melvich lots:

> The removals from Gorval etc. become a most difficult subject if you cannot provide for them at Melvich. The present temper of the Times, the condition of Ireland, all make it a puzzling question . . . The greatest care must be taken not to lay the grounds for any outcry at the present moment. Consider well before you take any step in advance. Consider whether they cannot be removed gradually.

In the course of these deliberations Lady Stafford received a representation from the people of Halladale:

> The Complaint and Petition of Twenty-Five Tenants, and Householders on the Estate of Bighouse, County of Sutherland.
>
> That your Lordship's Petitioners with their families who are in number a Hundred and Twenty Six persons of whom are twelve Female Widows. Your Lordship's Petrs in October last got a general warning of Removal from Mr Horsburgh who at the same time told your Lordship's Petitioners they were to get other Holdings in Ederachilles or Melvich, which is of late cut out in lots. Your Lordship's Petitioners in whole overlooked the said lots, and now your Lordship's Petrs considered it their duty in plain fact, to acquaint your Lordship's that they will sooner with pleasure throw themselves on the neighbouring Counties to beg their living, before they would take a grant of the said

lots of Ground which undoubtedly would soon put an end to our lives with Starvation and famine. Your Lordship's Petitioners who for the most part are frail old men [and] women, who mostly passed the days of their health and strength in the farming line need never be thought to earn their living from the waves of the Ocean suppose there could not be any other provision made for them in the world but to Harrass and drive them to the disagreeable lots of Melvich which is neither sufficient to sustain one man or one beast where never was any manner of living, unless it would come out of the sea. Therefore your Lordship's Petitioners will venture to hope and pray your Lordship again and again to grant unto them suitable possession as farmers in which occupation they and their forefathers were bred up to. May therefore the Petitioners Humbly beg and request that your Lordship would be graciously pleased to take the foresaid in to consideration and in respect thereof confer and grant the said Petitioners a favourable reply, in due time.

6 Jan. 1831

The petition was accompanied by a letter from a local landowner, Innes of Sandside in Caithness, an old friend of the Sutherland family. The people had thought that Lady Stafford would not read their petition unless Sandside vouched for them. He wrote:

I trust the Marquess and you will excuse me for pleading the cause of the Poor Highlanders. The offer made to them on their removal I cannot think reasonable nor can I think that the Marquess and your Ladyship would think it so, if you knew the situation and the whole circumstances of the case . . . Indeed to my view it is as unreasonable as if your Ladyship was compelled to steer a man of war through the Pentland Firth in a gale wip'd – do consider the view I have taken with the one proposed, before the time of removal. The Marquess and you have the hearts of the highlanders and I should be much grieved to see the day It was otherwise. As the old peoples sons grew up it might be proper to turn their thoughts to Port Skerry and Melvich as fishers, and the fathers and sons families might both thrive, but in the plan proposed neither of them can thrive.

Innes apologised to the Staffords for his intercession and asked them not to regard him as 'a Turbulent fellow and a bad neighbour'. The upshot was that the Gorval people offered to build a dyke to prevent their cattle damaging the river embankment and the clearance was postponed.[38]

The Gorval petition was written by people under the threat of clearance. A second example is provided by a petition written in February 1831 in which was heard the voices of people who had been cleared many years before. Addressed to Lord Stafford from people in the north-west parish of Eddrachillis, it was full of a sense of deprivation, and a sense of loss of former comfort and security because of the clearances. While it expressed an overwhelming antipathy to the factors, it contained also a certain vestigial deference towards the proprietor. The petition was probably penned by a school teacher or a minister. It stated:

> That your Petitioners have been urged by necessity to apply to your Lordship's Commissioners for a Reduction of Rent, and not having received any satisfactory answer they are compelled as a last resource to apply to your Lordship. That more than two thirds of the Parish in which your Petitioners reside have been laid waste by the sheep farming system, in consequence of which the part inhabited is overcrowded with the surplus Population. That your Petitioners formerly paid their rents by rearing Cattle and by fishing, but now that ten families occupy the place formerly inhabited by one, the rearing of Cattle was rendered unpracticable, and the fishing which at all times is precarious has this year in a great measure failed. That your petitioners are prevented from improving the little land they Cultivate, not only by not having leases on it, but above all by being prohibited from using the sea ware on the coast for manure. That in consequence of these hardships there are not in this parish nine families which can be supported for nine months by the produce of their lands, that the young men of the Parish, though much attached to their superiors and to their country are compelled by their grievances to emigrate to Foreign lands, but before they reluctantly leave their native soil they deem it their duty to make their case known to your Lordship.[39]

Notes

1 SCRO, D593/K/Sinclair to Loch, 17 August 1819.

2 On Dudgeon, see Bangor-Jones, op. cit., p. 37.

3 SCRO, D593/K/Dudgeon to Suther, 30 August 1819; Loch to MacGillivray, 18 August 1819.

4 SCRO, D593/K/Loch to Lady Stafford, 8 August 1819.

5 NLS Dep 313/1016 Letters relating to the removals in 1819.

6 SCRO, D593/K/Loch to Suther, 9 October 1819.

7 SCRO, D593/K/Suther to Loch, 7 December 1819.

8 SCRO, D593/K/Loch to Suther, 9 October 1819.

9 SCRO, D593/K/Gunn to Loch, 18 December 1819.

10 SCRO, D593/K/Loch to Suther, 22 January 1820.

11 On Culrain, see Eric Richards, 'Patterns of Highland discontent, 1760–1860', in R. Quinault and J. Stevenson (eds.), *Popular Protest and Public Order* (London, 1974), pp. 88–91.

12 SCRO, D593/K/Loch to Suther, 26 March 1820.

13 SCRO, D593/K/Suther to Lady Stafford, 8, 27 May 1820.

14 SCRO, D593/K/Gunn to Loch, 8 June 1820.

15 Richards, 'Highland discontent', pp. 91–3.

16 SCRO, D593/K/Gunn to Loch, 26 March 1821.

17 On the question of cottars see especially Bangor-Jones, op. cit., pp. 45–6.

18 See Bangor-Jones, op. cit., pp. 36–9.

19 SCRO, D593/K/Gunn to Loch, 22 July 1820.

20 SCRO, D593/K/Gunn to Loch, 12 January 1822.

21 SCRO, D593/K/Loch to Gower, 3 October 1820.

22 SCRO, D593/K/Mackenzie to Loch, 10 August 1820. James Loch, *Account of the Improvements on the Estates of the Marquis of Stafford* (1820).

23 SCRO, D593/K/Smith to Loch, 11 August 1820.

24 SCRO, D593/K/Mackay to Loch, 13 April 1821.

25 See Richards, 'Highland discontent', passim.

26 SCRO, D593/K/Loch to Suther, 24 February 1822.

27 Alexander Sutherland, *A Summer Ramble in the North Highlands* (Edinburgh, 1825), pp. 101–3.

28 See Ronald Miller, *Orkney* (London, 1976), p. 123.

29 SCRO, D593/K/Gunn to Loch, 23 May 1823.

30 Evidence of Purvis, factor to George Traill, MP, before the Commissioners inquiring into the Administration of the Poor Laws in Scotland, PP (1844).

31 Ibid., pp. 278, 286, 292, 305.

32 Teignmouth, *Sketches*, vol. I, Chapter XIV.

33 *New Statistical Account*, vol. XV, p. 159.

34 Bangor-Jones, op. cit., p. 12.

35 SCRO, D593/K/1/3/60/ George Greig to Henry Wright, 2 November 1882.

36 Charles H. Fernstein, 'Pessimism Perpetuated: Real Wages and the

Standard of Living in Britain during and after the Industrial Revolution,' *Journal of Economic History*, 58 (1998), p. 652.

37 James Wylie, *Disruption Worthies of the Highlands. Another Memorial of 1843.* (Edinburgh, 1877), p. 90.

38 SCRO, D593/K/Innes to Lady Stafford, 10 January 1831; Horsburgh to Loch, 2, 19 March, 12 May 1831; Loch to Horsburgh, 10 October. 1830; 28 January 1831.

39 SCRO, D593/K/Petition to Lord Stafford, 9 February 1831.

12

Sweeping the Highlands:
The Middle Years – Lewis, Rum,
Harris, Freswick and Strathaird
(Skye)

I. *Clearance by attrition and by stealth*

SOME OF THE HIGHLAND clearances were like an earthquake shattering the foundations of entire communities, displacing large numbers of people almost overnight, and sometimes executed with physical force. These events attracted publicity and outrage and live longest in the folk memory.

But the process which transformed the Highlands, though sometimes cataclysmic, was mainly gradual and occupied more than a century from the 1760s. Much of the agrarian upheaval was not entirely dissimilar to that in the rest of the British Isles, especially in the upland districts. People were eased off the land in small discontinuous shifts so that eventually the land was occupied by fewer people, with each generation retaining a smaller proportion of its people in the land of their birth. This erosion of the rural population was a defining characteristic of the age of industrialisation and the events in the Highlands should be seen in that wider context. As Devine says, 'Gradual and relentless displacement rather than mass eviction was the norm.'[1] A small farmer in Denbighshire or Roscommon or Wiltshire or Sussex experienced the same contraction of his local horizons as the man of Lewis or Caithness. The most important difference between them was the opportunity for alternative employment in the reasonably close vicinity. However much Highland landlords tried to generate new industry in the north – from Sir John Sinclair through Lord Stafford and Sir James Matheson to Lord Leverhulme – the outcomes always disappointed. So in the Highlands the trauma of change was greater, the poverty worse, the outrage more intense, the feelings most personalised against the landlord.

The velocity and scale of clearance in the nineteenth-century Highlands is difficult to determine because much of the process occurred in relative quiet and without publicity. Some of it is recorded only in the memory of descendants or in the laconic remarks of contemporary travellers. Neil M. Gunn, who portrayed the Sutherland clearances in his novel *Butcher's Broom* (1934), discovered only late in his life that he had been raised in a district which had once accommodated seventy-eight crofters.[2] They had been removed at some unknown past time to make way for one big farm, and the event had never been recorded.[3] Similarly, clearances in Skye in the 1820s passed virtually undocumented apart from a casual remark in the meandering reminiscences of Joseph Mitchell, the early nineteenth-century Highland roadmaker.[4] Yet this is not an exclusively Highland amnesia: every rural district in the British Isles has been subjected to population turnover, voluntary and coerced, and few families have exact historical memory of these past dislocations. Often the memory is distorted or confused.[5]

Contemporary newspaper coverage was mostly associated with anti-clearance demonstrations. It inevitably highlighted the dramatic part of the story at the expense of the slower and more widespread erosion of the old Highland agrarian structure. Most landlords avoided publicity and conducted their removals by attrition and by stealth.

II. The changed context

After the Napoleonic Wars the old Highland economy collapsed, especially in cattle and kelp production. Competitive conditions were severe also for the new economic enterprise that had been created since about 1780. Adverse forces, mostly beyond the control of the landlords (or anyone else) in the Highlands, made economic growth and social amelioration vastly more difficult. Even the sheep farmers complained loudly and urgently against the high rents that had been contracted during the wartime inflation. Suddenly their appetite for the logic of the free market was sickened and many of them begged for special favours from their landlords. Detailed accounts of individual sheep farms show unambiguously that failing sheep farmers were evicted with no more sentimentality than the smaller tenants they had themselves displaced.[6] Added to the calamitous fall in commodity prices was the greatest factor of all in the post-Waterloo Highlands: population continued to rise rapidly, especially in the west. It was a time of accelerating bankruptcy among landowners. Many lairds in the Hebrides failed to rein in their expenditures when their kelp revenues collapsed and they swiftly sank into debt: Grant of Rothiemurchus cut down his forests in a desperate effort to raise income but continued to slide into financial purgatory.[7] Even the most sympathetic and tender-hearted landlords tightened their squeeze on the small tenantry, now urging them to get off their estates. All this sharpened further the battle for the land.

Emigration became an obsession with many landlords. Where once they had banded together to implore the government to prevent the exodus of their tenantry, after 1815 they instituted every device to promote their departure. Many of the traditional tenantry, especially those with means, had been reading the signs for decades, some of them emigrating ahead of impending clearances. Thus, for instance, large departures from Loch Linnhe for Montreal in the first decade of the new century included families able to pay £10 each for the voyage, some of them anticipating the removals planned by Donald Cameron of Clunes.[8] Adverse economic circumstances had tightened around the neck of the economy and there seemed little hope for the small tenants of the interior glens, the most vulnerable element in the economy. Most of these people would be cleared from the old pastoral lands in the period 1825–60.

The reasons impelling landlords into policies of clearance altered as their circumstances deteriorated. Thus, added to the pursuit of extra gains by the introduction of sheep, was the argument that clearances had become imperative for landlords burdened with a redundant and poverty-bound peasantry. The population, by then swollen in numbers and placed at greater risk of famine by the decline of the economy, had become a millstone around the necks of the proprietors who had an acknowledged moral responsibility to supply relief during food shortages. Before 1820 it had appeared plausible that the people could be relocated on the coasts to establish them in a more secure alternative livelihood; after 1820 this idea lost most of its credibility. The retention of the cleared population was now a much lower preference. Clearance policies came to be linked less with resettlement plans and more with outright ejection and schemes for subsidised emigration. The idea of retaining the population in the region was now improbable; many landlords wanted to reduce estate populations to minimise the danger of massed poverty and recurrent fears of starvation. There was a conspiracy of circumstances, mediated by the landlords, which rang the death-knell of most of the interior peasantry.

The run-down of the old economy was registered by the ministers of the church, themselves often increasingly at odds with their landlords and the established church. They were the authors of the second great *Statistical Account Of Scotland*, which was written mainly at the end of the 1830s, recording, usually *en passant*, the coming of the sheep in many Highland parishes. This was often the only record of the transformation. In Argyll, for instance, it was mentioned that Glenshira had been taken over for sheep walks, and that in Glenorchy and Inishail the 'aboriginal population' had also been replaced by sheep; at Morvern the people had been pressed out to the very edges of the estate and at Kilfinichen the sheep had taken over totally.

At Lismore the population had begun to fall even before the introduction of the sheep, which may be a clue to the operation of other expulsive forces in the north which tend to be obscured by the drama of the Clearances. But mostly the decline of population was attributed directly to the invasion of the sheep: the minister at Gigha and Cara testified to this, as did the minister at Kilmore and

Kilbride. It was reported that the Mull of Kintyre had been converted entirely to vast sheep walks.[9] In many places the process continued over several generations, which witnessed the reallocation of the shielings of the old cattle economy into large sheep farms and then eventually into deer forests. Victor Gaffney's precise study of Strathavon provided a clear example of this undramatic shifting of the basis of the economy.[10]

In the central Highlands the sequential clearance of the small tenantry continued its slow determined progress. Thus Leanachan, south of Spean Bridge, was already opened up for sheep farming when the traditional tacksman became a sheep master and fourteen sub-tenants were removed in 1807. By 1847 Leanachan was 'devoted exclusively to pasture'. Meanwhile the Keppoch family developed its own sheep farming at Inch near the Roy Bridge.[11] In the south the process became more comprehensive: in 1824 there were large-scale evictions in north-east Perthshire at Rannoch, Atholl and Strathardle which were said to have created serious misery among the people. Also in the south, the Breadalbane estates were subjected to large-scale clearances under the fourth marquis who ended runrig and curtailed wintering for cattle. After some hesitation he actively encouraged Cheviot farming and it is claimed that he evicted some 2500 people from districts, including Glenorchy where the population fell from 1806 in 1831 to 831 in 1841, as well as Glen Quaich and the Braes of Taymouth. Even then, some of the evicted were resettled on the estate. The Marquis was a great spender in the district but was accused of being a clearer in the same league as the Sutherland family.[12]

Adding to the negative pressures on the land was the increasing demand for shooting rights and deer forests, the origins of which can be traced to the previous century and which were emerging commercially by the 1820s. Here there is considerable evidence of dislocation in many Highland districts. Glen Dee was cleared for deer as early as 1829; Glen Ey saw the eviction of nine families in about 1830 to make way for the same animals; Glen Clunie was first cleared for sheep and later converted into a deer forest in 1884; Balmoral seems to have been originally converted to sheep in 1833 and then in 1848 switched to deer. Upper Deeside was subjected to gradual clearance across the decades from 1780 to 1815 and the high glens of Braemar showed signs of depopulation too. In Speyside, Rothiemurchus was cleared of sheep in favour of grouse-shooting in 1827 and then of deer in 1843. Glen Avon was cleared in 1838 and the forest of Glenavon in 1841; deer were introduced into Glen Esk in mid-century. Deer forests were advertised for Glen Feshis in 1812, and Gaick was converted from sheep to deer in 1826.[13]

Consequently clearances in the middle period were not confined to the congested western districts of the Highlands. From the eastern and central Highlands there were recurrent reports of depopulation and emigration. Thus in 1825 Alexander Sutherland described an emigrant scene from the port of Cromarty. The people in question had recently been cleared and were embarking for America.

> At this time were only two vessels in harbour. One of these was a brig to carry emigrants to America: the baggage of the wanderers was piled in heaps on the quay. These men were natives of a district of Sutherland, one and all quitting their fatherland to seek an asylum in that of a stranger. Infancy, youth, manhood, and old age; the patriarch of the tribe and his unweaned grandchild were there, prepared for the voyage; but the dejected looks of those who had reached maturity declared, that to suffer in crowds scarcely lessens the poignancy of misfortune. Driven from the huts that had sheltered their fathers for generations, the victims of their prejudice, and that rage for speculative improvement which threatens to de-populate the Highlands, they had resolved on repairing in a body to the untrodden wilds of the new continent, resting their hopes solely on the possession of those simple acquirements enumerated in the Yankee song,
>
> > O, you can reap and mow, love,
> > And I can spin and sew,
> > And we'll settle on the banks
> > of the pleasant Ohio.

These people, according to Sutherland, had 'been ousted from the paternal hearth by oppression'. He believed that they would be subject to severe tribulation in America, and were destined to become 'bondsmen for life'.[14] Emigration was not always entered into in a spirit of liberation and hope.

But the picture is complicated by the ongoing migration out of the many districts which had not been affected yet by clearances. Thus the glens of upper Deeside were de-populated even where there was no displacement. At Upper Glen Gairn, Glen Feardar and Wester Morvern there were no clearances but they 'lost all their people by non-enforced emigration', which effectively emptied the glens.[15]

III. The Hebrides

In the Hebrides clearances in the 1820s and thereafter were usually associated with emigration, frequently on a large scale. From almost all the islands there were outflows of people to Canada, some of whom were in the most pitiful condition on arrival. In 1826 and 1827 well over a thousand people left Tobermory for Cape Breton Island, and there were comparable numbers from Lewis.[16]

In the Western Isles there was a demographic crisis apparently developing inexorably through the first decades of the new century. The population of Harris rose by 13 per cent in the 1830s alone, South Uist by 7 per cent, Stornoway by 13 per cent and Barvas by 27 per cent. Unlike other parts of mainland Britain, their numbers multiplied while their economic capabilities shrank. A Malthusian nightmare seemed to grip the region and commentators prophesied catastrophe.

The island of Lewis became a watchword for poverty and squalor and vulnerability. The proprietor, the Earl of Seaforth, was in financial disrepair before the collapse of prices. In 1801 he sold off Loch Alsh; in the crop crisis of 1817 Seaforth spent £6000 on grain relief.[17] Poverty was endemic across the island but the population rose astonishingly. Seaforth was improvement-minded and attempted development schemes in Lewis in the 1820s, including kelp-processing projects as well as new distilling and commercial fishing enterprises. His success was very limited and failure stared him and the people in the face. There followed evictions and rationalisation: before 1830 there were displacements which involved more than 100 families. Intense continuing poverty co-existed with intermittent evictions. Coastal settlements at Loch Roag were cleared in 1836, when some of the people were shipped off to America. The *New Statistical Account* said that the island was 'a full century behind other parts of Scotland, in agricultural and domestic improvements.'[18]

As J.I. Little puts it, there was a 'full dress rehearsal for famine in 1836–7'. The local minister reported, there was no meal, no money, no employment and no means of procuring subsistence. Virtually everyone in the parishes of Barvas and Lochs was destitute, and in Stornoway almost half of the 5491 people were in distress. Great imports of relief food were required on a charitable basis.[19] By 1838 Seaforth became involved in further assisted emigration to Canada. At that time fifteen families (seventy individuals) were provided with passages while their former holdings were made over to sheep walks.

In 1838 it was reported that 85 per cent of the entire Lewis population of 18 000 was in a desperate state, in part because their rents had been doubled in the previous dozen years. The estate was drowning in debt, barely able to pay interest on its capital. The heiress married into Lowland wealth in 1817 but the resulting injection of £75 000 simply entered 'the maelstrom and vanished', producing no permanent relief, so hopelessly were the estates encumbered. The Seaforth Estates in Lewis, despite every stratagem to extract more income, were headed inexorably for bankruptcy and sale.[20]

By the 1830s the people of Lewis lived in a state of increasing insecurity of tenure, and their individual and collective anxiety can only be guessed at. Nor do we know much about the traditional levels of welfare on the island. While the demographic Sword of Damocles swung above them they were increasingly conscious of the more immediate threat of eviction. A petition from the tenants of Airdintroine in Lewis to the Earl of Seaforth, in 1823, captured an early moment of collective anxiety. The tenantry were consumed with a fear of imminent clearance:

Your complainants were lately warned and that verbally, that your hon. had it in view to remove the complainers [at] the ensuing term of May first and in consequence of this notice your complainers are all of a stand not knowing what to do in such predicament, had your hon. given the complainers notice to . . . Flitting sometime in Harvest last, the Complainers would then have it in their power to make use of the Complainers Cattle as also exert their endeavours to turn everything to the best advantage and by that the complainers would have it in their power to settle with you now for all demands against the complainers . . . and moreover the complainers would have something of their own, to encourage the complainers to take up Lands somewhere else.[21]

These people asked for a stay of the flitting for one year, which would be to everyone's advantage because it would allow them to pay off their arrears. They did not question the landlord's right to employ his lands 'to the best advantage'. Unlike the people of Sutherland, they had been given little warning and no alternative accommodation. They were the authentic refugees of agrarian displacement.

By 1839 the Seaforth family was resigned to the loss of these estates, 'the last great remnant of the very extensive Estates of the Family'. They would have to be sold, partly because of the enormous expense of management, and 'there is little prospect of ourselves ever enjoying again the influence, or adding to the happiness of its population by residing in the Lewis'. The eldest son was indifferent to the retention of the island.[22] This paved the way for the sale of the estate in 1844.

Clearances on Lewis, executed mainly by graziers,[23] continued throughout these decades. A retrospective account described the manner in which the transformation usually occurred:

Many years ago most of the Lewis was held by tacksmen or middlemen who had a number of Crofters as sub-tenants under them. The tacksman paid a fixed rent to the Proprietor, his sub-tenants paying him at a somewhat higher rate than he paid to the Proprietor. In course of time these sub-tenants began to fail in paying the tacksmen, who by degrees gave up their holdings except such portions as they held in their own personal occupancy and it is now [1888] somewhat difficult to ascertain how long the present farms have been purely large farms free from crofting sub-tenants. This state of matters was nearly abolished by the time of Sir James Matheson's purchase of the Island in 1846, there being then only two tacksmen with subtenants.[24]

People dislodged in this way usually drifted to the Lowlands or emigrated.

IV. The Island of Rum

The popular and much respected Gaelic preacher Norman Macleod testified to various episodes of clearance during these years. In his evidence before the Select Committee on Emigration in 1841, he recollected the circumstances associated with the clearance of the island of Rum fifteen years before. The proprietor, MacNeil of Canna, on a rental of £300 per annum, found that he could not maintain the people. Macleod said:

> He could not afford to devote the whole island to the maintenance of the people, and he went to the island, and said 'I will give you all your cattle, I will give you £600 over and above to enable you to remove to America, for I cannot afford the present system'; they very cheerfully accepted. The emigration was conducted under the very best superintendence; we have very frequently heard from them, they are most comfortable, and the proprietor has let the island at £800 a year, which is paid to him as regularly as any bank bill is paid.

Macleod favoured this type of solution, and chose to emphasise the extraordinary humanity of many Highland proprietors who made financial sacrifices on behalf of their people. The common vilification of the Highland landlords in the Age of the Clearances rarely acknowledges the humanity of many of their class nor the restraint with which they often behaved. Whether they should have been invested with such proprietorial power over the people was, of course, a larger question still.

The brutal reality was that the people simply could not make a living nor a return on the capital yield, especially in the west. As John Bowie expressed this precise point:

> with reference to many districts, if the land was given rent-free to the population, the land is still insufficient for the support of the population.[25]

Some landlords, restrained by their own consciences and public opinion, refused to maximise their estate income by means of sheep farming and consequently many parts of the Highlands remained uncleared even in the 1840s.[26] Norman Macleod remembered how the late Duke of Argyll had shed tears over the distress during famine in Tiree in 1836–7. The Duke had said, 'These people wish to remain, they are undoubtedly attached to that island, and I cannot think of removing them; they are my fencible men, and I love them.'[27] Tiree would suffer equally again in the famine of 1846–7.[28]

V. Harris in 1841

It was rare for newspapers in Edinburgh or London to give any attention to the Highlands in the twenty years after Waterloo. In 1839, the island of Harris for once attracted southern notice solely because a large clearance was strongly opposed by the common people. The alarm excited by this episode was enough to cause the dispatch of troops and journalists to the island.

The story concerned the estate of Lord Dunmore. His agent, recounting the events before a parliamentary committee on emigration in 1841, described the great distress which had descended on Harris in the recent famine of 1836–7. Dunmore's estate was crowded, with 440 crofter families holding directly from the landlord, in addition to a further 2300 people who were, presumably, squatters or sub-tenants, the Highland underclass rarely sighted in most Highland history. During the years of the destitution Lord Dunmore had, as usual, supported the people at great expense, and had no expectation of recovering more than one-third of the costs of relief. According to the agent, the people were in a most miserable condition. They had no kelp, the land was useless for crofting, and the tenants were heavily in arrears of rent. Many of them lived in the district of Borve which possessed excellent grazing and was much coveted by Dunmore's one sheep-farming tenant who refused to renew his current lease (£600 per annum) unless the land of Borve was made over to him. This was the classic dilemma facing the west Highland laird; it was a contest for land in unequivocal form.

Sheep farmers in the 1830s could dictate terms to Highland landlords; their bargaining power had been increased by the fall in wool prices. Dunmore could not afford to lose his forceful sheep-farming tenant: he therefore gave the Borve tenantry three years' notice to quit, which expired at Whitsunday 1839. He offered the old and infirm people some allegedly better lands elsewhere on the island. All the other families were offered a free passage to Cape Breton Island or elsewhere in Canada. Dunmore also promised to forgo their rent arrears and to buy their cattle stock at prices determined by independent valuation. It was the west Highland equivalent of a modern 'redundancy package', and the terms were good by most contemporary standards in agrarian Britain.

At the time, according to Duncan Shaw the factor, the people regarded the offer as generous and made no objection. On Shaw's evidence, the subsequent altercations were caused by an 'infection' brought from Skye where some of the small tenantry had recently combined in an elaborate system of resistance to Macleod of Macleod, which included the maiming and killing of sheep, 'inflammatory proclamations' and threatening letters. The Skye 'outrages' had passed unpunished (and barely recorded) and, in emulation, the Harris folk decided not only to refuse Dunmore's offer of assisted emigration, but also to block the removal. In effect, Shaw believed, there had been an embryonic and widening conspiracy at work: it was designed to resist the law across the west Highlands. Dunmore's advisers decided to bring in troops to smother the opposition before it got out of hand. The revolt was quickly scotched, though Dunmore ensured that the guilty parties were dealt with leniently.[29]

The turbulence in Harris was reported in the *Glasgow Saturday Post*, which expressed surprise that a company of soldiers had departed from the city

for the purpose of ejecting some poor tenants from the island of Harris. It would appear that the proprietor of that island has recently let his ground in large divisions to opulent farmers, and the consequence is that the poor islanders are not now in legal possession of the land they and their forefathers have occupied for centuries. On receiving notice to quit in the usual manner, we are informed that they resolved they

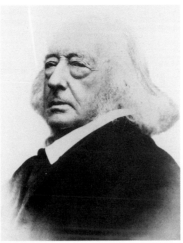

1. John Stuart Blackie(1809–1895), Professor of Greek at Edinburgh, 1852–82, who founded and endowed a chair of Celtic in 1882. Blackie championed Highland causes and wept for the cleared Highlanders. He also publicly attacked the memory of Patrick Sellar, the clearer whose own son occupied the chair of Latin in Edinburgh in the years 1863–90. Erudite and eccentric, with 'a cawing, cackling voice', Blackie possessed 'a rich fund of Scottish prejudices'.

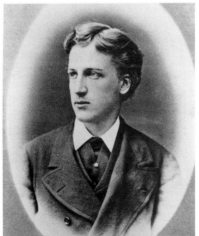

2. The Marquis of Lorne (1845–1910), son of the ducal families of Argyll and Sutherland, Governor-General of Canada, and ninth Duke of Argyll from 1900. His father was the 'fiery little Duke' who asserted that all progress in Scotland derived from the replacement of the 'old Celtic character' by 'those higher customs which came from the Latin and Teutonic races'. Lorne believed that the Highlands were capable of great productive improvement but witnessed little in his own lifetime.

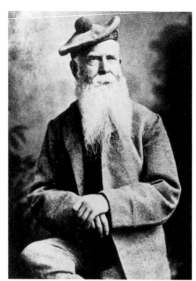

3. Charles Fraser-Mackintosh, Highland antiquarian and Liberal Member of Parliament. He was a passionate advocate for Highland societies and the Gaelic language. Fraser-Mackintosh was a somewhat selective chronicler of the Clearances.

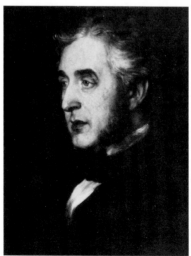

4. Francis, Lord Napier (1819–1898), the highly experienced diplomat who dealt with large-scale famine as Governor of Madras and was sometimes regarded as overly socialistic in his political views. He showed great sympathy with the poor, urban and rural. In 1883 he presided over the Royal Commission into the condition of the crofters and cottars. He drafted the final Report and became the target of the vehement criticism of the Duke of Argyll. (Portrait by G. F. Watts, reproduced by permission of National Galleries of Scotland.)

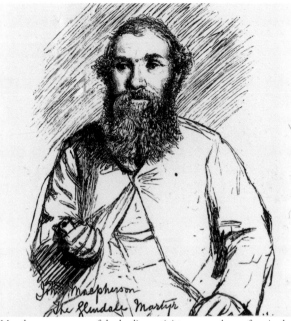

5. John Macpherson was one of the leading activists among the crofters in the 1870s and 1880s. He was imprisoned in Edinburgh after the Glendale Riots in north-west Skye in 1883. He then became a prominent advocate of land reform and an itinerant lecturer to large gatherings across the Highlands at the time of the Crofter Commission.

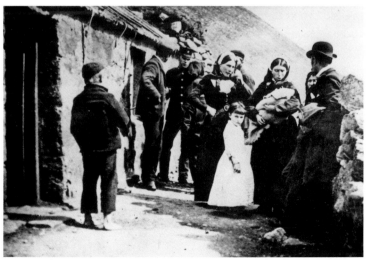

6. A scene from Population and Settlement Clearances 1870–90. (Scottish Life Archive)

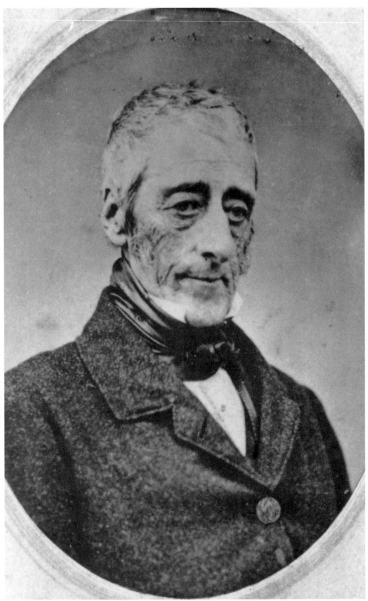

7. Patrick Sellar (1780–1851), the Elgin lawyer/factor who, as estate agent and
sheepfarmer, was the rigorous instrument of mass clearance in Strathnaver in the
1810s. He was tried and acquitted for 'culpable homicide' in Inverness in April 1816.
From a photograph late in Sellar's life, by courtesy of Christopher and Valerie Lang
of Titanga, Victoria, Australia.

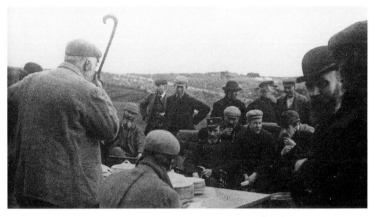

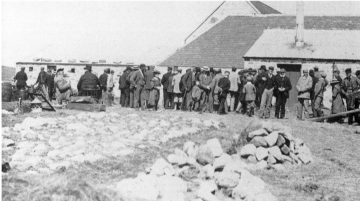

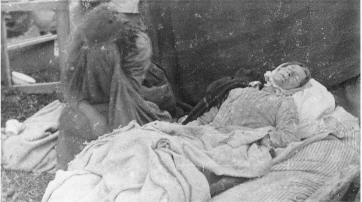

8, 9, 10. Eviction scenes from the late nineteenth century, long after the great age of the Highland Clearances.

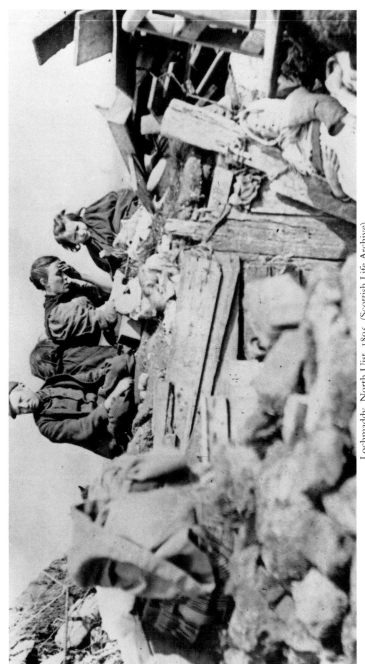

Lochmaddy, North Uist, 1895. (Scottish Life Archive).

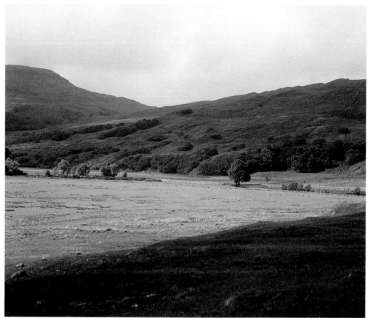

12. Acharn (© Iain Thornber)

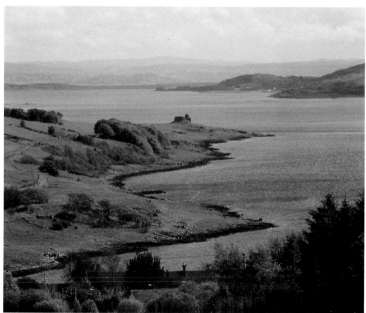

13. Ardtornish Point and Farm (© Iain Thornber)

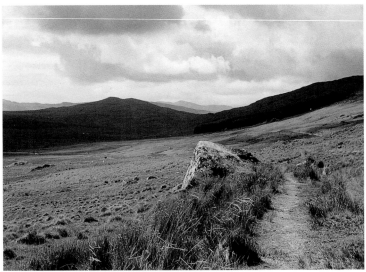

14. Sellar's Stone (© Iain Thornber)

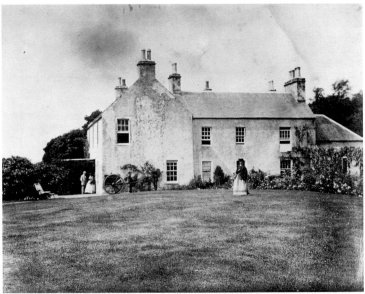

15. Ardtornish House (photographed in 1865) in Morvern acquired by Patrick Sellar in 1844. He and his family returned to Ardtornish for the late summer and autumn each year. After Sellar's death it remained a popular resort for family and friends including Tennyson, Palgrave and Herbert Spencer. Ardtornish symbolised their version of Victorian success, culture and respectability in a remote setting. (Reproduced by permission of Faith Raven.)

would not do so with their lives. Seeing that peaceable means were of no avail, the military have been resorted to, and they, with the aid of the preventative service, will, no doubt, accomplish the severing of the poor people from the land of their nativity.[30]

The military action, as always, was immediately effective. The people's resistance was quickly quelled and five 'leaders' were captured and sent to Portree. The people were reported to have given 'unconditional compliance'. The *Inverness Courier* commented, 'We trust the proprietor will render their emigration from the island as favourable as circumstances will permit.'[31] According to the factor of the estate, the people remained at Borve for a further twelve months and then were removed; they resettled in other parts of Harris or elsewhere, but refused to accept the emigration assistance. It was some time later that they began to petition Dunmore to renew his offer of a passage to Canada, and eventually more than 600 of them at last crossed the Atlantic. Another group departed the Dunmore estate for Australia in 1854.[32] It was a further case of clearance dislodging the people and, after a time, precipitating their emigration. Emigration was often a staggered response to the initial displacement.

VI. The tenacity of the small tenantry

Landlords became more urgent about reducing their small tenantry, but the people seemed to become less pliable as their plight deteriorated. In the Western Isles they seemed to cling onto the land even as their total numbers accumulated in the middle decades of the century. As conditions worsened so the tenacity of the lowest strata seemed to strengthen, sometimes using income from seasonal employment outside the region to sustain the family back home in the townships and the crofts.[33] Thus the Highland problem became the more resistant. Mid-century saw a convergence of two factors which, together, came to darken the reputation of Highland landlords as a class. One was their increasing desperation for financial salvation in a context of worsening prospects. The other was the countervailing power of the press and public opinion, which sought increasingly to restrict the excesses of the landlords.

The clearances were, of course, the final expression of the immense discretionary power which resided in the hands of the Highland landlords. Their licence to evict their tenantry gave them almost unlimited authority in the community. It could be employed not merely to re-arrange the use of the land, but also as a weapon to control and discipline the people as circumstances arose. It was a permanent threat hanging over the people, invoked at the will of the proprietor whenever he or she chose to make an example or to remove any undesirable element. Moreover landlords often acted together informally, as a class. Thus a person evicted from one estate, and given a black name, might be refused accommodation of any kind on a neighbouring estate. Even the church might be under landlord pressure to deny asylum to an evicted tenant, especially where the position of minister was in the gift of the proprietor. It was said that the people of Glencalvie (see Chapter 2) were refused settlement on several adjacent estates, and that they depended entirely on the good offices of the Free Church ministers.

By the 1840s the augmentation of population was generally feared by almost all Highland estates. It is true that refugees from earlier clearances on the Sutherland estates sometimes found a welcome in Caithness, but in the later period few landlords were prepared to build up dense estate populations, regardless of the plight of such displaced people. It was more likely that they would persuade their own tenantry to leave altogether; if they had the resources they might subsidise their emigration, though they had to be careful not to appear to be using coercion. The approach of a compulsory Poor Law added greatly to landlord apprehensions.

VII. Sinclair of Freswick

Far from the Hebrides, in the north-east corner county of Caithness, another landlord, Sinclair of Freswick, demonstrated the methods of arbitrary and hard-minded proprietorship. In 1835 Sinclair undertook a relatively conventional clearance at Dunbeath in order to rearrange his lands and increase rents. The clearance was barely even mentioned in the standard sources in Caithness but it left a legacy of soured relations between landlord and people.

Caithness is not normally regarded as part of the Highlands at all. It is largely low lying and arable. It was a place of refuge for evictees from the clearers to the south. Nevertheless Caithness itself witnessed substantial clearances in many places in the nineteenth century. These were generally undramatic and, for the people displaced, there was usually alternative employment nearby in the fishing villages or in the comparatively labour-intensive agriculture of the county.[34] William Sinclair of Freswick, who had trained as a doctor in Edinburgh, purchased the Lochend estate in 1778 and inherited Freswick in 1794. In 1835 he tried to clear some of his Dunbeath tenantry from pasture at Badfern to make way for sheep. The removal affected 107 families who were dependent on the pasture designated for clearance; they claimed that they had occupied the land for centuries and paid their rents from the sale of cattle which they grazed on this pasture. Consequently several hundred people were at risk in this turmoil.

Sinclair's action was unpopular among the people and there was rudimentary resistance, including the destruction, by arson, of some peat stacks at Achnachy. The opposition to Freswick's Dunbeath clearance exhibited signs of co-ordination: there was rumour of threatened violence, of armed resistance, and of the creation of 'a committee of insurgents'. The tenantry were alleged to have written threatening letters, and to have been involved in 'riotous and threatening behaviour'. It was claimed that Angus Henderson had been commissioned to manufacture 'lead balls' and to borrow a gun from a man in neighbouring Latheron. The people of Dunbeath had been told to meet at the Brae to prevent the introduction of sheep. It was also alleged that Robert Sutherland, a tenant and military pensioner of Balnabroich, had offered

> an Anker of Whisky to the people to go to Achnachy and bring down Douglas [the incoming sheep farmer, whose peatstack had been sabotaged] and send him across the Ord . . . but the people had not the courage to accept the offer.

There were additional allegations of housebreaking and robbery during the disturbances.

The targets of the threatened violence in 1835 were the landlord, his property and his agents. At the same time some of the tenantry began a manoeuvre to negotiate a settlement with the landlord. They formed themselves into a committee and drafted petitions to Sinclair of Freswick, in which voices of some of the common people were heard. The first petition spoke of the 'unfortunate' arson and violence that had been perpetrated, and the petitioners undertook to

> voluntarily bind and oblige ourselves, individually, not only to preserve the Public Peace on this Estate to the utmost of our power, but also to prevent any disturbance or violence from any other tenants to the Proprietors person, his family, Gear, and Effects, and also to his servants . . . and while we thus unite ourselves for the Preservation of the public peace, we rely on the Proprietor's goodness to deal with his Tenants with his former tenderness and mercy.

It was, of course, an effort to pressurise the landlord by a guarantee of protection. The petition was headed 'Guarantee'.[35] It was close to collective bargaining by blackmail.

The April petition had been preceded by a much more specific and less literate petition, dated 3 March 1835. It was from 'the humble tenantry of Dunbeath', and it too was couched in terms of a bargain: they offered an end to violence in return for security of tenure, they requested:

> That your honour shall not remove any more of your tenants on purpose of the placing of any more sheep but that you will grant them their lands at a rent that may be put on the lands by three men, one from the County of Ross, one from the County of Sutherland and one from Caithness, to judge the quality of the lands and likewise the quantity, and that the rents may be laid on the land according to the times, that the tenantry may have a small living after paying their rents according as their fore father had, not that we wish any thing else but to be humble subjects and wish to wocke within the [compass?] of the law of King and Contry and wishes nothing else but that your honour shall say if you are to grant the above petition or not.
>
> We your humble petitioners expects that your honour will take things to a consideration and loke with an eye of peaty on your humble Tenents and grant to fore said petition for if your honour were to know

the poverty of the place it would melt a heart of stone for their was deforant individuals lost their livis by the want of cloths all in point of poverty that they had not cloths to keep them warm when they went to sea and by that means they cane home lifles corps.[36]

Another petition from the Dunbeath community, altogether less threatening in content, but no less anxious in tone, stated that if the land were denied them, the people would not be able to

> keep or water a Beast in any other part of the hill – and what is intended to be left is of no use summer or winter. *Therefore* as your Petitioners had always experienced such *tenderness* and enjoyed such *tranquillity* besides [i.e. compared with?] some of the neighbouring Estates, They the old *Residenters* of the Place would never wish during their lives to seek shelter from any other neither do they know what to do or where to go if your Honour shall be pleased to withdraw your Protection from them. May it therefore be pleased to take their case of so many poor creatures which are born to no inheritance but in slavery and the most part of which can neither work nor [?] and has no means for support them.

The people acknowledged that the landlord was able to 'turn the ground to the best advantage or to any purpose you deem proper'. The Dunbeath petitioners said they were prepared to pay any rent he asked. They dissociated themselves from their fellow tenants who had resisted by 'detestable actions', and described themselves as 'honest and innocent people', who threw themselves on their landlord's mercy.[37] The fate of these petitioners is not known, but the entire episode was subjected to a precognition in August 1835, which suggests that the landlord offered no compromise.

The attitude of fellow proprietors in the district was expressed in a letter written to another Caithness landowner in March 1835 by William Sinclair of Barroch, who had already advised Freswick to reduce the changes he intended to lay upon his tenants.

> I very much suspect it will not be an easy matter for Freswick to carry his views on Sheep Farming into effect. I know that some persons in his employment and confidence are opposed to his extending his sheep . . . It is further to be regretted that such gentlemen as Lord Duffus and Sandside and many others deprecate Freswick's proceedings and this

gives the people confidence in resisting. I mention this in confidence to you. I know it to be the fact. Freswick is exceedingly unpopular and I am confident he will have trouble in this affair.[38]

This was another indication of the disquiet which attended clearances even among fellow proprietors.

There was a sequel to the Freswick Clearances. In 1836–7 hunger descended on the district and the people endured their plight with great stoicism and peaceability, for which they were publicly commended.[39] William Sinclair of Freswick died in 1838. His successor, W.J.J.A. Sinclair, was a man of equal resolution. Near-famine conditions returned in the last months of 1846 and food riots erupted along the east and north coasts of Caithness in the following February and March. The rioters made desperate efforts to prevent grain exports and some of Sinclair's small tenants were involved in the dramatic turbulence. Sinclair was inflamed by the insubordination and the indiscipline of his tenantry. He sought retribution by way of new evictions. The local minister, the Revd Peter Jolly, interceded on behalf of the people and entreated Sinclair to be merciful.

Sinclair remained firm in his resolution to punish the people by clearing them, and Jolly again begged for a reconsideration of the question. He put the people's case in the strongest terms. A clearance, he pointed out, would be a very unpopular act; it would create 'very unpleasant consequences . . . The very idea of turning out forty-one individuals in such a year as this is very far from being agreeable in contemplation and will appear almost inhuman in realisation'. More subtly, Jolly alluded indirectly to the odium that had been poured on the public name of the owner of Glencalvie only eighteen months before:

> I suppose the poor creatures must just adopt the way of some of our neighbours a little farther South and set up Tents in the Churchyard. If Freswick would only leave them this year and acquaint them with his firm purpose of removing them at Martinmas, he would avoid much of the odium that must attach to the matter.

In virtually the same breath, Jolly emphasised that Freswick had a perfect right to do what he wished with his land.

Jolly pointed out that, because of their crime, the people would be unable to obtain alternative accommodation. If the clearance were delayed a year it would give them the opportunity to find somewhere to settle, and the whole case would be more humane. If they migrated to a town they would be reduced to poverty and starvation. He remarked, 'Indeed I pity the poor creatures, and I fear their young families will be the principal sufferers.' He gave pathetic detail of the circumstances of the families, the awful dependency of many of the relatives, and the severe invalidity of some; they would in effect become an impossible social problem. A removal, he warned, would produce a 'scene of wretchedness and misery'.[40]

The Sinclair of Freswick clearances exposed the sheer power vested in landlords in an abjectly poor community. The events showed also the informal powers of retribution possessed by landlords, and the use of evictions as punishment and social control. It was a society which concentrated authority in the hands of men whose personal temperament determined the welfare and security of the common people. Sinclair of Freswick was not necessarily typical of Highland landlords: his estate was only marginally Highland in character and the people were already technically crofters. The timing of the eviction was unusually inauspicious – it was midwinter and mid-famine. The fact that neighbouring landlords, in both 1835 and 1847, showed sympathy with the people suggests that the Freswick case lies at the more severe end of the spectrum of clearances in the nineteenth century.

VIII. Potato famine

The potato famine in the west Highlands and Islands brutally exposed the vulnerability of the population, cleared or not. Congestion, rapid population growth and a high dependence on the potato had created a cruel susceptibility to the onslaught of the potato blight. The human suffering in the west was severe and prolonged. The harvest was very poor from 1846 until the early years of the 1850s. But the rigour of the famine in the west was less extreme, and associated with far less mortality, than the concurrent privations of the Irish. Nevertheless in 1846 it was claimed that three quarters of the population of the Highlands and Islands were entirely without food. Even as late as 1851 in Lewis half the crop was destroyed by the same blight. Desperate hunger and poverty were general and the gravity of the crisis was clearly reflected in the renewed and rapid increase of emigration. A cardinal aspect of the crisis was the orchestration of relief measures in the region.[41]

As the scale and intensity of the crisis emerged philanthropic bodies galvanised themselves to provide immediate succour as well as assistance for the subsidisation of emigration. Special relief committees operated in Edinburgh and Glasgow. Within the region the response of the Highland lairds to the famine varied. There is good evidence that some rich proprietors, for example the Duke of Sutherland, were able to support their dependants (usually on credit or with a work test) throughout the crisis. Others, for example, Clanranald and Macleod in Skye, bankrupted themselves in relief measures for their people. Most landlords were glad to accept outside support for their people, and this undoubtedly mitigated the worst consequences of the food emergency.

On the other side of the balance sheet, there were widespread allegations that some landlords took advantage of outside support to avoid their own responsibilities and to rid themselves of their small tenantry by coerced emigration. Nevertheless it is generally accepted that the relief measures, in their different forms, were remarkably successful for, despite the severity of the famine, there was no perceptible leap in mortality rates in the region.[42]

The financial impact of the famine on landlords was overwhelming. Income from rent fell while expenditure on estate management rose. Some landlords sold up altogether; others decided that they must adopt firmer measures with regard to the disposition of their lands. Famine, according to one view of the world, provided the ultimate and irresistible justification for clearances: the land simply could not support the people at a tolerable level of security and welfare. In some parts of the Highlands the tragedy of the potato famine was, therefore, entangled with the renewed anguish of clearance. Strathaird was the best example of this melancholy convergence.

IX. The Strathaird evictions

Strathaird was a large estate in the south-west of Skye, thickly populated and desperately poor. It had been bought by Alexander Macalister, who decided to clear the land in 1850 for the purpose of sheep farming. The people, who were suffering badly from the continuing destruction of their blighted potato crops, numbered 620. Most were crofters and cottars, located mainly at Elgol and Keppoch. It was a comparatively large-scale, and therefore a potentially hazardous, clearance. The people were known to be in a state of turmoil and resistance to the announced intentions of the landlord. The scene was set for collision.

Knowing the disaffection amongst the Strathaird people, Sheriff Fraser of Portree decided to address them about the situation facing them and their landlord as well as the law which he himself represented. He wrote a long public statement. It was a careful and compassionate effort to make the best of a tragic choice. Addressing 'My Friends', Fraser told the people that the landlord of Strathaird was 'firmly resolved to have the removings obtained against you carried into effect by ejectment'.

The people had been given proper legal notice by Macalister. Fraser knew that they had made no attempt to prepare for their clearance; they remained as a stark obstruction to the process for which Fraser had little stomach. He feared that they might be foolish enough to think of resisting the legal process. His duty in law was to maintain the peace of the community. He told the people that he was aware of 'the bitterness of feeling that compulsory removings are fitted to excite'. But 'as a private individual, anxious for your welfare', he begged them to desist from such thoughts. He pointed out that, between them, they paid a total rent of only £150 and yet they were currently already £450 in arrears. This was the typical position for small Highland tenants in the famine years. Exposing his own sympathies, Fraser then remarked that

It will not be considered strange that a proprietor should think of removal of a population in such miserable circumstances expedient for their interest and his own. But it is not for me to say whether this opinion is right or wrong.

It was the common paradox that the more desperate the condition of the people the more rational became their expulsion.

Sheriff Fraser emphasised that Macalister had full legal sanction to take this action and that the magistrates were bound to give it effect:

> He has a perfect right to turn you out of your dwellings and possessions, and to call upon me and other authorities of the country to aid him with the force of the country in so doing.

Fraser, thus caught invidiously between landlord and people, then outlined in blunt terms the meaning of his obligations at law, should the people resist the eviction:

> I should have to proceed to your lands with such officers and constables as I deemed necessary to turn yourselves, your families and property out of your lands, and to protect the persons employed by your landlord while they unroofed and destroyed your dwellings.

These, of course, were the ruthless realities of clearance in the Highlands. Any obstruction by the people would lead inevitably to imprisonment. If the constabulary were inadequate to the task, the militia would be called in. This was the inexorable sequence. Fraser clearly recoiled from the entire business, but he was required to impress upon the people that resistance would be folly in the extreme.

Sheriff Fraser reiterated the terms which the proprietor, Macalister, had offered with regard to removal and emigration. The people, though they were to be ejected, would be treated with 'great leniency and liberality'. Macalister's factors would not confiscate their effects in lieu of arrears (to which he was entitled). And although the law required him to make no provision for their future welfare after the eviction, Macalister was

> willing, if you consent to emigrate to Canada, not only to forgive you all your arrears of rent, and allow you to dispose of your crop, stocking and effects for your own advantage, but also to advance to you a sum of £1200 to be divided among you according to your necessities, for the purpose of helping to pay your passage and providing your outfit.

The landlord was prepared to pay about ten times the current annual rent to rid himself of his small tenants. This was a precise measure of the economic issues involved in the clearances. Fraser described this offer as 'liberal', but emphasised that the landlord 'has no right to compel you to emigrate to Canada, or force you to leave your native land at all. Whether or not you will do so is a matter for yourselves to determine.' There was a fine line between coercion and persuasion; the people in these circumstances had Hobson's choice.

Fraser himself was opposed to 'compulsory emigration'. It was the subject of great controversy across the Highlands at the time. But Fraser could not ignore the poverty and wretchedness of the people, nor the fact that the relief schemes in the south had virtually exhausted their subscribed funds. Nor could he discount the likelihood that the people would fall into starvation if their present circumstances in Skye continued. Fraser pointed out that, even if the people possessed the land rent free, it could not support them: emigration had become virtually inevitable. He recom-mended that the Strathaird people accept their landlord's offer.[43]

The plight of the Strathaird people was confirmed by reports in the northern newspapers. The *Inverness Courier* pointed out that the people paid virtually no rent and that the public burdens on the estate, which was strictly entailed, were £275 per annum. The Destitution Fund associated with famine relief in the west Highlands had ceased to provide assistance to the people. The potato crop had failed for four seasons in succession. Macalister had offered to forgo all arrears and to expend a large sum to assist their emigration. Yet the newspaper reported:

> The people were unwilling to remove – a cry of expatriation and cruelty was raised – and the proprietor having tacitly abandoned his intended process of ejectment, the people remain in their miserable huts and holdings on the brink of starvation, while the proprietor continues without rent, and his land is unimproved.[44]

It was the familiar litany of the intractable and tragic problems of the west Highlands and Islands in mid-century.

The condition of the Strathaird people was soon corroborated by their own words. In October 1850 seventy of the 'cottars and others' drew up a document described as 'a lamentable and humiliating Memorial', which was originally sent to the *Daily Mail* in Glasgow, and subsequently reprinted in the northern newspapers. The signatories claimed to represent 620 people of Strathaird. They wrote:

> We have to inform you that our potatoes have almost entirely failed; the relief given to us by the Highland Relief Fund is discontinued; and many of us and our children will suffer severely during the next winter and spring unless some food is offered to us. We have been prevented from going to any employment at a distance during the summer season, as the proprietor and his factor, and the Sheriff, always threatened to put ourselves and our families away by military force. The heads of families could not leave their wives and children unprotected, and they waited hitherto with them so that they might be together wherever kind Providence would be pleased to cast their lot. We are very ill off for clothing, and we suffer death in consequence for the loss of the potato. We have no prospect how to sustain life during the next six or seven months, and we know not what to do. We are on the brink of starvation.[45]

In their own words they thus confirmed in detail the views of the landlord and the Sheriff. It was the corollary that they could not accept.

The offer made by Macalister to the people of Strathaird can be seen in different lights. By contemporary British standards, a Highland proprietor such as Macalister was placed in an unenviable position. Most other landlords (in England, for instance), or capitalists in industry or trade, were normally able to deploy their property as they wished. The idea that a man should, at considerable expense, subsidise arrangements to secure the future of an unwanted and dependent tenantry or workforce, would have been an unacceptable obligation to any industrial employer or, indeed, any proprietor.

On the other hand, the people were victims of famine and in desperate straits. They chose emigration under extreme duress. The landlord offered them compensation if they acceded to their own clearance: if they agreed not to resist they would be treated liberally. It was a squalid set of choices for everyone concerned. In the long run, however, there was a case for saying that all the parties would be better placed by mass emigration. Certainly the landlord would derive a higher rent, and no longer be faced with requests for famine relief; for the people, Canada usually offered a material life fuller and more secure than that in Strathaird.

The initial response of the Strathaird people to Macalister's offer was negative and they made no move to comply with their notices to quit. It was reported that they had resolved not to shift unless 'compelled by superior force'. Fearing resistance, the landlord postponed the clearance, but maintained his pressure upon the people to emigrate to Canada.

Meanwhile, a report in the *Scotsman* reaffirmed their extreme privation. The support of the Destitution Fund, upon which they had depended for the previous four years, had come to an end. Macalister's action to remove them was, in part, occasioned by the new situation: as the *Scotsman* pointed out, 'If so large a body of people were thrown on the poor rate (the burden of which would fall on the proprietor), it is obvious that the value of the estate would be wholly destroyed.'[46]

In the last months of 1850 the *Northern Ensign*, a newspaper highly critical of clearing landlords, and edited by the volatile and voluble Thomas Mulock, reported that:

> The quiet and peaceable people of Strathaird had been visited by self-seeking emigration agents, and have been flattered and cajoled to emigrate.

Though the subsequent events attracted little publicity, the people of Strathaird appear to have emigrated in 1851–2, and were replaced by sheep.[47] In this way the Strathaird clearance, which for many months threatened to burst into violence, passed in relative quiet, and the people were finally expatriated.

The Strathaird clearance exposed the most fundamental problems of the local economy. The prolonged impact of the famine, the undeniable symptoms of overpopulation, the excruciating poverty of the people, the burden on the poor rates, the limits of charity, and the awkward economics of Highland landownership, all conspired towards eviction. By contemporary standards the response of the people was not violent, nor was the behaviour of the landlord unusually lacking in humanity. It was, in all, a good example of the economic predicament in which the west Highlands had become entrapped. It challenged everyone, then and since, to conjure alternative solutions.

In general, landlords appear to have adopted a rosy view of the effects of sheep farming in the Highlands. The manner in which most proprietors assimilated the moral implications of the change was probably typified in the words of Sir George Mackenzie of Wester Ross in 1844. The common people, he thought, initially suffered considerable hardship by the introduction of sheep farming. Eventually they came to realise that they could live better as wage labourers in the service of sheep or as corn farmers than as independent landholders. Meanwhile, as a consequence of sheep farming, the entire region had become vastly more productive. In the old order, said Mackenzie:

> the vast extent of moorground did not yield a thousandth part of the human food that it does now for cattle and sheep. I should say that for one animal that was produced under the old system, perhaps fifty or a hundred are now produced.[48]

Sheep were effectively a new product of the soil.

Mackenzie's was a Panglossian view of the world, undisturbed by the imminence of famine or by the continuing rural squalor of the Highlands. It ignored the social tragedy of the clearances, the literal dislocation of lives. It took no account of the detestation with which the common people viewed the substitution of the status of day labourer for that of landholder. Mackenzie's argument, ultimately, balanced local costs against the gains to the nation, a painful calculus for all victims of change.

Notes

1 Devine, *Clanship*, op. cit., p. 37.
2 See Sherrie A. Inness, ' "They must worship industry or starve": Scottish resistance to British imperialism in Gunn's *The Silver Darlings*', *Studies in Scottish Literature*, 28 (1993), pp. 133-49.
3 Neil N. Gunn, 'The tragedy of the Highland Clearances', *Radio Times*,

10 (December 1954), p. 5.

4 Mitchell, *Reminiscences*, vol. II, p. 110.

5 See for example Paul Basu, 'Narratives in a landscape. Monuments of the Sutherland Clearances', M.Sc. thesis, Social Anthropology, University College, London, 1997, passim.

6 Iain S. Macdonald, 'Alexander Macdonald Esq. of Glencoe: Insights into early Highland sheep-farming', *Review of Scottish Culture* 10 (1996), p. 62.

7 See Mitchell, I, p. 170.

8 See Somerled MacMillan, *The Emigration of Lochaber MacMillans to Canada in 1812* (Paisley, 1958).

9 *New Statistical Account*, vol. VII (Argyll), pp. 26, 186, 245–6, 309, 407, 435, 528, 918.

10 Gaffney, 'Summer shealings', op. cit.

11 Iain S. Macdonald, op, cit., p. 59.

12 See C.J.A. Robertson, 'Railway mania in the Highlands: The marquis of Breadalbane and the Scottish Grand Junction Railway', in Roger Mason and Norman Macdougall (eds.) *People and Power in Scotland*, (Edinburgh 1992) pp. 189–91.

13 This section draws freely on Adam Watson and Elizabeth Allan 'Depopulation by clearances and non-enforced emigration in the North East Highlands', *Northern Scotland*, vol. 10 (1990) pp. 31–46.

14 Sutherland, *Summer Ramble*, pp. 81–2.

15 See Watson and Allan, op. cit., pp. 31–43.

16 See J. S. Martell, *Immigration to and Emigration from Nova Scotia 1815–1838* (Halifax, Nova Scotia, 1942), pp. 61 et seq.

17 Mitchell op. cit. I, p. 210.

18 Ibid., p. 16.

19 Conditions on Lewis are well summarised in J.I. Little, *Crofters and Habitants* (Montreal, 1991) pp. 11–27.

20 Mitchell, op. cit., I, pp. 232–4.

21 SRO, Seaforth Papers, GD46/L/294/Petition of Airdintroine Tenants to J.A. Stuart Mackenzie Esq. of Seaforth, 12 February 1823.

22 Quoted ibid., p. 18.

23 See Caird, *Park*, pp. 2–3.

24 SRO, Stewart and Stewart Papers, AD/56/5/ Memorandum of information with regard to farms in the Lewis threatened to be taken possession of by Crofters or sought to be handed over to them (1888).

25 Ibid., p. 9.

26 Ibid., pp. 148–9.

27 PP, 1841, VI, p. 71.

28 See Richards, *Leviathan*, p. 262.

29 Ibid., pp. 198–200.

30 Quoted in *Scotsman*, 24 July 1839.

31 Quoted in *Scotsman*, 31 July, 7 August 1839.

32 The emigration to Australia in the 1850s is discussed in Eric Richards, 'The Highland Scots in South Australia', *Journal of the Historical Society of South Australia*, no.4 (1978), pp. 33–64.

33 See T.M. Devine, 'Temporary migration and the Scottish Highlands in the nineteenth century' *EcHR* 32, (1979), pp. 344–59.

34 See Donald Ormond, *The Caithness Book* (Inverness, 1972), p. 143. See also 'A Philanthropist', in *Northern Ensign*, 28 September 1854.

35 SRO, Sinclair of Freswick Papers, GD136/956/6 Papers concerning agitation of tenantry of Dunbeath against the clearance for sheep of the hill pasture of Badfern, [and] disturbances including the burning of the peat stack at Achnachy.

36 Ibid.

37 SRO, GD136/956/6/ Copy of a paper from John Sutherland (undated).

38 SRO, GD136/587 Letters to James Traill of Ratter, James Sinclair of Barroch to Traill, 11 March 1835.

39 *New Statistical Account*, vol. XV (Latheron Parish).

40 SRO, GD136/997/Jolly to Henderson, 7, 12 March 1847. See also Richards, *Scottish Food Riots*, passim.

41 See Devine, *Clanship*, op. cit., p. 153 and Chapter 4, and *The Great Highland Famine*, passim.

42 Flinn, *Scottish Population*, pp. 35–6; see also Devine, op. cit. Chapter 11.

43 *Inverness Courier*, 25 July 1850.

44 *Inverness Courier*, quoted in *Northern Ensign*, 31 October 1850.

45 Quoted in *Northern Ensign*, 31 October 1850.

46 *Scotsman*, 6 June 1850.

47 *Northern Ensign*, 21 November 1850; Cooper, *Skye*, p. 134.

48 Quoted by C.S. Loch, 'Poor relief in Scotland: its statistics and development 1791 to 1891', *Journal of The Royal Statistical Society*, vol. LXI (1892), p. 291.

13

Colonel Gordon,
Barra and the Uists

I. Headlines

AGGRAVATED CLEARANCES CAPTURE THE historical headlines. The Glencalvie evictions in 1845 (see Chapter 2) set new standards of landlord ruthlessness which were matched by several large-scale and heavily publicised events in the middle of the century. Some of the most tragic and dramatic clearances were perpetrated by landlords of the old order, those who inherited their estates finding them smothered in debt and on the brink of extinction. The heir could sell out and retire to the suburbs of Edinburgh or London (as did Lord Reay) or even emigrate to Australia (like the hapless Glengarry in 1840).[1] The possible alternative was to try a once-and-for-all modernisation of the estate to bring it to solvency and profit. This almost invariably meant the dismissal of many of the old population and their replacement by modern graziers who could run their animals at a profit and pay a decent rent. It was a wrenching dilemma either way. If a landlord took the latter course then he could increasingly expect the scathingly critical attention of the southern press which welcomed colourful stories from the exotic Highlands. They were much more newsworthy than, for instance, the plight of the urban people summarily cleared from the path of the new railways as they ploughed their tracks into every city of the south.

The strong-arm methods of some of the old class were equalled by the behaviour of the new men who bought up estates in the Highlands, anticipating the free use of their lands without restraint. The incoming owners tended to be homogenised in local perception as 'Englishmen' or, in Henry Cockburn's dismissive phrase, 'base but wealthy Saxons'.[2] Many of the parvenu landlords were inadequately briefed on the expectations of Highland landownership or indeed of any kind of landownership. Some of them regarded their new estates as prime investments; others thought of them as self indulgence, a place to display and celebrate commercial success. Either way they often did not realise the can of worms into which they had bought.[3]

Cockburn was especially aware of the changing pattern of ownership in the Highlands. In September 1841 he mused: 'We shall see what the English purses and the English comfort of the southern supplanters of our banished, beggarly, but proud lairds, will do.'[4]

II. *The reputation of Gordon of Cluny*

Colonel John Gordon of Cluny was an incoming millionaire landowner. He bought several large islands in the Outer Hebrides and then cleared them with minimum regard for their inhabitants. In the demonology of the Highland clearances Gordon of Cluny ranks high, along with the names of Patrick Sellar, James Gillanders and the Countess of Sutherland. He was responsible for some of the most widely publicised acts of inhumanity that disfigured the life of the Highlands in the years around the great famine of the 1840s. His clearances were as thoroughgoing and single-minded as had ever been seen in the north.

Cluny's unsavoury reputation related most notably to his treatment of the tenaciously Catholic island of Barra. Charles Fraser Mackintosh, the Highland antiquarian and member of parliament, subsequently described Cluny as

> the unlamented Aberdonian who . . . wished to turn the isle [of Barra] into a convict settlement, and was ready to dispose of it as such to Government, no doubt first by clearing off the whole population as was done in Clan Ranald's other islands of Rum and Canna.[5]

Cluny's Barra evictions in the late 1840s were the most sensational model of a Highland clearance. They combined violence, forced emigration, landlord trickery, starving peasants, conniving factors, premature deaths and the fawning collusion of the minister of the established church. This was the basis of Cluny's extraordinary infamy. Later in the century the radical propagandist, Alexander Mackenzie, described Cluny's clearances in Barra in these terms:

> He was confronted with the perplexing problem of dealing with the surplus population of Barra. For the deceitful promises by which the people were induced to assemble at Loch Boisdale; for the scenes which occurred when the disillusioned peasants fled to the mountains and were dragged on board the transports [to Canada] by main force; for such acts as these, Colonel Gordon must share the responsibility with his agents, the chief of whom was a minister, who seems to have been a disgrace to his cloth.[6]

A standard modern reference guide sums up the tradition in a few words: 'The population of Barra suffered grievously at the time of the late Highland Clearances, but the indomitable spirit they showed has won them their reward. They are still there. They have not forgotten their sufferings, but are quite embittered.'[7]

III. A Hebridean investment

Adversity on the island of Barra was not new. Its population grew alarmingly, partly under the stimulus of kelp production in the French Wars. But then kelp prices collapsed and, in 1816, the local minister bemoaned the rising 'spirit of emigration' from the island. The current owner Colonel MacNeill had mixed feelings about emigration:

> It is no doubt distressing to my feelings, that People to whom I am so much attached, should leave me; but if it is for their good, I should regret it less.

Cheap fares to Canada and the blandishments of emigration agents were effective spurs to voluntary evacuation. MacNeill remarked that 'such a traffic is not congenial to my feelings' and in May 1817 he again voiced his ambivalence:

> I am sure you are heartily tired of Emigrants concerns: the loss of so
> many very decent people, is much to be regretted; at the same time,
> those that remain, will in time, be much better; this reflection always
> offers us something consolatory when one reflects he has seen for the
> last time, those he has been accustomed to from early infancy.

MacNeill was the last Barra proprietor to utter any regret regarding
emigration from the island. Even under his regime the old townships were being enclosed into crofts and most likely this stimulated
further emigration.

Economic conditions on the island were primitive. In 1827 the
crops failed generally and, according to the minister, some 350 of
the population resorted to the beaches in search of cockles without
which 'there would have been hundreds dead this day on Barra'. It
was reportedly a 'scene of horror', exacerbated by the influx of even
more miserable people from North Uist and Tiree. Yet there was
also reported a sense of stoical acquiescence in hardship, of a people
inured to privation. They made good soups from the cockles and
'under all these destitutions, it is surprising how contented they are
with their lot'.[8] Spectacles of worsening poverty were exposed recurrently in near-famine conditions which descended on the island on
several occasions in the 1830s.

The estate was tied up in entails and marriage settlements,
labouring under the weight of mountainous debts. The new
MacNeill, in 1823, complained in bitterness that he was 'literally tied
to the stake' by his inherited debts. His frustration kept him in 'a
permanent state of rage'. He tried to repair his finances by putting
pressure on his tenantry. He wanted them to become much more
efficient. He even used the threat of emigration '*in terrrorem*'. He said,
'I must have fishers and kelpers who will cheerfully do my bidding . .
. if one set of servants (tenants at will are nothing else) wont do it, the
master must try others.' MacNeill failed in his efforts and soon he was
bankrupt and trustees were appointed. The church ministers were
unable to collect their own fees from such a poor place. An attempt to
introduce kelp manufacturing processes sank without trace.[9] In 1836
the trustees of the estate recommended that two-thirds of the population be transported to Canada. Eventually the estate was
sequestrated and then sold off to Gordon of Cluny in 1841.[10]

The Gordons were a well-established landed family in Aberdeenshire, heavily committed to the new improved agriculture of the age; they had been at the cutting edge of the modern movement in the north-east and had made large financial gains. The Gordons were renowned for their extraordinary acquisitiveness. Of Colonel Gordon's grandfather it was said 'every shilling he got within his fingers stuck to them'. Gordon's own father accumulated property and nurtured his wealth:

> As he advanced in years the passion for saving became a perfect disease. He declined moving about for fear of incurring expense, and latterly he refused even to get up out of bed, on the ground that he could not afford it.

Colonel Gordon himself was distinguished solely for his wealth; when he died in 1858, he was thought to be the richest commoner in Scotland, leaving property worth between one and two million pounds. Altogether an oddity like his father, Gordon displayed exaggeratedly miserly habits. He felt a compulsive need to supervise the entire populations of his estates and it was said that he signed, with his own hand, virtually every rent receipt issued from his estate offices. His detestation of toll bars (which he shared with Patrick Sellar) was legendary and he would travel great distances to avoid such payments. He was a figure of Scrooge-like eccentricity and meanness.[11]

Most of this notoriety arose from Gordon's dealings in the Hebrides. In the east, in Aberdeenshire, he was apparently reckoned as a 'faithful' and reliable landlord, firm rather than severe. It was

> a feature in the management of his estate . . . that he liked to have about him the old tenantry, seldom parting with any who had occupied his land for any considerable time and were willing to remain on it.[12]

His move into the Western Isles was prompted by 'no apparent reason other than that he was dissatisfied with the interest and dividends that he obtained from his capital elsewhere'.[13] He probably regarded the very low price of land in the west as remarkably attractive, suggesting a better return on his capital. The differential between land prices in the north and the south of Scotland always attracted venturing capital since it seemed a promising avenue for higher returns.

Altogether Gordon of Cluny spent £163 799 on property in the Western Isles, which yielded £8223 rent per annum. Here was the successful agricultural entrepreneur, heavy with capital accumulated on the efficient eastern margins of the region, swallowing great territories in the west. In three years Gordon thus acquired Clanranald's islands of Benbecula, South Uist and Barra which he bought in 1841. It was a rational channelling of capital to a new zone ready for modern enterprise. The former factor of the South Uist estate, however, publicly advised Gordon to remove 2500 of the people immediately. It was the only way to reduce the cost of meal imports for the recurrent destitution among the population.[14]

At the time of the sales of Clanranald's property the advertisements drew special attention to its financial potential. The clear assumption was that, under a new owner, sheep would have to be introduced.[15] However, in an article published in 1842, it was reported that Gordon's prime concern in the islands was to maintain the level of population. He apparently believed that the islands represented a great prospect for agricultural development without depopulation. As he gathered together his new empire in the Western Isles he entertained grandiose plans for improvement and profit for everyone concerned. It was in the tradition of delusion that connected the Duke of Argyll in the eighteenth century through to Lord Leverhulme in the twentieth. In 1842 his attitude to the resident population was announced clearly enough:

> Colonel Gordon . . . wishes to keep them all . . . in doing so he acts judiciously for his own interest, as well as most humanely with a view to the real interests of the people.

When he acquired Barra, Gordon announced spectacular plans for its development. They included a clearance in reverse – that is, a redeployment of the 'redundant population of the coast' into the interior of the island. His policies were heralded at the start with enthusiasm:

The prodigious improvements already effected in this parish, under the most favourable circumstances, afford a powerful guarantee to the full accomplishment of his most sanguine hopes.[16]

Gordon thus embarked on a plan which, in essence, was the conventional improver's answer to the pessimists who believed that there was no solution to the Highland problem other than mass emigration. In the early 1840s, the auguries of Gordon's intervention in the islands were all positive.

IV. Clearance and famine on Barra

Within a few years each of these initial anticipations of Gordon's arrival in the west was reversed. The new landowner came to an opinion diametrically opposite to his original views. As early as 1843 Gordon was recorded as notably tight-fisted in his treatment of his tenantry. Seventy people from Barra received 'no assistance whatever for the purposes of emigration' to Canada at that time. This contrasted unfavourably with the relative generosity emigrants received at the hands of the estates of Lords Macdonald and Breadalbane.[17]

Gordon's optimistic plans soon faded and he immediately changed his tune when the returns on his capital proved derisory. He first attempted to sell off his island estates, and, when this failed, he instituted a policy of full-blooded clearance and forced emigration. As a student of the period has said, 'It would thus appear that while Gordon might momentarily have thought it possible to maintain the population on the islands, he soon realised that economically he could not afford to operate the estates with their growing populations'. The massive programme of clearance and subsidised emigration eventually instituted produced great hardship and widespread recrimination.[18] The population of the island had increased by 13 per cent in the 1830s but fell by 21 per cent in the following decade.

Gordon, of course, had bought into the Western Isles only a few years before the onset of the potato blight on the west coast in 1846 and this magnified all the problems he faced as a strictly rationalising landowner. It was during the years of the great famine that Gordon of Cluny caused the emigration of several thousand tenants from his estates in the western islands. He ran foul of public opinion and then became the object of severe criticism from government officials who supervised and inspected relief arrangements, both private and public, during the famine emergency. One of the most able and humane of these was Sir Edward Pine Coffin who pursued Gordon with considerable vigour on account of his neglect of the people in his charge in the Hebrides.

It was acknowledged that Gordon had expended considerable capital on improvement to his estates, and that these works had employed many of the people. It was also recognised that the material condition of the people of Barra had generally improved since he took possession of the island in 1841. Nevertheless in the famine year of 1847 the people had been reduced to pathetic impoverishment and their plight had been unattended by the landlord – rather, their condition had been exacerbated by Gordon's continuing clearances. It was reported from Barra that

Colonel Gordon has lately created several farms, turning the people for that purpose off their small holdings, and locating them on the sea coast, where they received coarse land which would grow potatoes and nothing else.

The people of Barra were, therefore, appallingly at risk in the potato blight. Some of them were actually without food. Major Haliday told Coffin that when Gordon received a representation about the state of destitution on Barra

he returned a very harsh, indeed inhuman reply, the terms of which I will not repeat, that in any period demanding an outlay of money, it is vain to appeal to him. At the same time, he owns that the extreme laziness of the crofters, and their dislike to move off the spot they were born upon, furnishes some excuse for a landlord's apparent harshness.

Early in 1847 it was reported by Captain Pole that:

Every week for the last two months they have been expecting a supply of food from Colonel Gordon, but have been disappointed. The very poor must live as they can, and die as they can, unless speedily relieved.

The poor ever were and now are perfectly willing to work, if work is provided. No idea can be formed of the wretched state of the poor in these islands, as respects food, clothing, and accommodation. It is quite heart rending. They are nevertheless very patient. Has heard of two deaths at Barra from starvation, but cannot say how true it may be. Many cases have occurred in which the poor have come to say they have killed their last hen, and some have gone to tacksmen to confess they are eating the turnips which they have from want taken from the tacksmen's field. The Revd Mr Chisholme concluded his tale of distress by adding that he had lately attended the death bed of a parishioner, whose only nourishment was an uncooked turnip by the bedside.

Coffin's report of the distress across the west Highlands in 1847 concluded that the most wretched conditions were found on Gordon's estates in Barra, where extreme isolation caused the people to be more dependent on their heritor than anywhere else. The clear verdict of the officials was that the landowner had neglected his duties during the time of crisis. Gordon, who lived mainly in Edinburgh, received a series of severe and castigating letters from Coffin during these months. He was told categorically that the Barra people were starving and that his factor on the island had received no authority from Gordon to relieve them. Coffin gave Gordon an unadorned warning:

> I cannot suppose that you intend deliberately to abandon to such a condition a large population, whose fate is in a great measure dependent on your proceedings; but I am, nevertheless, bound to forewarn you, that if such a determination were possible, it would become my duty to interpose in favour of the sufferers, and to take those measures on your behalf which are at present neglected by you, leaving to Parliament to decide whether or not you should be legally as well as morally responsible for the pecuniary consequences of this just and necessary interference. I hope to be spared such an obligation; but I am quite prepared to fulfil it, if needful.

Gordon, it is not surprising, found Coffin's letters profoundly 'menacing' and protested vehemently. He blamed the people them-selves who, even robust young men, simply refused to work, 'alleging that the proprietor of the soil is by law bound to feed them'. He was infuriated at the odium heaped upon him by his enemies, as he termed them. He contended that he had treated the people of Barra far better than any previous owner, and declared that he fully acknowledged his responsibility to feed the people during the crisis. In so many words Gordon told Coffin, Sir John McNeill and Sir Charles Trevelyan to mind their respective businesses. Coffin, however, was not convinced that Gordon could be properly trusted with the care of his people. Nor did Pole's close inspection of Barra give any support to Gordon's accusations that the people were indolent.[19]

Through all the years of the famine Gordon of Cluny executed policies combining eviction with emigration. He was not alone in adopting such a root-and-branch solution to the problem of famine: Lord Macdonald's estates followed a parallel plan. But no other landlord attracted as much denunciation as Gordon. In mid-1848 the Scottish newspapers reported that he had organised an emigration from North and South Uist to Quebec, whence the people would rejoin relatives already settled on Cape Breton Island. The people were under great pressure from Gordon to leave the Uists.

A vessel was arranged to arrive at Lochmaddy on North Uist in July 1848. The people had readied themselves, and Gordon, in conformity with his usual policy, had paid their passages and forgiven their arrears. On 15 July they were reported as

> encamped or squatted with their wives and children in the neighbourhood of Lochmaddy and elsewhere; but after long waiting, the emigrant ship did not make its appearance, and they were then told by Cluny's agent that a vessel would be provided for them at Glasgow.

Two contingents reached Glasgow by ship. 'Few of them were blessed with the possession of sixpence.' Only two or three out of the 150 Barra folk knew any English; many were children, and some were more than seventy years of age. Few could afford accommodation in Glasgow; the rest were turned into the streets. Of these, many became ill with measles and whooping cough and were taken to the Night Asylum. Yet, although they were penniless, they generally seemed hale, honest and respectable people, decently dressed in homespun. Their plight in Glasgow produced further adverse comment on Gordon and his factors.

V. *Internal refugees*

In all the confusion Chisholm, Gordon's agent, offered the Barra people immediate conveyance to New York, but they refused because they thought it was too far from their ultimate destination, Cape Breton Island. After further delay Chisholm promised to pay their accommodation in Glasgow until their ship arrived. He blamed the ship's agents for the delays and inconvenience.[20] Even at the best of times emigration was a trauma for the departing people; in times of famine and clearance it became a nightmare.

Gordon of Cluny continued to promote emigration from all his Hebridean properties. In some cases the pressure of famine was enough to make the people eager for their own expatriation; in others, the landlord could apply various measures of compulsion by way of reinforcement. In August 1849 there were large emigrations from several estates in the western islands. From Lochboisdale, South Uist, two vessels picked up 750 souls and sailed for Quebec. Gordon of Cluny continued to assist his people by purchasing their stock at valuation, and the Glasgow Destitution Board provided them with further financial assistance. The *Scotsman* reported that 'The people go away quietly, and are most anxious to leave, offering to sell their clothes, and to do anything to get away.'[21]

With or without emigration, clearances continued on the Gordon estates; the consequences were felt in other parts of Scotland when the refugees tried to gain relief and settlement. In 1850 Gordon's clearance policies once more caused a national outcry. By December that year further groups of refugees who had been cleared from Barra had reached the mainland. Some arrived in Edinburgh 'in a state of absolute starvation'. That city had long been apprehensive of the dangers of attracting large numbers of the poor of Scotland to become burdens on its relief system. In 1841, for instance, it had been pointed out that a very high proportion of the out-pensioners in the Edinburgh Charity Workshop were drawn from distant counties, especially the Highlands. This almost certainly reflected the impact of clearance and the consequent internal migration.[22]

The situation on Gordon's properties in Barra was denounced by the vehement journalist Thomas Mulock. He described the extreme privation on the island where, he said, there were 168 families who did not possess a single morsel of food, a condition he attributed to Gordon's total neglect and inhumanity. 'Sickness and death will ere long mow down the miserable people of Barra, while Col. Gordon is gloating over his banker's book, and living as if he were never to die!'[23] It was ironic that, at the same time as Mulock's denunciation, Gordon was also accused of creating the crisis on Barra through his earlier kindness, that is, by his excessive indulgence at the time he first acquired the property. At that time, said the *Scotsman*, he had not charged his small tenants any rent – 'If Colonel Gordon had compelled his tenants to improve their land, he would have shown that much more real kindness than by remitting their arrears and spending thousands of pounds besides in feeding them.'[24]

In December 1850 the pathetic band of Barra refugees arrived in Exchange Square, Edinburgh, where, it was reported:

> they have just been served with an allowance of bread to prevent them from starving. They came to this city to throw themselves on the compassion of the public; for, if this were not granted to them, they must perish.

The city fathers attempted to improvise some relief, and yet prevent the recurrence of such an inflow. They sought information about the causes of the Barra people's plight. An eyewitness account from the island described the great distress that had prevailed there. A total of 132 families had been deprived of their crofts but had been sustained by the Highland Relief Fund until that body suspended its operations in the spring of 1850.

> The unfortunate people received notice to remove from their houses in March, but they were allowed to remain in them till May, when they were ejected from them. The only resource in the circumstances was to erect tents by means of blankets raised upon sticks, while some of them took refuge in caves and in their boats. From these places also they were subsequently warned to remove, and shortly afterwards, under the warrant of the Sheriff Substitute, their tents were demolished and the boats broken up.[25]

As soon as the Destitution Fund had ceased to support the people Colonel Gordon had acted to eject them, an operation 'which was accompanied by demolishing their cottages, and then, after they were cast out destitute on the fields, getting them shipped off the island'. No one in Barra or the Uists would speak up for them, even with regard to parochial relief. The 132 families got to Tobermory and, of these, thirty-seven families travelled on to Glasgow, and some others to Edinburgh, 'and more were on their way, with the idea of seeing Colonel Gordon, who resided there'. The Edinburgh authorities feared that if they gave the Barra people much encouragement, the city would find itself inundated with Highland refugees.[26]

From Glasgow came a similar report on its contingent of Barra people who had arrived in the city late in December 1850. Among them were two widows and five children in a state of extreme debility; they were sent immediately to the Town Hospital. Their clothes were so appalling that they were burned. It was reported that they had been driven from the island by extreme privation, and that, although they had been on the poor roll, they had received only a peck of oatmeal for each family per week, and in return even the women were required to break stones for road repairs.

> They have come to Glasgow as they state with the intention of seeking justice. As they are paupers, of course, the expense of their maintenance, while here, will be charged against the place of settlement, which is Barra.[27]

There was public and civic outrage at the condition of the Barra people. It was established that they had little English, and that the factor had cleared them on the express instruction of Gordon. While it organised some immediate relief, the Edinburgh Council felt that Gordon of Cluny should be prevailed upon to accept responsibility for his people.

There were similar outbursts of indignation in other cities in Scotland, and Donald Ross (another prominent anti-eviction writer) added this cause to his campaign against Highland landlords. On a different note, Thomas Mulock was typically caustic about the 'newborn zeal on the subject of Highland

Destitution' displayed by the Edinburgh newspapers and civic leaders; it was, he implied, only proportional to the financial burden likely to be placed on the ratepayers. 'What columns of indignant invective against tyrannical proprietors! What floods of compassionate concern for maltreated Celtic serfs! ' He also turned on fellow critic Donald Ross and denounced him as a showman who was gaining cheap personal publicity from the sufferings of the Barra folk in Edinburgh.[28]

While his critics bickered Gordon of Cluny found himself under a deluge of public censure. He responded crisply and unambiguously:

> Of the appearance in Glasgow of a number of my tenants and cottars from the parish of Barra I had no intimation previous to my receipt of your communication; and in answer to your enquiry – 'What do I propose doing with them?' – I say – *Nothing*.

Gordon simply denied that the Barra people had been 'mercilessly turned out of their dwellings by me . . . at this inclement season of the year'. He had no knowledge of anyone leaving the island, and if they had, they must have left of their own accord.

> And I am not sorry they did so . . . It should be borne in mind that the majority of the present inhabitants were not originally natives of Barra, but brought there by the late proprietor, without regard to the characters they brought with them, the disadvantages of which I have dearly experienced – for they have uniformly thwarted all my efforts to put them in the way of maintaining themselves and their families by their own industry, and have rendered the property of no value, but rather a heavy incumbrance.

This then was the authentic voice of the successful east-coast proprietor bursting with impatience to rid himself of his intractable and uneconomic western islanders. Cluny also pointed out that he had spoken to the government in London about the impossible position of landed proprietors in the west Highlands. He himself had derived income of only £1273 16s 5d during the last three years from the island of Barra, in exchange for an expenditure of £3117 2s 6d. He continued to feel compassion for the people, and he had recently sent a cargo of Indian corn for their relief, but his philanthropy was exhausted. The people had not responded to his assistance, and he was simply not prepared to do any more for them.[29]

The circumstances on Barra were subsequently investigated by Sir John McNeill in his Report on the western Highlands in April 1851. He received evidence from 'eight gentlemen of Barra', including three tacksmen, one factor, a Roman Catholic priest and a merchant. They considered five particular cases of complaint. Three of them concerned individuals who were 'notoriously indolent', another was a thief, and the last was, in all probability, 'the mother of a bastard'. The Barra gentlemen were also of the opinion

> that the eleemosynary relief afforded to the people has had a prejudicial effect upon their character and habits; that it has induced many to misrepresent their circumstances with a view to participate in it; that it has taught the people generally to rely more upon others, and less upon themselves.[30]

Another group of Barra refugees arrived in Inverness aboard a steamer from Glasgow, and squatted themselves 'down on the Exchange, to the great amazement and no little alarm of the community. An immense crowd soon collected about them.'[31] There were about sixty-five of them; they were in a wretched condition, and spoke only Gaelic. They too claimed that they had been ejected. They had first gone to Tobermory where the local people, apprehensive of their dependent state, paid for their onward fares to Oban and the mainland. From Inverness it was reported:

> The sight of these creatures, old men hugging their children to their bosoms to protect them from the weather, and women sitting on the cold wet stones on a winter night suckling their infants with perhaps little nourishment to give them, and all without a single morsel of food, was sufficient to raise the sympathies of the most hardened.

In Inverness the Barra folk obtained private charity and food, and were taken to the Poor House. The local reporter expressed some scepticism about the eviction stories retailed by the Barra people, and noted that Gordon had denied that any clearance had taken place. But he also observed:

> It may be true that neither Colonel Gordon, nor any of his underlings ever actually took them by the shoulders and drove them out of his dominions, but the same end may be accomplished in a different manner. The short and simple truth is that Col. Gordon, years ago, contemplated getting rid of them. Two years since, he deprived them of their crofts, subsequently their huts were gradually pulled down, and finally all means of shelter and sustenance were cut off, and then, as a matter of course, they must seek a living somewhere else.

Nevertheless, the reporter found the people were perfectly idle and highly unco-operative: 'they will prefer sucking their thumbs in the Poor house to handling the pick and the spade'.[32]

In the meantime, in Edinburgh, a public subscription was raised for the Barra people, and they were transported to Lawrencekirk where work was found for those among them who had not been struck down with smallpox or fever. Gordon of Cluny, apparently, made no further contribution to the public debate, but one correspondent described him as a 'most indulgent landlord' who had done much good for the people by way of relief employment. Gordon of Cluny, he contended, had reached the end of his capacity to support the people, as had the Destitution Board. The west Highlands had come to a crisis 'and it is perhaps expecting too much that even a rich man is to expend what he gets from other and better paying properties to maintain those from which he has probably never got anything'.[33] This, of course, was a common theme of Highland ownership in the mid-century.

The Barra people who went to Inverness remained there for two more years, living in extreme wretchedness until church ministers made representation on their behalf in London. Sir Charles Trevelyan of the Treasury made provision for them to be given free passages to Australia. It was reported in 1853 that 'Strange to say, although they are in a wretched state of poverty, only two families have hitherto been induced to avail themselves of the benefit.'

The Barra account, of course, was a perfect juxtaposition of extreme wealth and poverty, of the power of the landlord and the impotence of the peasantry; it also provided the sharpest focus on the extreme frustration which faced the improvement mentality in the context of the recalcitrant economy of the west Highlands and Islands.

VI. Coerced emigration

The story of the Barra refugees in Inverness and Edinburgh was sensation enough, but was soon dwarfed in scale by further events on Cluny's island estates in the summer of 1851. On this occasion the landlord engineered the emigration of at least 1700 people from South Uist and Barra.[34] These were numbers reminiscent of the great Sutherland clearances of 1819–21.

Gordon of Cluny was now accused of usury, bribery, trickery and violence in his plans to coerce his people onto the ships for Canada. A modern account retells the particular story of the boarding of the vessel, the *Admiral*. The people

> were seized and dragged aboard. Men who resisted were felled with truncheons and handcuffed; those who escaped, including some who swam ashore from the ship, were chased by the police and press gangs.[35]

These dramatic scenes were derived from accounts published later by Donald Macleod and Alexander Mackenzie. Macleod, who frequently employed hyperbole for passionate emphasis, claimed that 'under the protection of . . . law, Colonel Gordon has consigned 1500 men, women and children, to a death a hundred-fold more agonising and horrifying' than the deaths of Napoleon's prisoners-of-war. Macleod argued that the government had co-operated in the atrocity by granting public money to facilitate the crime. The people, he said, were

> in a hopeless condition at their embarkation, decoyed, in the name of the British Government, by false promises of assistance to procure houses and comforts in Canada, which were denied them at home – decoyed, I say, to an unwilling and partial consent – and those who resisted or recoiled from this conditional consent, and who fled to the caves and mountains to hide themselves from the brigands, look at

them, chased and caught by policemen, constables, and other underlings of Colonel Gordon, handcuffed, it is said, and huddled together with the rest on an emigrant vessel. Hear the sobbing, sighing, and throbbing of their guileless, warm Highland hearts.

Macleod continued further in this fashion, and was able to add more substance to his account by quoting from an eyewitness account of these episodes in South Uist and Barra in the summer of 1851. The essence of these allegations was that the people had been 'tricked' into promises to emigrate, in the same way as the victims of 'old-fashioned slave traders'. Like many would-be migrants, before and since, the people changed their mind when the plan took more palpable and immediate shape. Thus when the emigration ships arrived at Lochboisdale the people were summoned to a public meeting, on the threat of a £2 fine for absence:

> At this meeting, some of the natives were seized and, in spite of their entreaties sent on board the transports.

One large islander was collared and brought on aboard only after being handcuffed. The eyewitness recounted that

> One Morning, during the transporting season we were suddenly awakened by the screams of a young female who had been recaptured in an adjoining house, she having escaped after her first capture. We all rushed to the door, and saw the broken-hearted creature, with dishevelled hair and swollen face, dragged away by two constables and a ground officer. Instrumental in these events was the Revd H. Beaton who gained a black name in the memory of the migrants.[36]

These descriptions are melodramatic and sensational. They were, nevertheless, given considerable if not complete corroboration in three other separate sources, two contemporary and one retrospective. Between them they suggest that Macleod's witness did not greatly exaggerate the circumstances of the clearances.

First, a Canadian newspaper, the *Quebec Times*, reported the condition of the people on their arrival in Canada. Some 1100 had arrived from the Gordon estates. The newspaper printed a statement made on arrival by Hector Lamont and seventy other passengers; it was in the form of a petition and was a rare and direct expression of the people's attitude. The petition recorded that they had embarked on the *Admiral* from Stornoway, and were among many hundreds of Gordon tenants who had been sent to Canada in that year. Gordon of Cluny had instructed his factor to take 450 aboard the *Admiral* at Lochboisdale on 11 August 1851. All the signatories and most of the others had embarked voluntarily,

> but . . . several of the people who were intended to be shipped . . . to Quebec, refused to proceed on board and, in fact, absconded from their homes to avoid the embarkation.

The factor had then ordered a policeman, a ground officer and some constables to pursue the people into the mountains, where about twenty were captured. Handcuffs were applied and the people forced back to the ship. Several families were divided by the incident.

The signatories had volunteered to emigrate only on the understanding that their passage to Quebec would be paid by Gordon, and that the government emigration agent would deliver them to Upper Canada where they would obtain work and land. But in Quebec they found themselves utterly destitute and their promises only half-honoured. Unless they received immediate relief, they warned, 'the whole will be liable to perish with want.' The *Quebec Times* waxed indignant at the monstrous treatment meted out by Gordon of Cluny, and at the abject condition of the people. Other Canadian newspapers carried similar stories about the pitiable condition of Highlanders recently disembarked at Canadian ports.[37]

The official correspondence relating to these emigrations also corroborated Donald Macleod's ostensibly histrionic account. A stream of reports was despatched from the Chief Immigration Officer in Quebec in the autumn of 1851; they contained damaging statements about the plight of the 2000 people Gordon had sent across the Atlantic. In part, the problem was the result of usual confusion: orders for the clothing and provisioning of the people on arrival in Canada had not been fulfilled. The people could speak no English and were in desperate straits. But two years before, 1000 people from the Gordon estates had been relatively successful in Canada, and Gordon had provided them with free passage, clothing and shoes. The 1851 emigrants were, by contrast, totally destitute, 'without the means of leaving the ship, or of procuring a day's subsistence for their helpless families on landing'. The medical reports on the people were comparatively favourable (only five out of 1686 had died), and the transatlantic journey had been well provisioned. However, the Medical Superintendent at Grosse Isle quarantine station, Quebec, reported:

> I never, during my long experience at the station, saw a body of emigrants so destitute of clothing and bedding; many children of nine or ten years old had not a rag to cover them. Mrs Crisp, the wife of the master of the *Admiral* . . . was busily employed all the voyage in converting empty bread bags, old canvas, and blankets, into coverings for them. One full-grown man passed my inspection with no other garment than a woman's petticoat.

Unflattering contrasts were drawn between these people and those assisted from Lewis to Canada by Sir James Matheson (see Chapter 14). The colonial authorities tried to induce Gordon to pay for the provisioning and transport of the people between Quebec and Upper Canada: the correspondence was full of acid denunciation of his methods of expulsion. And amid this tragedy was the unsavoury pantomime which saw the correspondence from Canada being returned to Quebec by both Gordon and his agent because the letters had been addressed to the wrong party.[38]

The third confirmation of the case against Gordon was produced three decades later. The events were recalled before the Napier Commission in 1883 when evidence was taken at Castle Bay (Barra) and Lochboisdale (South Uist). A great deal of the testimony at that time related to the still raw memory of factorial oppression during the emigration from Lochboisdale in August 1851. A beneficiary of the clearances was D.W. McGillivray, a surgeon and farmer, then aged seventy-four, who spoke approvingly of:

> the emigration promoted by Colonel Gordon which relieved the property very well. The people of South Uist and Barra petitioned in a

body to be helped away. He sent a vessel to South Uist and a vessel to Barra to take them. He also sent clothing for scores of families.

McGillivray said that their subsequent experience in Canada had been mixed, but he did not think that any of the emigrants had become destitute.

Set beside McGillivray's testimony, the evidence of the crofters was in total contradiction. John Mackay of Kilphedar, aged seventy-five, recited a full litany of the allegations made against the Gordon estate; he told of the people being driven and compelled to emigrate to America: 'Some of them had been tied before our eyes, others hiding themselves in caves and crevices for fear of being caught by authorised officers.' He said:

> I saw a policeman chasing a man down the macher [a sandy slope] towards Askernish, with a view to catch him, in order to send him on board an emigrant ship lying in Loch Boisdale. I saw a man who lay down on his face and nose on a little island hiding himself from the policeman, and the policemen getting a dog to search for this missing man in order to get him on board the emigrant ship.

He told of another man who had been put on board the ship by force – 'he was caught and tied, and knocked down by a kick' – despite the fact that he had 'four dead children in the house', who were buried before his wife joined him on board. From Benbecula, Angus McKinnon described the fate of the migrants in Upper Canada: 'I heard that they were so poor after landing, without food or clothing, that they died upon the roadside, and were buried into holes where they died.' The Revd Donald McColl recalled that

> many were bound hand and feet, and packed off like cattle on board the vessel to America. The recollections of ill-treatment and cruel evictions towards many in those days operates unfavourably on the minds of the present generation towards emigration.[39]

Almost all the evidence relating to the Gordon clearances is, therefore, mutually corroborative: it is virtually certain that there were scenes of hysteria and cruelty during the mass emigrations of 1851. The condition of the people on arrival in Canada was certainly appalling. Gordon of Cluny had attempted to apply a radical and crude solution to a problem to which he could see no other answer. His estates had been totally uneconomic by any conventional criteria; he had spent many thousands of pounds trying to develop a firmer economic foundation in the islands, but without success. His tenantry was famine stricken and dependent on charity. Gordon therefore decided to spend further large sums of money on the subsidisation of emigration in order to break the vicious grip of overpopulation. However, in its practical details, the solution had the appearance of an atrocity arising not so much from famine as from the wanton cruelty of a millionaire landlord.

In 1883 the factor of the Barra property was asked to provide the rental statistics for the previous half century. He said that the boundaries of landholdings had not changed but that all income from kelp production had ceased.

	Crofters' rent	Large farms
1836	£1950	£950
1883	£550	£1500

The factor said that the crofters simply could not pay any higher rent. The total return on the estate had not improved, though the impact of falling farm prices was the most critical factor in the 1880s.[40]

The bitterness against Gordon of Cluny was imperishable. Even in the 1890s, he was remembered as 'a most tyrannical landlord'. It was a reputation sustained with some vigour by his successors on Barra. Sir Reginald Cathcart, in particular, continued the reign of terror and, according to the local priest in 1897, 'ground down the tenants until they were little better than slaves'.[41] Yet, in defiance of landlord and perhaps Malthus too, the population of Barra regenerated and in 1881 was greater than it had been in 1831.

Notes

1 See Eric Richards, 'The highland passage to colonial Australia', *Scotlands* (1995), pp. 28–44.

2 Cockburn, *Journals*, op. cit., p. 136.

3 For a useful survey of new landowners in the Highlands see Devine, *Clanship*, op. cit., Chapter 5.

4 Lord Cockburn, *Circuit Journeys* (Edinburgh, 1983 ed.) pp. 67–8.

5 J.L. Campbell, *The Book of Barra* (London, 1936), pp. 34–5.

6 Quoted in Campbell, *Book of Barra*, p. 35.

7 Moray McLaren, *Shell Guide to Scotland* (London, 1972), p. 96.

8 Ibid., p. 205.

9 See British Parliamentary Papers (Shannon: Irish UP 1968), Emigration, vol. 3, Q 697.

10 This section is based on the evidence presented in John L. Campbell, *Songs Remembered in Exile* (Aberdeen, 1990), pp. 61–71 and 156.

11 *The Times*, 23 July 1858; *Gentleman's Magazine*, vol. V (1858), pp. 310–11.

12 Campbell, *Book Of Barra*, p. 34.

13 John Malcolm Bulloch, *The Gordons Of Cluny* (Buckie, 1911).

14 BPP, Emigration, vol. 3, Q 2687.

15 SRO, GD201/1235/16/Particulars of the Clanranald Estate.

16 William Yorstoun, in *Journal of Agriculture*, 1842 , p. 541, quoted in James M. Cameron, 'A study of the factors that affected assisted and direct Scottish Emigration to Upper Canada 1815–1855' (University of Glasgow Ph.D. thesis, 1970), p. 346. On the high hopes of the new owner see PP Emigration, op. cit., Q184.

17 Quoted in Ian Leavitt and Christopher Smout, *The State of the Scottish Working Class in 1843* (Edinburgh, 1979), p. 248.

18 Cameron, *Scottish Emigration to Upper Canada*, p. 356.

19 Correspondence from July 1846 to February 1847, relating to the measures adopted for the relief of the distress in Scotland, PP, LIII, 1847, pp. 294–300.

20 *Scotsman*, 5 August 1848.

21 Ibid., 11 August 1849.

22 William Wallace, 'Statistics of the poor in Edinburgh parish', *Scotsman*, 16 January 1841.

23 *Northern Ensign*, 19 December 1850.

24 *Scotsman*, 5 February 1851.

25 Ibid., 21 December 1850.

26 Ibid.

27 *Perthshire Courier*, 2 January 1851.

28 Newspaper cutting, dated December 1850, in *Historical Pamphlets in Inverness-Shire* [An unpublished scrapbook edited by J. Maidment, in Inverness Public Library].

29 *Scotsman*, 25 December 1850.

30 Report to the Board of Supervision by Sir John McNeill on the

Western Highlands and Islands, PP, XXVI, 1851, pp. 127–9.

31 *Perth Courier*, 20 February 1850.

32 *Banffshire Journal*, quoted in *Scotsman*, 5 February 1851.

33 *Scotsman*, 25 January 1851; *Inverness Courier*, 6 January 1853.

34 *Scotsman*, 20 September 1851.

35 Murray, *Islands of Western Scotland*, p. 226.

36 Donald Macleod, in Mackenzie, *Highland Clearances*, pp. 218–22.

37 Quoted in Mackenzie, *Highland Clearances*, pp. 218–22. See also Richards, *Leviathan*, p. 265.

38 Papers relative to emigration to the North American Colonies, PP, XXXIII, 1852, pp. 566–98.

39 Napier Commission, Evidence, pp. 680, 704, 708, 711, 779.

40 Ibid., p. 693.

41 Aberdeen University Library Archives, MS 897, Diary of William Carson, 1897, pp. 51–5.

14

Trouble in the Islands:
The Macdonald Estates in North
Uist, Benbecula and Skye

I. Famine relief

COLONEL GORDON OF CLUNY was not the typical Highland landlord – he became the caricature figure of the monstrous evictor, unresponsive either to human feeling or public outrage. But it would be a mistake to suppose that he was alone in thinking that comprehensive emigration was the essential solution to the Highland problem at the time of the famine. By 1850 public opinion became impatient with the limitless begging on behalf of the Highlanders. Charity seemed to encourage indolence and dependence. Public subscriptions for the relief of destitution in the Highlands declined. At the same time rigorously Malthusian doctrine cast a pervasive influence over public opinion.

Though no lives were lost by starvation in the Highlands,[1] the effects of the Great Famine were deeply depressing. There was a widespread air of disenchantment and impatience. The *Inverness Courier* expressed the ruling mood at the end of 1850:

> That the Highlanders, after having had a sum of little short of £200 000 expended in their relief, and that under the auspices of a body of philanthropic and highly intelligent men, with the assistance of a corps of officers of high character, energy and ability, should at the end of the relief operations be in a worse condition than at the commencement, is so very startling and mortifying a fact as to call for inquiry and explanation.[2]

The corollary of this failure of relief measures to provide long-term solutions was, in the eyes of the landlords (and many of the people themselves), emigration. The famine, which dragged on for half a decade in many places, stretched the resources of the local economy to the point at which much of the population seemed to be in danger of becoming permanently dependent on charity. Rental incomes declined and estate finances worsened. There was a further stimulus to clearance.

In some places landlords reaped negative returns at a time when sporting tenants were beginning to offer large rewards for cleared land. Many of the small tenantry in the west appeared increasingly to favour a final capitulation to combined pressures of famine and rent, and sought, sometimes besought their landlords for, assistance to emigrate. The belief that mass emigration was the only true answer now became almost irresistible. Sir Charles Trevelyan from the Treasury spoke in terms of channelling 100 000 people out of the Highlands to Australia, and organised a great scheme to effect the proposal (which eventually expatriated one-twentieth of that number). There was little opposition to the sponsorship of emigration as such: controversy surrounded the manner of its execution, but hardly in any plausible way its necessity. Emigration accelerated dramatically at the time of the famine and, as always, there were examples of voluntary and coerced departures. Overhanging the process was the duress of circumstances which meant that even the willing migrants were victims of expulsive forces. The choices open to the people were narrow and most, of course, choose to remain. At least one philanthropic organisation was left with unspent funds in 1855 because it could no longer raise recruits for free emigration. Yet, meanwhile, the population resumed its growth in many of the most impoverished districts of the west and the islands.

Few voices were raised against the diagnosis that led to emigration, even from the conservative side of northern opinion. One, however, was the minister of the established church in Sleat, on Skye, a parish wickedly ravaged by the famine, who made no bones about the clearances that had continued in his district, nor about the morality of the proceedings. He remarked in 1851:

I could at this moment point out places from which upwards of sixty tenants were ejected within a short space of time, and not one of them in a penny of arrears. All their land is now in the hands of four or five men, and these small tenants have been driven up the hillside to trench more ground, to be at some future period pounced upon by a large farmer; or you will find some of them in lanes or closes, or dark areas in Edinburgh. Let a more equitable distribution of the land be made in the Highlands, and the causes of destitution will cease.[3]

In these words the minister described a process which had been witnessed on arable lands across the Highlands, from Lewis to the Black Isle, and from Perth to Caithness. He was one of the radical conservatives who believed that the redistribution of land could solve the population problem in the Highlands, and that emigration was unnecessary.

II. Lord Macdonald and Sollas

North Uist, the central island in the Outer Hebrides, witnessed sensational clearances between 1849 and 1852, and they matched in every department the crude methods employed by Gordon in Barra. The North Uist clearances were set in a context of famine and induced emigration. These conditions always gave eviction an especially hard edge, and the best publicised and most emotional episodes in this category were the Sollas evictions, on the property of Lord Macdonald. And here the struggle for the land reached its cruellest extreme, the peasantry declared redundant by economic forces which outreached the power of either the people or the landlord.

The Macdonald estates in the Hebrides had followed the classic pattern of economic boom and decline over the previous half century. The landlord had made excellent profits from kelp and had trebled his rents in the years of the French Wars to 1815. Kelp was valuable especially in glass manufacturing; as Joseph Mitchell remarked, it was 'like a gold mine to the whole Hebrides'.[4] To supply the labour demanded in kelping he had encouraged the growth of population by the sub-division of holdings, and

Macdonald had taken active measures to deter emigration at the turn of the century.

By 1820, when kelp entered its long catastrophic decline, Macdonald found himself burdened with an excessive population. This was the recurring irony and tragedy of economic development during industrialisation in the south. Kelp was superseded by new industrial processes and imports. The factories in the south of Scotland quite suddenly sent a reverse message to the producers in the west Highlands, and the people were, within a very few years, anonymously declared surplus to requirements as the great pantechnicon of industrialisation changed direction and changed its suppliers.

Clearances on Macdonald's Skye estates were executed in the 1830s, and between 1838–43 the landlord assisted the emigration of 1300 people from North Uist, who were replaced, in the familiar way, by sheep. During the famine the Macdonald administration, like that of the odious Gordon of Cluny, was heavily criticised for its inactivity in relief work. This was despite the claim that Macdonald spent most of his personal resources on the relief of destitution during these years.

Lord Macdonald of Sleat (1809–63) was a man of slight distinction though he had the advantage of marrying, in 1843, the co-heiress of George Wyndham of Cromer Hall in Norfolk. By the late 1840s, however, Macdonald's finances were in serious disarray. His debts now amounted to the astonishing sum of £218 000 and he was pressed by his creditors on all sides.[5] How much of this enormous debt can be credited to his humanitarianism in the destitution, and how much to conspicuous consumption, remains unclear.

In 1849 Macdonald advertised the island of North Uist for sale, but it attracted no offers. It was necessary to raise large loans on the estate, and to place the estate under the control of trustees who accepted the responsibility of retrieving the position. The local chamberlains were replaced by Edinburgh law agents. 'A trustee on a bankrupt estate, you know, cannot afford to be generous,' said J.S. Blackie later in the century, 'women may weep and widows may starve; the trustee must attend to the interest of the creditors.'[6]

Trusteeship was the prelude to an inevitable and rigorous rationalisation following the full logic of Highland poverty without further delay. As the *Scotsman* observed at the time:

> When the lands are heavily mortgaged, the obvious, though harsh resource, is dispossessing the small tenants, to make room for a better class able to pay rent, and this task generally devolves on south country managers or trustees, who look only to money returns, and cannot sympathise with the peculiar situations and feelings of the Highland population.[7]

The trustees of Macdonald's estates decided to clear much more of his territory in Skye of the population, and to convert the estates to sheep farms. The policy would be conducted in conjunction with emigration.

North Uist encapsulated the tragic conjunction of west Highland conditions. There had been a simultaneous decline in economic activity and a rise of population. For at least twenty years estate officials had repeatedly spoken of the central contradictions in local finances. In 1839, for instance, the rent arrears of the small tenants had already accumulated to a figure of £1171, and yet their economic condition continued to deteriorate. The collapse of the kelp industry had long since obliterated the main source of income which had paid the rent. The tenantry were not self-sufficient and their landlord was on the brink of bankruptcy. As the North Uist factor put it:

> Kelp is not now a productive manufacture. The population on the Estate is greater than the Land, kelp being abandoned, can maintain. Tenants are so small that they cannot maintain their Families and pay the Proprietor the rent which the Lands are worth if let in larger Tenements. It becomes necessary therefore that a number of the small tenants be removed; that that part of the Estate calculated for grazings be let as grazings; and that the allotments, on that part better calculated for small tenants, be so enlarged as to enable the Tenants to raise a surplus of produce for the payment of the rents. In *this way the yearly rent of the Estate will not be materially, if at all,* diminished.[8]

The position was as plain as a pikestaff. It was a way of saying that structural change in the local economy necessitated clearances.

Similarly, in 1851, the factor, Balligall, called for a further remodelling of land occupation and the clearing of small tenants, but he advised caution, in view of the recent changes in the provisions of the Poor Law of Scotland. In the event of a clearance, he said:

> many of the poorer lotters possessing a few sheep on the common hills . . . would undoubtedly become paupers were the Test removed whereby an Inspector can allow their admission to the Relief board.

There could have been no clearer statement of the impact of clearance on the poorest members of the crofting community, or of the impact of the Poor Law burden on the Highland proprietor. Moreover the large farmers regarded the crofters as a nuisance. At Snizort, for instance, Balligall observed:

> When Mr Martin took the farm there was a number of crofters settled on it whom he was never able to get quit of, they constitute a barrier to all improvement and in the event of relet in 1858 they should be cleared away; if this were done the Rental might be maintained.[9]

This was the Highland tragedy in a nutshell. The potato famine in 1846–51 multiplied the dilemmas facing both the landlord and the people; melancholy and failure overwhelmed North Uist. In 1849 the Macdonald estate administrators decided to clear Sollas in the north of the island and also offered the people assistance to emigrate. It was the final solution to what otherwise appeared an intractable situation.

The Sollas clearances occurred in stages. Until the final blow of the clearances the population of the island, destitute since 1846, had been supported by the landlord, with assistance from the Drainage Act Commissioners and the Famine Relief Committee. The new estate policy in 1849 was designed to diminish the population by emigration and to enlarge the size of the remaining crofts by amalgamation with vacated holdings. It was a root-and-branch solution, and inevitably coercive because the broken people were paralysed by their poverty and fear.

III. The moment of clearance

In March 1849 a hundred cottars at Sollas were ordered to remove with their families by the approaching Whitsun. They were offered free passages to Canada, the Relief Board agreeing to pay most of the cost. Macdonald agreed to forgo all outstanding arrears, and to purchase clothes for the most destitute of the emigrants. None of the people would agree to these terms: they were resolutely and unambiguously opposed to the idea. It was an offer of emigration under duress, eviction and charity working in tandem.

Patrick Cooper, the landlord's agent, prepared the necessary legal steps for the Sollas ejectment. An eviction party was organised, and proceeded to Sollas. Substantial resistance was offered: 'Immediately on their appearing in sight a black flag was hoisted, and a great number of people assembled', probably in excess of 100. The Sheriff decided to withdraw, to give the people time to cool down. In the event this was a mistake since several hundred people now joined the throng, and the resistance was redoubled:

> The most prominent of the leaders declared that the people would neither go away nor pay rent; that they would not allow sequestration of their effects, but keep their cattle for sale at the markets . . . One man said that before they would be turned out, they would do as the Hungarians did with the Austrians.

Even while the clearance remained incomplete, the newspapers turned the fire of their indignation on Lord Macdonald. The *Scotsman* wrote: 'The extraordinary power possessed by one individual in such circumstances is certainly anomalous, and ought to be exercised with great moderation and humanity.'[10] No mention was made of the fact that Macdonald was himself in the iron grip of his trustees, but the case in his defence was put by the Revd Thomas Grierson, Minister of Kirkbean, who had travelled the Highlands regularly since 1811. He wrote:

> Lord Macdonald has been blamed for his conduct to the inhabitants of North Uist, but if they who blame him reflect on the extreme poverty of the people, and the enormous expense to which his Lordship has been exposed by supporting them, while in many instances he receives not a

shilling of rent, fault finders may see cause to alter their opinion. Like the Irish, the Highlanders are indolent and inactive at home but in almost all cases are industrious and excellent workers abroad. Emigration therefore seems the only effectual remedy for the evil, and in such an emergency, there is much to reconcile them to the prospect, provided whole families remove from the same district, and are not separated beyond seas.[11]

The *Inverness Advertiser* would not swallow this line of argument and was openly critical of the landlord, pointing out that the population of North Uist was large precisely because the Lords Macdonald had encouraged in-migration and sub-division during the days when kelp-making had been lucrative. Rents had not been reduced, despite the decline in incomes, and this, combined with the ruin of the potato crop, had caused arrears to mount. The Sollas district, reported the *Advertiser*, had been afflicted severely in the famine and contained 600 people now threatened with forcible ejection. They had asked for a delay while they sold off some of their cattle to pay their arrears, which would allow them to renegotiate their rents. Macdonald had ignored petitions for delay:

Every three of four tenants have had their goods hypothecated, and many fires have been put out, and the furniture thrown out of doors, and the doors sealed up. Very great is the distress, and heartrending the cries and sobbing of the helpless children. His Lordship bids them, by his servants, to be off to Canada; alas! at this late season, without money, without friends! The passage money will be paid by his Lordship; aye, it will, but out of the proceeds of their cattle and crops! But what of the unbedded and cold shed on the quays of Quebec and Montreal, and the weary way to the interior, and bread for the coming severe winter? Is all this enacting so near home, and none to interfere? no voice to be lifted to expose to merited obloquy such oppression – such a trampling on the rights of so many of our countrymen?

The people, said the *Advertiser*, faced this choice: either they signed a document to commit them to emigration, or their houses would be destroyed.[12]

But Whitsun passed and the Sollas people remained. To break the impasse, Patrick Cooper assembled a reinforced eviction party comprising thirty handpicked men of the Inverness-shire

Constabulary at the end of July 1849. They were accompanied by some of the 'gentlemen of North Uist'. In Cooper's own words, the eviction party descended on the township, facing practically the entire population of the island:

> they found a mob of more than two thousand waiting for them. On the evictions being proceeded with, the mob, after a time, attacked the party with stones.[13]

Eyewitness accounts described the actual confrontation. There was the destruction of furniture, the unroofing of houses and the desperate alarm of the people. Between four and five hundred people of the district's population of over 600 were due to be evicted and emigrated to Canada. Cooper 'expressed his intention to proceed with the ejectment of the whole population of the district of Sollas, unless the offers previously made by him to the people as to emigration were agreed to.' The constables entered the village:

> The moment the force was seen from the houses three signals were successfully raised from the roof of one of the bothies, and the people from all the neighbouring towns were seen crowding along the paths leading to the house from which the signals were flying and around which a large crowd of men, women and children had already assembled.

The crowd followed the eviction party in high excitement. The leader of the evictors came to a householder and asked him if he would go to America by a vessel which was due to arrive at Lochmaddy within a few days: the proposition was translated into Gaelic for him. He flatly refused, saying that it was too late in the season, and that he had no friends in Canada nor any money. Cooper responded that he could not allow the man to stay until the following spring, unless he provided a large bond to remove at that time. An accompanying minister agreed to provide this. It was at this point that the ringleaders of the previous deforcement were captured:

> Moments afterwards the women raised a continued yell, and seizing stones rushed down the hill to intercept the officers.

The ministers managed to calm them, and the prisoners were marched away.

The following day the process of clearance at Sollas continued. The people were now each given a choice of being evicted there and then, or signing a pledge to emigrate. Ejections were undertaken amid scenes of pathetic sorrow. In some of the worst cases, the Sheriff refused to execute the summonses despite pressure from Cooper. The Sheriff also called for the Inspector of the Poor to take care of the most needy families. Hostile feeling continued to mount among the people and there were repeated outbreaks of stone throwing.

The police officers lined up in two groups to protect the ejecting party as it went about its work. At one point it was engaged in removing the furniture and a loom from the house of Mrs Mackaskill when the woman rushed out crying 'My children are being murdered'.

This precipitated a stampede of women at the police, who had raised their batons. After a scuffle the women retreated, there was a pause for explanation, and then a further volley of stones was aimed at the police. The ammunition was replenished from a stream-bed. The police then charged in two divisions, which sent most of the crowd scurrying away, though several were caught. These scenes erupted repeatedly as the ejectments continued. When houses were demolished the women became increasingly agitated, flinging themselves to the ground or at the police. Cooper came to the view that the clearance would have to be postponed and that troops would be necessary for its completion. He also saw that the action would create a great burden for the poor law administration.

After the tenth ejectment Cooper, concerned that the clearance was becoming a shambles, decided on another compromise. He agreed to let the Sollas people stay until the following spring, but still on the condition that they sign a pledge then to emigrate. A conference was arranged for the next morning, when Cooper and the other officials met a number of the leaders of the people. Although there was still opposition to this idea Cooper seems to have been successful in cajoling most of the people into a promise to emigrate. Having achieved this limited objective, Cooper and the evicting party departed. Cattle were taken in lieu of arrears.[14]

The subsequent history of the Sollas people is fragmented and less clear. Many eventually emigrated to Canada under the terms of the agreement with the Macdonald Trustees. There were further scenes of clearance in 1850 but when a reporter of the *Inverness Courier* visited Sollas in September of that year, he found that seventy families remained and were still under notice to quit. They were in an extremely wretched condition and unable to sustain themselves, their plight having been investigated by charitable relief bodies in Perth and Glasgow. They continued to resist the Macdonald emigration offer, and a new plan was hatched to resettle them on wastelands near Loch Efort, South Uist, on an allotment of twenty acres per family. The Perth and Glasgow committees provided a capital of £1700 to develop the sites and Lord Macdonald agreed to the plan despite the loss of rent that was entailed. It was pointed out that the maintenance of the Sollas people would otherwise cost him £500 a year. In the event, the scheme failed and some of the people followed their compatriots to Canada, an emigration which Cooper described as 'safe and comfortable'.

Most of the remainder eventually, after much agonising delay, departed for Australia under the auspices of the Highland and Island Emigration Society, just before Christmas 1852. They were shipped to South Australia and Victoria aboard the *Hercules* in a voyage of almost unprecedented misery, which turned the already melancholy story into high tragedy.[15]

The contemporary accounts of the Sollas clearances were clear enough: that there was hysteria, violence, the destruction of homes and extreme poverty, is beyond doubt. Nor is there any question but that the Sollas people harboured feelings of detestation towards Cooper and his agents for many decades. Their hatred rings through the evidence taken by the Napier Commission in 1883, when the 'Battle of Sollas' was remembered as:

> Victory for the nobles, and the defeat and utter discomfiture of the peasantry. As is always the case, this battle was fruitful of immense sufferings, hardship and loss to the defeated.

Giving evidence before the Commission in 1883, Charles Shaw, who had been the principal law officer during the Sollas affair, testified to the violent abhorrence of clearance which had been displayed by the people, both in 1849 and 1852, when some of them were removed for the second or third time. Shaw himself had been generally popular throughout Sollas

> both on account of his own merits and those of his father. The people emphatically said that they would not hurt a hair on his head, but they threatened with instant death any officer who should attempt to eject them.

During the actual clearance at Sollas in 1849 Shaw had reaped his share of abuse. Nevertheless, he recounted that within a few years of their emigration to Australia, some of the expatriated Sollas folk had sent money through him to their friends still in North Uist. As Shaw recollected:

> So much had their tempers changed, and their feelings towards me, that they put a sum of money together, and remitted it to me, with a request that I would purchase my wife a ring with it as a token of their gratitude to me for all the trouble I had from first to last taken in their matters; and in writing me they begged on no account to return the money as they would not accept of it. I felt gratified, after all the ill-feeling they had all shown, that they at last appreciated my disinterested efforts to improve their condition, though these efforts had not at first met their approval but very much to the contrary.[16]

Though there was probably an element of self-advertisement in Shaw's remarks there was evidently some healing of old wounds and even a suggestion of repentance.

IV. The Sollas trial

The Sollas rebels of 1849 – those who had resisted the eviction – were ultimately vindicated in court. The trial of three Sollas men, two labourers and a farmer, charged with mobbing and rioting, took place in Inverness before a jury under the presidency of Lord Cockburn in September 1849. Cockburn had a long acquaintance with clearing episodes in the Highlands – he had been a junior defence counsel for Patrick Sellar in his famous trial in the same town as long ago as 1816.[17]

A great deal of publicity had attended the clearances in North Uist and the trial attracted even more attention, both in the town and in the rest of Scotland. Many witnesses were called and Cockburn instructed the jury on points of law. He observed that a riot had certainly occurred, and that the accused men of Sollas had unquestionably participated in the riot. He also made clear to the jury that Lord Macdonald had proceeded in a perfectly legal manner: the question of the legality of the removals was not a matter for the jury to consider. Indeed, Cockburn pointed out, Macdonald had been in the same position as a house proprietor who wished to remove a tenant. Cockburn instructed the jury to purge itself of all presuppositions about the circumstances of the case.

The jury took little time to agree that the prisoners were guilty of the charge. More significantly they

> unanimously recommended the prisoners to the utmost leniency and mercy of the court in consideration of the cruel, though it may be legal proceedings adopted in ejecting the whole people of Sollas from their houses and crops, without the prospect of shelter or a footing in their fatherland, or even the means of expatriating them to a foreign one.

The last statement was curious since Macdonald had undoubtedly given the people an option of emigration. Cockburn, passing sentence, said that a heavy punishment was not appropriate, and sentenced the men to four months' imprisonment.[18]

The light penalty imposed on the Sollas rioters was vastly popular with the people in the court. Privately, Cockburn wrote, 'The popular feeling is so strong against these (as I think necessary, but) odious operations, that I was afraid of an acquittal.' The statement made by the jury, said Cockburn, 'will ring all over the country . . . the slightness of the Punishment will probably abate the public fury.'[19] Cockburn said that Lord Macdonald was blameless, 'he was in the hands of his creditors, and they have their doer, a Mr Cooper, their factor. But his lordship will get all their abuse.'[20]

Henry Cockburn wrote two accounts of the Sollas trial, both of which were strongly sympathetic to the people charged. He observed that 'even the law has no sympathy with the exercise of legal rights in a cruel way.' His own interpretation of the events suggests that Cooper's arrangements for the people had been far less adequate than any other report had indicated:

> It was established 1) that warrants of ejectment, that is, of dismantling hovels, had been issued against about sixty tenants . . . nearly 300 people, warrants which the agents of Lord Macdonald had certainly a right to demand and the Sheriff was bound to grant; 2) that the people had sown and were entitled to reap their crops; 3) that there were no *houses* provided for them to take shelter in, no *poor house*, no ship. They had nothing but the bare ground, or rather the hard, wet beach, to lie down upon. It was said, or rather insinuated that '*arrangements*' had been made for them, and in particular that a ship *was to have been* soon on the coast. But, in the meantime, the people's hereditary roofs were to be pulled down, and the mother and her children had only the shore to sleep on, fireless, foodless, hopeless. Resistance was surely not unnatural, and it was very slight. No life was taken, or blood lost. It was a mere noisy and threatening deforcement.[21]

A discordant note on the Sollas verdict was struck by a correspondent of the *Inverness Courier* who, in a few words, summarised the essential case for the application of radical solutions to the Highlands. He regarded the surge of public feeling for the crofters as puerile: 'Sympathy is a cheap virtue.' He argued that everyone was subject to the rights of property. It was splendid that clanship and feudalism had passed away and that 'the tie which now connects landlord and tenant is purely commercial'. It was a much fairer system:

> A pity it was that the tenants [of Sollas] did not apprehend so plain a matter as that trustees are bound to make the most of the property under their management – that this is competent to even the proprietor of an estate unencumbered. In large towns blocks of buildings are gutted and transformed in every way, so that the proprietors may derive a better income from their subjects. In Edinburgh whole streets have been swept away to form *termini* to railways. In neither case are landlords and trustees or railway directors held up to public

opprobrium. Why the proprietors of land should be differently treated I cannot perceive, unless reproach and vituperation comports with the maudlin sentiment or sinister interests of certain fussy people.'[22]

'The public fury' to which Cockburn referred was directed against Highland landlords. It deterred some of the less robust landowners from policies of eviction and forced emigration. But the reality was that, between 1846 and 1855, the pace of clearance had accelerated and produced a further series of human tragedies, most especially in Skye.

V. Boreraig and Suishnish in 1853

Public outcry did not restrain the administrators of the other Macdonald estates. On Benbecula the small tenants could not believe that the trustees would treat them so badly by forcing them to remove to even poorer land than they already occupied. In disbelief they appealed directly to Lord Macdonald himself. A petition, in broken English, was prepared by five Airdeon crofters in January 1852. It declared that their conditions were already appalling; they would not remove to the 'worse place where we cannot get any seaweed nearer than a mile' until they had heard directly from Lord Macdonald. They warned that the removal would cast them on to the parochial board. It was evidently an example of a small tenantry being further marginalised by evictions. They pleaded finally: 'We hope your honour will have pity on us for it is said by the factor that we will be sent away from your estate at Whitsunday because we refused to go to the bad place they want [us] to.'[23] In reality Macdonald had already lost control of his estates to the trustees.

The trustees were responsible for the further and equally infamous clearance at Boreraig and Suishnish in south-west Skye in 1853.[24] It was, in winter, bleak country: the people involved were, like those from Benbecula, the remnants of previous clearances on the Macdonald estates. They had been shifted at least twice before, in 1849 and 1852; they were greatly in arrears of rent and unable to support themselves by their crofts. In 1853 the tenants were offered the choice of assisted emigration to Australia or removal to yet another part of the estate. None of the people would accept emigration, but eight out of eighteen families chose to shift to the other location on the estate. The remaining ten families were ordered out in October 1853.

Some opinion at the time believed that the Macdonald estate had behaved reasonably and had given the people full opportunity for their own amelioration. Whatever the case, Macdonald's factor, Balligall, removed the people from Suishnish and Boreraig in the last part of 1853. Resistance was quickly suppressed, prisoners were taken, and the old dwellings were razed to the ground to prevent their return. It was a time of snowfall, and one man, who returned to his home in Suishnish, was found dead the following morning at the door of his ruined house, having perished in the night from exposure and cold. It was one of a small number of deaths directly attributable to the Highland Clearances.

Another report at the time provided more detail. It described the

unfortunate people – many of them tottering and trembling on the verge of the grave – [evicted] from humble cottages which they have inhabited, perhaps for their whole lives.

They blamed not the landlord, Lord Macdonald, whom they thought sympathetic to his people, but the Trustees, notably a 'Mr Brown of Edinburgh'.

During the actual clearance the officers had first removed the furniture from the houses 'to which the people offered considerable resistance', but 'no positive violence' according to a journalist. Some of the people were more than eighty years old, and one was ninety – but 'all were turned to the door, penniless and homeless, without so much as a refuge, at a very inclement season.' This indeed was the scene in which a partly bedridden woman of ninety-six was excluded from her home, and remained homeless for several weeks. With so many dependent persons amongst those removed in this way it was inevitable that they would become candidates for poor relief. There was much criticism of the fact that the evicting ground officer was also the Poor Law inspector.[25] Pluralism of this sort, with its attendant allegation of corruption, was rife in the

Highlands in the mid-nineteenth century. It reflected the sparsity of the middle ranks of Highland society, much diminished by the clearances over the previous three quarters of a century.

Resistance during the Suishnish and Boreraig Clearances had been relatively slight but three of the people were brought to trial in November 1853. They were charged with deforcing and obstructing the officers of the law in the execution of their duty. The Skye people were defended with unusual eloquence by an Inverness lawyer, Rennie. The *Northern Ensign*, a radical anti-landlord newspaper published in Wick, commented:

> It was one of a fearful series of ejectments now being carried through in the Highlands, and it really becomes a matter of serious reflection how far the pound of flesh allowed by the law was to be extracted from the bodies of the Highlanders.[26]

Rennie's defence provided specific detail of the events at Suishnish. There had been thirty-two families, perhaps 150 people in all, who were driven from 'their happy homes'. He claimed that they had virtually no arrears of rent despite the repeated failure of their potato crops. Nevertheless Brown and Balligall had decided to eject them. Making reference to concurrent clearances at Knoydart which were still warm in everyone's mind, Rennie said that they were extremely cruel, but at least some refuge was provided for those who were evicted. At Suishnish no such provision had been made.

As for the accusation of 'deforcement', Rennie maintained that it required evidence of active 'striking or pushing'. In fact the people had remonstrated without any resort to force; they had not even spoken loudly. Rennie pointed out the irregular status of the officer named Macdonald: he appeared before the court in three roles – sheriff officer, ground officer [that is, local estate agent] and inspector of the poor. Rennie contended that it was a mockery to describe the passive resistance of the Suishnish people as a 'deforcement'. The moral character of the people, he declared, was beyond reproach. In the dramatic outcome the jury returned a verdict of 'not guilty' by a majority decision. The clearance itself was, course, irreversible.

One week later there was a further report of the continuing plight of the people evicted from Suishnish. One of the evicted families had moved into

> a wretched hovel, unfit for sheep or pigs. Here six human beings had to take shelter. There was no room for a bed, so they all lay down to rest on a bare floor. On Wednesday last the head of the wretched family (William [Matheson], a widower) took ill, and expired on the following Sunday. His family consisted of an aged mother (ninety-five years) and his own four children – John seventeen years, Alex fourteen, William eleven, Peggy nine. The old woman was lying in, and when a brother-in-law of Matheson called over on Sunday to see how he was, he was horror struck to find Matheson *lying dead* on the *same pallet of straw* on which the old woman rested; and there lay also his two children, Alexander and Peggy, sick! Those who witnessed this scene declare that a more heart rending scene they never witnessed. Matheson's corpse was removed as soon as possible; but the scene is still more deplorable. Here, in this wretched abode, an abode not fit at all for human beings is an old woman of ninety-five, stretched on the cold ground with two of her grandchildren lying sick, one on each side of her.

It was alleged that the Parochial Board had totally neglected these people, that the responsible officials were land agents and that 'many of the Inspectors are mere tools in the hands of greedy and unfeeling heritors'.[27] For the poor, it was all a cruel farce.

In January 1854 the Macdonald estate officials proceeded once again to Suishnish to evict the few remaining cottars. On the day of this new eviction there was a violent storm accompanied by drifting snow. It was a small episode. The people involved were Neil MacInnes, his young daughter-in-law and her month-old infant:

> She had never crossed the door from the time of her confinement; but not to give offence, she went to the well and brought a drink to the officers of the law. Yet she and her infant were turned out in all the horrors of the fearful storm.

During the following days there was a series of small evictions and there were more public allegations of rough handling by the officials of the estate. Once more, people with small children were driven out of their houses and into the snow. It was further ammunition for the critics of Highland landlords, notably for Donald Ross who emphasised the gross anomaly which permitted the evictors of the people to act simultaneously in the role of inspectors of the poor. He reported his own observations of several cases in Skye. One related specifically to the scene of the recent eviction:

I found Flora Robertson or Matheson, a widow, aged *ninety-six* years, at Suishnish, in the parish of Strath, Isle of Skye, suffering from the infirmities of old age, and only allowed by the parish the sum of *two shillings* and *sixpence per month*. Anything more wretched than the appearance of this old woman I never yet witnessed. Her bed, a pallet of straw and some pieces of old blanket, was on the bare floor. Her appearance, as she lay on this collection of straw and rags, with a thin threadbare dirty blanket over her, was enough to have excited pity in any breast. Her face and arms had the colour of lead – she was evidently starving. She was evicted by the *Inspector of Poor* for the parish of Strath in September last, when the rest of the people of Suishnish were turned out. The Inspector showed her no mercy. He then acted as ground-officer for Lord Macdonald, and assisted by a few similar characters with himself, he carried out that shameful clearance in Suishnish and Boreraig, without regard to age or sex, details of which occupied so much of the attention of the public, through the country newspapers. After the poor old woman was ejected from her son's house, she was assisted to a neighbouring sheep-cot by two of her grandchildren – Peggy, aged eight years and 'Willie', aged eleven years. These poor children helped the old creature up the brae – sometimes they tried to carry her; but their strength was not equal to the task, and they had just to help her as she *crawled on her hands and feet*. The cot into which she crept was a miserable place – cold, damp, and dilapidated – yet there she was all owed to remain, the Inspector all the while carrying out the Trustee's and Lord Macdonald's instructions in turning the whole inhabitants of Suishnish, together with their furniture or effects, out on the heath, and locking up their houses and barns in name of these authorities!

Widow Matheson had received from the parish a sum of two shillings and sixpence per month, with no allowance for food or clothing. She was entirely in the hands of her eleven-year-old orphan grandchild. The Inspector had repeatedly rejected applications for more help. She was in a state of emaciation and literal starvation. Ross said that she was merely one of a hundred such cases.[28] It was, of course, part of a wider indictment of the landlords and of institutional neglect.

VI. Islands of clearance

At Strathaird, Barra, Sollas, Benbecula, Suishnish and Boreraig the scale and suddenness of the mid-century clearances were reminiscent of the great Sutherland clearances in the 1810s. But there was a significant difference: in the later events there was no local facility arranged for the resettlement of the people on the estates whence they were cleared. The entire purpose of Colonel Gordon's exercises, and Macdonald's too, was to expatriate the people – to remove the burden once and for all.

The events had been characterised by anger and panic, rough handling and pitiful suffering. The physical dislocation was matched by psychological trauma. These clearance episodes were the visible and human expression of the Highland tragedy. To use Malcolm Gray's evocative phrase, this was an economy 'in travail', a society undergoing one of the most painful adjustments in modern British history, comparable with the difficulties of western Ireland. But by contrast with the Irish catastrophe, the loss of life was small on any Irish scale.

Behind the specific episodes of clearance wider changes in the islands were continuing. Ownership of land turned over faster than ever. This was registered in a minimal fashion in a letter written in 1853 from Skye to a kinsman on the other side of the globe, in Tasmania.

> There has been many sad changes in Skye, by deaths and otherwise. The Island of Skye has been reduced to the lowest pitch within the last three years, and credit and value proceeding from Bankruptcy and pauperism. All our first rate people have failed, and their estates in the hands of Edinburgh lawyers, and the others secured by Parochial Boards I have upwards of £80 a year to pay for the poor . . . It is supposed that no person in Skye could hold out . . . Lord Macdonald

left the country with a determination of selling most of his property to get clear of his Law Agents in Edinburgh . . . Macleod of Macleod is similarly situated if not worse.[29]

Macleod of Macleod was one of the many proprietors who had reached the end of the long road of insolvency: the 'old potentate of Skye' had been £40 000 in debt at the time of Boswell in 1773; Macleod lands in Harris and Glenelg were sold off to liquidate debts to an English banker paid £100 000 in 1811. In mid-century the remaining estates were seized by creditors and Macleod eventually sought employment in London, where he lived by his own labour.[30] All the news from Skye was gloomy, even when the harvest improved after 1853.

In the Western Isles emigration had risen to a flood in the years about the famine. Between 1841 and 1861 Uig lost 50 per cent of its population, Jura 33 per cent, the Small Isles 50 per cent and Barra 33 per cent. There was also a fall in the number of marriages and births and an increase of temporary migration.[31] This was demographic adjustment with a vengeance, and only partly attributable directly to clearance, though everywhere there was the generalised duress of hard times to urge people away. More surprising was the recovery of some of these populations in the later nineteenth century before decline was again resumed in the twentieth.

Across the smaller isles the demographic shifts were not exactly synchronised though the long-term outcomes were much the same everywhere. The islands once accounted for 8 per cent of Scots population but eventually fell to only 2 per cent. Total numbers rose until 1861, followed by a continuous decline. The movement of people in the islands charted the effects of clearance. The small islands between Barra and Uist acted as refuges for people removed from townships in South Uist who had been moved on to Barra. Scalpay in Harris received people removed from North Harris; evictees from Skye went temporarily to Raasay and Soay. Soay's population rose from a few families in 1823 to 158 in 1851. Paabay was cleared of its population 'soon after' 1841 to make a sheep farm and its population was thereby reduced from 338 in 1841 to 25 in 1851.

Depopulation in the islands, it is clear, sometimes followed the
heavy hand of landlordism, poverty and eviction. But there were
also telling and instructive exceptions. Some of the later
evacuations from the islands, from Boreraig, North Uist in 1922–3
and Mingulay, were self-generated, triggered not specifically by
poverty but by the idea of resettlement on the mainland.[32] The
story of the most remote of all the islands, St Kilda, suggests that
the younger generations sought escape from isolation and social
constraints. A third of the people of St Kilda took assisted
emigration to Australia in 1852–3. Their landlord was left weeping
on the quayside in Glasgow, imploring them to desist.[33]

Notes

1 See Trevelyan quoted in Mitchell, I, pp. 298–9.
2 Quoted in *Scotsman*, 18 December 1850.
3 Quoted in William Pulteney Alison, *Letters to Sir John McNeill, GCB,
on Highland Destitution* (Edinburgh, 1851).
4 Mitchell, op. cit., I, p. 205.
5 See James Hunter, *The Making of the Crofting Community* (Edinburgh,
1976), pp. 29, 46, 62, 74.
6 J.S. Blackie, *Altavona* (1882).
7 *Scotsman*, 25 August 1849. See also, Mitchell, op. cit., I. pp. 212–13.
8 SRO, Lord Macdonald Papers, GD221/38/ Report of North Uist
Factor as to arrears, 14 December 1839.
9 SRO, GD221/51/View of the Rentals of Lord Macdonald's Estates on
Skye and North Uist 1852; GD221/77/ Copy of Report by Mr
Balligall, 1851.
10 *Scotsman*, 28 July 1849.
11 Thomas Grierson, *Autumnal Rambles Among the Scottish Mountains*
(Edinburgh, 1850), pp. 104–6. See also *Scotsman*, 5 October 1850,
report of the Skye correspondent. Patrick Cooper gave his own defence
in *An Old Story Retold, The So-Called Evictions from the Macdonald
Estates in the Island of North Uist, Outer Hebrides, 1849* (Aberdeen,
1881).
12 *Historical Pamphlets In Inverness-Shire* 'Disturbances in North Uist',
July 1849; *Scotsman*, 28 July 1849.
13 Cooper, *An Old Story*, p. 10.
14 *Inverness Courier*, quoted in *Scotsman*, 11 August 1849.
15 *Inverness Courier*, 12, 26 September 1850.

16 Napier Commission, Evidence, pp. 787, 801, 2736; see also Richards, 'Highland Scots of South Australia', pp. 47–8.

17 See Eric Richards, *Patrick Sellar*, op. cit., chapter 6.

18 *Scotsman*, 19 September 1849.

19 Henry Cockburn, *Circuit Journeys* (Edinburgh, 1888) p. 221.

20 Ibid.

21 *Journal Of Henry Cockburn 1831–1854* (2 vols., Edinburgh,1874), vol II p. 247.

22 *Inverness Courier*, quoted in *John O'Groats Journal*, 25 November 1853.

23 Copy from J.L. Campbell provided by the late Dr Ian Grimble.

24 See Geikie's description of part of these events, quoted in Chapter 1.

25 *Inverness Courier*, 5 January, 2 February 1854; Alexander Nicolson, *History Of Skye* (Glasgow, 1930), p. 366; *Historical Pamphlets In Inverness-Shire*, 'Heartless Proceedings'.

26 *Northern Ensign*,10 November 1853.

27 Ibid., 24 November 1853.

28 Ibid.,19 January, 2 March 1854.

29 Allan Macdonald quoted in J.F.M. Macleod, 'Notes on Waternish in the nineteenth century', *Transactions of the Gaelic Society of Inverness* LIX (1994–6), pp. 516–7.

30 Mitchell, op. cit., I, p. 222.

31 See T.M. Devine, 'Why the Highlands did not starve; Ireland and Highland Scotland during the potato famine' in Connolly, Houston and Morris, op. cit., p. 78. See also Charles W.J. Withers, 'Destitution and migration: labour mobility and relief from famine in Highland Scotland, 1836–1850', *Journal of Historical Georgraphy*, 14 (1998), pp. 128–150.

32 See H. A. Moisley, 'The Deserted Hebrides', *Scottish Studies*, 10 (1966) pp. 44–68.

33 See Eric Richards, 'St Kilda and Australia: Emigrants in Peril, 1852–3', *Scottish Historical Review*, LXXI (1993), pp. 129–55; *idem.*, 'The decline of St Kilda: Demography, Economy and Emigration', *Scottish Economic & Social History*, vol. 14 (1992), pp. 55–75.

15

Frustrated Lairds and Bloody-Minded Crofters: Lewis, Durness and Coigach

I. Highland poverty

IN THE 1840S AND 1850S the serious economic condition of the Highlands affected the subsistence sector more severely than the graziers or the sportsmen. Sheep and wool prices improved but the small tenantry faced recurrence of crop failure and sharpened competition in the cattle market. They had virtually lost the kelp trade and illicit distilling was almost certainly less lucrative in the face of legal production in the great distilleries of the region and in the south. Meanwhile, in the rest of the mainland the benefits of industrialisation were beginning to accrue even in the lower echelons of the population. The Highlanders appear to have been passed by, clinging on to a redundant system of production which continued to fall behind.

The realities of Highland poverty, in both cleared and uncleared districts, were inescapable. Henry Cockburn knew the Highlands throughout the Age of the Clearances and described a recurrent Highland scene on his circuit journey in 1841 at Glengarry:

> We saw mud-hovels today, and beings with the outward forms of humanity within them, which I suspect the Esquimaux would shudder at. And this, as usual, close beside the great man's gate.[1]

In many places, the evicted people found themselves dumped on the coast in congested crofter communities, dependent on a patch of potatoes, a few beasts and an unreliable fishing. An observer writing in 1828 about the condition of some recently resettled lotters in the Aird of Tong, Lewis, remarked:

> It was worse than anything I saw in Donegal, where I always considered human wretchedness to have reached its very acme.

He went on to describe the appallingly decrepit state of the houses:

> The poor people at the new lots there, are suffering the greatest hardship, many of them dead, I am told, from disease brought on, I have no doubt, from the unwholesome situation in which they had been forced to plant themselves.[2]

It was a devastating contemporary indictment addressed directly to the landlord responsible. The congestion in Lewis was the product of the combined effects of clearance and the doubling of population on the island between 1801 and 1841.

Lewis was the most intractable district of poverty and congestion. The island was eventually bought by Sir James Matheson who was born second son of a tacksmen in Lairg, Sutherland, the very class which produced much of the opposition to the clearances and also many of the personnel of Empire in the early nineteenth century. He left Sutherland, prospered in business, and in 1828 he established the firm which became Jardine Matheson and Co., the greatest tea and opium merchants in the China trade, the basis of his spectacular fortune. On his short return home in 1835 he bought the estate of Achany in Sutherland; he finally retired from trade in 1843 with colossal accumulated profits which he used to buy up Highland property including Rosehall and the Gruids, and the estates of Ardross, Pitcalnie, Cadboll and Corriemony on the west coast.[3] Matheson entered political life as an MP and two years later bought Lewis. Thus, once more, exotic profits of Britain's booming industrial and commercial economy were diverted to the Highlands. Matheson's wealth was already a legend and he could afford to continue the modernising improvements inaugurated by Seaforth.[4] By 1851 Matheson owned 400 000 acres of the Highland estates. But Lewis had passed into famine in 1846 and its population was growing at more than 16 per cent per decade. Matheson shouldered immense famine expenditure and very low rents. He spent £102 000 on employment programmes (though he recovered some of this, possibly even a third). But the catastrophic harvests continued and even in 1851 half the crop was destroyed in Lewis. Charitable relief supplies were again indispensable.

As the crisis slowly waned Matheson and his management decided on a rigorous policy of population reduction and the rationalisation of rent and land distribution. The landlord campaign to rationalise the crofts began – by reorganisation and emigration; there were 382 summonses of removal in 1849 alone. This was a formula for clearance and emigration though the estate insisted that neither force nor coercion was employed. In reality a carrot and a stick were brought to bear; the idea was to cull the population of Lewis. The tenantry were offered relatively generous terms to emigrate; but if they stayed they would be treated with the formal demands of the law. In other words if they fell into arrears they would be summarily evicted. Estate policy was spoken of in terms of 'clearing out' entire villages. Thus would Matheson cut through the problem: it was emigration and clearance at great cost, and under the whip of famine.

There followed a mass exodus from Lewis, mainly in 1851, to Lower Quebec and Ontario; it is claimed this was achieved 'without the intervention of a single soldier or policeman, with no civil disobedience of any sort.'[5] The policy was implemented by the estate Chamberlain who toured the villages explaining the problem to the destitute people, outlining to 'them the conditions offered them if they emigrated, their desperate [sic] prospects if they remained there, and the good prospects before them in America etc etc.' There was clearly a great deal of persuasion and pressure applied. Many of the people were literally without food and certainly lacked the ability to pay rent.[6] They were offered passages to Canada and clothing supplies too, having been told that they could expect no further assistance if they refused the offer and that they would be evicted if they fell behind with their rents. The response among the people varied and many declined the offer.

In the community there was great debate about whether Matheson was being benevolent or tyrannical; the Free Church minister and local merchants condemned the policy.[7] The Chamberlain answered the Stornoway critics thus:

> I state that no one c'd compel the people to emigrate, and that they need not go unless they please, but that all those who are in arrear for rent two years and upwards, would be deprived of their land at Whitsunday next if not paid up by then, giving them the option of emigrating if they cannot pay. That the proprietor can do with his land as he pleases and other parties have no right to interfere or dictate to him what he is to do. That those who do not pay their rents cannot be allowed to remain in possession of lands.

Matheson was effectively challenging his critics to specify an alternative solution to those of clearance, emigration, reduced population and commercial farming. Between 1851 and 1855 Matheson despatched 2337 persons to Canada at the cost of £10 000. As Dr Little says, 'These families had little choice but to submit to Matheson's dictates'. They could either emigrate or be evicted. Moreover the policy was selective – the landlord rationally chose to press into emigration those in particular whose rents were furthest in arrear; all subdivision was fully prohibited. It was a clinical and expensive exercise in the assertion of landlord power to diminish the population and the burden.[8]

The policy pursued by Matheson was adopted in many parts of the west Highlands in these years though the scale of the Lewis removals was larger than the average. The long-term results were remarkably equivocal, for though emigration accelerated, the total population of Lewis continued to rise in the following decades. The riches of the Orient, in the outcome, had not solved the demographic dilemmas of the west Highlands and Islands.

II. Rich and poor

While poverty proved extraordinarily intractable in the Highlands the embarrassment of the landowners was heightened by the increasing number of tourists and journalists visiting the north of Scotland. Spectacles of poverty were exposed repeatedly in the middle decades, usually during clearances, or emigrations or famines. As we have seen, new owners like Gordon of Cluny and Matheson of Lewis tried to cut through the problem like a Gordian knot.

The Victorian Highlands attracted some of the most spectacularly successful families of the age, setting up in considerable splendour, from the Queen downwards. It was the invasion of leisured capital seeking acres of space. The tradition had emerged as early as the 1770s with the return of Nabobs from India and successful colonials from the West Indian trade, some with fine wealth derived from slave plantations. The Marquis of Stafford and his son channelled their legendary wealth to the northern Highlands from some of the best profits of the early phase of the Industrial Revolution, from canals and railways in particular.

The velocity of land transfer seems to have been faster in the Highlands than elsewhere.[9] Joseph Mitchell remembered the sale of a great number of Highland estates including Hilton, Gare, Dundonnell, Mountgerald, Ardross, Letterewe, Letterfearn, Inverinate, Culrain, Dalmore, Braemore, Tarlogie, Culrossie, Applecross, Tarradale and Redcastle. Morrison the great linen draper of Fore Street in London had already spent £700 000 in land before he bought the Isle of Islay in 1847 for £450 000.[10] The story of Belladrum was another variant: the lairds became planters in the West Indies and brought home great profits from their slave estates to build a handsome mansion and distribute largesse across the neighbourhood. When the West Indian wealth evaporated Belladrum was sold to Stewart, an East India merchant, for £65 000, and still later to a Glasgow ironmaster.[11] The island of Eigg was sold in 1828 for £15 000 to Hugh MacPherson, formerly Surgeon in the Indian Medical Service and later Principal of King's College, Aberdeen.[12] The haemorrhaging of imported capital in the Highlands continued decade by decade. The Duke of Gordon was forced to sell Durris for £100 000, and in 1828–9 Ballidalloch was sold to Sir George Macpherson Grant, while Kingussie went to Baillie of Bristol. Only a few Highland families, like the Baillies of Dochfour, retained and expanded their territories by sensibly investing in the south and cross-subsidising their Highland properties.[13]

The tradition of capital inflows continued and English entrepreneurs followed – men such as Octavius Smith, the wealthy London distiller who became laird in Morvern. Later still was Andrew Carnegie, the great Scottish-American steelmaster who, among other conspicuous outlays across Scotland, established himself as a latter-day laird in Sutherland. Australian wealth also returned to the Highlands. The following century continued the tradition, spectacularly in the case of William Lever who was no less captivated with the mirage of Highland profits and development.

Most conspicuously, millionaires sprang from the south, eager to display their new wealth in the newly magnetic north. They sought a new theatre for their success, a playground – and they sometimes looked to the old social leaders for a model of upper-class indulgence. Following royalty and aristocracy, some of the industrial magnates turned to the Highlands for investment and pleasure. If they were Scots, or indeed Highlanders, the north was fashionable. If they were English they too saw vast territories going for a song – with scenery and fishing and shooting. In this way a keen juxtaposition emerged: the greatest beneficiaries of industrialisation came face to face with the losers in that very process. Clearances continued and in some places hastened. A few of the new plutocracy in the Highlands came from Highlanders returning to their native land; one or two, such as Patrick Sellar at Morvern, reinvested profits from the new-sectors of the Highland economy. But most of the opulence – Scottish, Highland, English, colonial and American – was new money, fully imported.

The infusion of external capital did little to reduce local resentment when the affluent immigrants used their capital to induce yet more clearances in the Highlands. Moreover the capital flowing into the Highlands did little to solve the long-term problem of Highland poverty, though it created some local employment and helped to make more likely the introduction of railways in the 1850s and 1860s. But mostly the Highlanders were simply not generating income or exchangeable products to the outside world; and meanwhile their numbers continued to rise and they became more dependent on charity and subsidies from landlords who were less prepared to pay. Their economic base shrank while the rest of Britain moved forward, and consequently some of the worst poverty in Britain co-existed with extraordinary wealth.

III. Contrasting landlords

Landlords by mid-century were, therefore, heterogeneous and their responses to the problems of the Highland economy, and to the management of the dependent small tenantry, were likewise also extraordinarily varied. There was, it is true, a uniform pressure towards clearance but even within the policy of clearance there were wide differences among lairds, in terms both of motivation and of humanitarian concern for the people.

The fate of the people who had been subject to clearances depended largely on the resources of the clearing landlord. It also depended on the opportunities for reasonable resettlement in the vicinity. For many cleared tenantry, the flitting was only the first step along the road towards the Lowland towns, or else emigration overseas. But, in the first instance, many, of course, resettled within the Highlands, probably on the very skirts of the estate whence they had been cleared. If elaborate resettlement facilities were provided by the landlord, particularly where they were associated with new employment opportunities (as in Sutherland, for instance), the prospect of a better standard of life was not impossible. But even in the best-planned estates there were uncontrolled elements at work which undermined the grand plans of aristocratic improvement. In Sutherland the best example was Durness, the village and parish, located near Cape Wrath in the far north-west of the county.

The Durness case cuts against the grain of the conventional history of the clearances. It shows the modest control which even the most powerful landlord could exert once the law had established its framework. The people of Durnesss erupted into resistance in 1841. Their landlord, the second Duke of Sutherland no less – son of the most notorious of the clearers – sided with the evicted in trying to prevent a clearance.

Sutherland was always a special case in the story of the Highland

Clearances. After the greatest transplantations of people on the Sutherland estate in the decade ending in 1821, the Countess/Duchess initiated no new large-scale clearances. This was not from a want of urging by some of the sheep farmers who were keen to oust the remnants of the inland peasantry from their fastnesses in the west. When the great bankrupt estate of Lord Reay was acquired in 1829 there was a grand debate among the estate managers and the new owner about whether clearances should be executed. The debate ran on for several years and expired without further changes.[14]

A rising fear of further inflaming public opinion caused the Sutherland family to be cautious about any fresh action, and it adopted a cautious and gradual approach to the problems of estate management. Financial incentives were offered to the small tenantry on the west coast to emigrate. Moreover there were occasional rationalisations of landholding, on a small scale, executed with the minimum of fuss. But, on the whole, the landlord now chose to live with any remaining uneconomic or illogical arrangements of his lands. Most of the estate was under sheep farmers, and the outstanding problem was the congested population residing on the west coast (a problem which was partly the consequence of earlier clearances).

The clearance at Durness in 1841 was undertaken entirely at the behest of a large tenant and leaseholder, James Anderson. He wanted to rid himself of a large number of small sub-tenants in order to convert his operations more fully to sheep farming. His landlord, the second Duke of Sutherland, wanted no part in the clearance, and was positively and angrily opposed to the tenant's action. The whole episode was regarded by the landlord with excruciating embarrassment, especially because it generated widespread publicity against the estate. The events in Durness reopened twenty-year-old wounds from the Sellar era in the Sutherland clearances.

The events owed their origins to arrangements contracted at a time when Durness had been in the ownership of Lord Reay. In 1818, Anderson, a substantial entrepreneur in the district, took a lease from Reay for a considerable stretch of the northern coast in the parish of Durness. The lease did not run out until 1846, which therefore gave Anderson a free hand until that time. Anderson, who was engaged mainly in cod-fishing (an industry strongly advocated by all Highland improvers), employed a large number of his sub-tenants in the enterprise. Anderson, until the expiry of his lease, was immune from the Sutherland estate regulations which strictly prevented sub-letting.

For many years Anderson's ventures in fishing were successful, and in 1829 he offered local people enough incentive to dissuade them from migrating to the larger fishing centres to the east, in Caithness. He expanded his operations along the west coast of Sutherland. He was, however, critical of the west-coast folk in Assynt, whom he regarded as undisciplined: they were, he claimed, qualified only in the business of procreation. In the late 1830s the fishing fell into decline and, in 1839, Anderson decided to cut his losses and quit the trade. He believed that it was rational, in the new circumstances, to switch out of fishing into sheep farming. This however required the removal of his sub-tenants, who were in the way of the sheep. These were the people he had encouraged to commit themselves to his enterprise over the previous twenty years. Anderson now set in motion a series of evictions. Great distress descended upon his sub-tenants. They lost their employment in the fishing and then, into the bargain, they lost their land.

The Anderson clearances were executed in two phases: between 1839 and 1841 he evicted thirty-two families, comprising 190 people. Some of them migrated, but most dispersed into the surrounding Sutherland estate. Four families went to Upper Canada, two to Caithness, three to Ross-shire and one to Inverness-shire; twenty remained in Sutherland. The first ejection apparently passed without resistance.

In September 1841 Anderson planned to eject a further thirty-one families, comprising 163 people. Among these people were shoemakers, coopers, fishermen, boat builders, farmers, cottars, 'weak children', 'a sickly weak family', one affected by paralysis, and 'an indigent old man, disabled and bent by rheumatism'.[15] Anderson was a man of business and felt no obligation to make provision for the resettlement of these people. They naturally turned to their minster and to the Duke of Sutherland, their ultimate landlord, to intercede on their behalf. They pleaded with him to prevent the clearance, begging him to provide 'shelter against the threatening and expected storm of tyranny'. It was an ironic twist that the most notorious clearing landlord in the Highlands should be thus petitioned for protection against clearance.

Anderson, acting fully within his legal rights, attempted to evict the people on forty-eight hours' notice. The stage was set for a classic eviction and the drama was played out in the predictable pattern. The evicting party, attended by the Sheriff, arrived in Durness where it met the energetic resistance of a body of women and faced the 'menaces and threats of an angry mob'. Then the 'large body of officers were deforced and expelled at midnight from the parish of Durness by a ferocious mob.' The resistance of the people was much more spirited and implacable than anticipated. Local proprietors now feared that a general mutiny might develop, supported by reinforcements from Assynt, and even from distant Culrain (both scenes of vigorous resistance in the period 1810–23).

Only when military intervention was mooted was a compromise negotiated by which the Durness people achieved an extra six months' notice before their ejection. The negotiations were mediated by the minister, Findlater who had interceded on behalf of the people. Shocked by Anderson's action, Findlater wrote to the Duke of Sutherland at the time of the disturbance:

> Two days ago, on the summons of ejection at forty-eight hours' warning, being about to be executed, or rather served, by the officers on entire families . . . they were resisted by almost all the females of the district. I dreaded the consequences might be serious. It was in vain to persuade in the present excited state of feeling. When no prospective opening was provided for so many destitute people, public sympathy could not possibly be suppressed, and the indomitable love of country must be felt more ardent in proportion to their being mostly allied to each other.[16]

The people of Durness recognised Findlater's advocacy and were 'so grateful . . . for their pastor's interposition, that they gave a public dinner for himself and another gentleman who had also taken their side.'[17]

Anderson, having pursued his clearance in the teeth of the landlord's opposition, was severely chastised by the Sutherland regime and the factors tried in vain to persuade him to abandon his clearance. Anderson simply mocked the estate officials for their naïvety: the people of Durness, he asserted, were indolent; they had become a dead burden on the estate and now had

> content[ed] themselves with the idea, that as they have no employment nor the means of being employed, the Duke will supply them with meal, rather than let them starve.[18]

But the Sutherland estate would not be a party to the eviction. The factors said that the fundamental cause of Anderson's action was 'that wretched system of sub-letting', which had been abolished everywhere in Sutherland except in Durness. Although the Duke of Sutherland, as landlord, had the power of buying out the lease, it was assumed that Anderson would demand extortionate compensation. James Loch, the Sutherland commissioner, angered by Anderson's intransigence, specifically refused to give Anderson the right to clear any land that he held on annual tenancy. He castigated Anderson relentlessly, and told him that he was under the strongest moral obligation to see that the evicted tenants were secure in their future livelihoods, were given ample warning, and should be fully compensated. These were Loch's unwavering rules of removal, but they had no authority over Anderson.

The Durness clearances illustrated the widespread pressures at work in the Highlands. The divergence of view about moral responsibility between the landlord and the entrepreneurial tenant was striking. In most clearances the feelings of landlord and tenant were in close accord.[19] At Durness the tenant was uncontrollable, fully protected by the law. The people of the parish, despite their noisy collective protest, their unusual solidarity and broad support in the district, achieved only a short delay to their ejection. And the greatest landlord in the kingdom was virtually powerless to curb his over-mighty tenant.

IV. Coigach and the naked clearer

The events at Coigach a decade later offered the reverse case in the annals of the clearances; this was to be the best known of the rare triumphs of the people over the landlord. At Coigach popular resistance was sustained and ultimately successful. The authority of the landowner was set at nought. Here, for once, primitive pre-industrial methods of protest and obstruction prevented the eviction of the common people from the land. The crofters could claim victory over the hated agents of the landlord. The clearance of Coigach was resisted five times during a period of eighteen months, and eventually the landlord gave up the struggle in a mood of exasperation.[20] The attempted clearance at Coigach on the Cromartie estate in Wester Ross in 1852–3, therefore, offers another exception to the general pattern of clearance.

How did the crofters of Coigach succeed where all others failed? Coigach was a remote peninsula on the extreme western mainland, heavily peopled and very poor. Its population had increased by 50 per cent in the first four decades of the nineteenth century, but the local economy showed no signs of growth. The local fishing industry, close by Ullapool, crumbled after the high hopes of the 1810s, mainly because the capricious herring shifted away from local coasts. Local subsistence had never been secure even when the population had been much smaller; now the problem grew with human numbers. Famines in 1837–8 and 1846–51 stretched the welfare and morale of landlord and people alike. The laird of Cromartie was John Hay Mackenzie, a benevolent but debt-ridden commoner who died in 1849. At that point the finances of his deceased estates were chaotic.

In normal circumstances the Cromartie estates would have been sold off to meet debts, and the fate of its tenantry thrown into the hands of a more capable or ruthless landowner. But the lottery of inheritance produced a different throw of the dice. Just twelve days before Hay Mackenzie's death, his daughter (the only child) married the heir to one of the richest fortunes in the kingdom: Anne Hay Mackenzie's husband was Lord Stafford, eldest son of the second Duke of Sutherland. They married in July 1849 and soon discovered the financial plight of the Cromartie estates which they had inherited shortly after the wedding. The rents were already largely committed in annuities and other inescapable annual payments to various family dependents hanging from the Hay Mackenzie estate. And, although Lord Stafford would eventually, in 1861, become one of the richest men in the country, he could not meanwhile count on any large-scale cross-subsidisation from the coffers of the Sutherland fortune. The management of the Coigach estate remained autonomous throughout the attempted clearance of 1852–3.

Old Hay-Mackenzie had possessed neither the energy nor the capital to indulge in improvement or clearances; this was part of the problem his daughter inherited. In the 1840s the Cromartie estate was well regarded because it had provided asylum for refugees from the Strathconan clearances (see Chapter 2). But, in 1852, under the pressure of financial stringency, the estate factor, the Lowlander Andrew Scott, decided that the time was ripe for the rationalisation of land use in Coigach. Specifically, there was a large farm at Achiltibuie and Badenscallie which was densely packed with small tenants. The tacksmen of this farm, who had held it on lease since 1838, were 'complaining so loudly of their sub-tenants' that Lady Stafford agreed to terminate the lease. At the same time, she was advised that the small tenants, some ninety families in all, were unable 'beneficially either to themselves or the Proprietor from want of Capital to stock the hill ground'.

The factor persuaded most of the people to relinquish their hill grazings and resettle on lots at Badentarbat. However, there remained a hard core of eighteen families who refused to budge. In Scott's angry words, the recalcitrant 'stirred up all the other people in their Townships to resist the removings in any way or under any modification whatever'. Scott wanted urgently to reorganise the Coigach grazings. He remarked that 'were they not burdened with so dense a population, they undoubtedly would be worth more rent than at present they are let for'. It was a classic Highland scene: the existing tenants were not able to pay the going rent and the landlord was financially frustrated by their immobility. But the people were in possession and would obstruct any change.

Lady Stafford found herself in a quandary – she had
contemplated the sale of some of the land in order to repair her
crippled finances. But even this course was blocked by the sitting
tenantry. It was clear that any potential capitalist buyer would be
loath to invest:

> seeing the Lot tenants are so numerous on that portion of the Barony,
> and are besides so turbulent and evil-disposed that a person induced to
> invest money in land might fear he would not be able to keep
> possession or get his rent paid.

The rights of property were under threat. Additionally, the estate
managers entertained high hopes of letting the shootings at
Coigach to sportsmen, to usefully add £400 per annum to the
otherwise stagnant rental. Several interested parties for the
shootings had been identified in the south, but each specified
awkward requirements concerning the removal of common stock.
The Cromartie estate was thwarted at all turns. In February 1853
Andrew Scott reported dejectedly:

> I am sorry to say Lord Dupplin [a prospective tenant] has given up
> thought of taking the Coigach shootings because he could not have a
> Hill on the Farm of Inverpolly cleared of Stock.

At every turn the landlord's financial interests were obstructed by
the presence of a super-abundant, uneconomic and recalcitrant
tenantry. The small tenantry had suffered badly in the recent
famine and had been relieved by the landlord through their
difficulties. Scott's proposal to clear the remaining eighteen families
at Achiltibuie and Badenscallie was, evidently, an attempt to gain a
reasonable return from one section of the land at Coigach.
Nevertheless the effort was sufficient to raise a furious resistance
among the ordinary people.

The actual opposition replayed the recurrent pattern of
Highland resistance. First, the officers serving the writs of removal
were met by a large body of people (many of them women); their
papers were destroyed, and they were packed off in a decidedly
humiliated state. Several such incidents followed and Scott
exclaimed: 'As no punishment followed on the back of these lawless

proceedings . . . I am persuaded the people think they may do anything they please short of destroying life.' Scott was much alarmed: the continuing resistance endangered the rule of law and order, and it also implied a general threat to the exercise of landlord property rights. Another attempt to shift the Coigach people was made in February 1853; this time the officer was comprehensively humiliated:

The summonses were forcibly taken from him and destroyed and himself grossly maltreated though fortunately without any serious injury to his person . . . The officer was entirely stripped of his clothes by these rebels, and was put into the Boat in which he went to Coigach in a state of absolute nudity.

The landlord and the authorities were now fixed in a dilemma. The local police force was obviously inadequate for the business of executing the clearance; it was possible to bring reinforcements from Glasgow but, even then, success could not be guaranteed. The landlord faced a choice: the military could be called in, which would inevitably attract highly undesirable publicity, or the clearance could be abandoned, which would constitute a capitulation by the landlord.

The managers of the Cromartie property were at their wits' end. Lady Stafford wanted the full force of the law to be employed against what she termed 'the refractory people'. Andrew Scott also urged the strongest action, and the Edinburgh legal adviser to the family advocated securing 'submission . . . first . . . and a proper demonstration of authority'.

In these inflamed circumstances James Loch, the Sutherland commissioner, intervened to restrain both Scott and Lady Stafford. Loch, of course, had presided over much larger clearances in Sutherland thirty years before. Loch had no direct responsibility in the Coigach affair but recommended conciliation. His advice guided the inexperienced Staffords into a position which was defensible in terms of prevailing public opinion.

Loch, true to his old principles, was critical of Scott's failure to provide adequate resettlement facilities for the sub-tenants who were to be removed at Coigach. It had always been a cardinal principle of the Sutherland clearances that every evicted tenant should be offered a coastal lot, some timber, some free trenching on the new lots, remission of arrears and a period of rent-free occupation for their new lots. Scott's preparations for the Coigach removals fell a long way short of these high standards. Loch concurred in the view that the law ought to be upheld but, he pointed out:

> One must consider well when you have got troops that hesitate to fight, and it must be well considered what your case is to go to the public on, if a resistance is the result.

The troops, he implied, would have no stomach for putting down Highland peasants threatened with eviction. Loch also rejected the idea that a visit to Coigach by the proprietor, Lord Stafford, would calm the situation: Stafford had no personal or hereditary influence among the Coigach people; worse still, he was English; and the family connection with the Sutherlands was even more embarrassing.

A final effort to serve the writs on the Coigach people was made in March 1853 with identical results. Once more the Sheriff's party was put to flight by a large body of people, mainly women. Although it was thought that another effort might be made in the following year, the Coigach clearance was, in the event, now abandoned. The entire affair had been the subject of a great deal of polemical discussion in many of the Scottish newspapers, especially from the pen of David Ross. There developed a public debate on the morality of landlords' pursuit of clearance policies, whatever the state of the law. It was a debate which questioned the very basis of landowning and caused grave disquiet among estate administrators. James Loch, a sober and much experienced observer of public opinion in the Highlands, felt that Highland society was in turmoil, even running out of control. He said despairingly:

> There is a prevalent feeling over all the West Coast, north and south, that the landlords are not cognisant of what is going on in their names, and that the Government are not serious in their desire to enforce the law.

At Coigach, therefore, the landlord found that the local resources of law and order were too weak to execute the clearance. There was also a weakening of the landlord's nerve: the fear of public opprobrium frightened him into surrender. Only two years before, the Duke of Sutherland had been enraged by a bungled attempt at clearance on his own estate in neighbouring Assynt, when the factors had arranged to clear people from Elphin and Knockan either to the coast or to take free passages to America. In fact the removal was resisted by the people who became 'very violent – quite proud of their illegal conduct, and not one of them would admit they did wrong'. When told of the events, the Duke expressed his anger with the local factor for having misled him about the probable consequences, and forbade any further action against the people. The Coigach events of 1852–3, though more violent than those of Assynt, followed an almost identical sequence, with the same outcome.

Underlying the attitude of landed proprietors was a fear of Highland radicalism and also a widening sensitivity to public opinion. Conversely there was also a developing confidence among the crofters, and the episodes at Elphin, Knockan and Coigach were part of a continuum of crofter resistance which was increasingly encouraged both in radical and respectable newspapers and in pamphlets. These events in the early 1850s were a distant prelude to the 'Crofters' War' of the 1880s, when resistance to Highland lairds became much more sustained and better co-ordinated. But, despite these omens, the most important element in the Coigach story was the fact that the landowner was not prepared (or strong willed enough) to weather the storm of public abuse that was raised against her clearance. The people of Coigach had defeated the richest and most powerful family in the Highlands.

Notes

1 Henry Cockburn, *Circuit Journeys* (1888) p. 67.

2 Quoted in Macdonald, *Lewis*, op. cit., p. 164.

3 Mitchell, *Reminiscences I*, chapter xxxi.

4 See Chapter 12.

5 John Munro Mackenzie, *Diary, 1851* (Stornoway, 1994), p. 9.

6 Ibid., p. 32.

7 Ibid.

8 J.I. Little, op. cit., pp. 22–5.

9 See Devine, *Clanship*, op. cit., pp. 64–5.

10 Mitchell, *Reminiscences I*, p. 301, p. 257.

11 Ibid., II. p. 19.

12 Camille Dressler, *Eigg: The Story of an Island* (1998), p. 68.

13 Mitchell, *Reminiscences I*, pp. 55–7.

14 See Richards, *Patrick Sellar*, op. cit., chapter 10.

15 SCRO, D593/K/Findlater to Duke of Sutherland, 4 September 1841.

16 Ibid.

17 Wylie, *Disruption Worthies*, p. 66.

18 SCRO, D593/K/Anderson to Loch, 2 August 1841.

19 See Richards, *Leviathan*, pp. 250–2.

20 This section draws upon Richards and Clough, *Cromartie*, passim. See also Eric Richards, 'Problems on the Cromartie Estate, 1851–3', *SHR*, vol. 52 (1973), pp. 149–64.

16

Landlords Unrestrained: Knoydart and Greenyards

I. Power and opinion

SOME HIGHLAND LAIRDS WERE keenly responsive to public opinion. The Sutherland family in mid-century was close to the Royal Family (Lady Stafford became Lady-in-Waiting to the Queen) and was at the very centre of liberal aristocratic society in London. They entertained Garibaldi and Harriet Beecher Stowe and conspicuously supported humanitarian causes through the middle decades of the century. They had become sensitive to the good opinion of mid-Victorian England and were in no mood to sully their reputations with further embarrassing rancour from the Highlands. Other proprietors were no less squeamish of protest and unpopularity and blenched at the idea of estate rationalisation, regardless of their continuing financial losses.

The editor of the *Inverness Courier*, Robert Carruthers (1799–1878), was said to have prevented a series of clearances in Ross-shire in 1844 by drawing the facts to the attention of the government which then dissuaded the erring landlord from his intended action. But there is no reliable evidence of this claim nor of the government's taking any positive role at any time in the course of the Highland clearances.[1] There were always men in the Highlands who were prepared to wear the badge of oppression in the pursuit of economic returns on their lands. Malcolm of Poltalloch, unlike his forbears, was fully prepared to risk riot and obloquy when he forced though a clearance at Arichonan on his Argyllshire properties in Knapdale in 1848, famine or not. He also tried to coerce some of his small tenantry to emigrate to one of the least hospitable spots in settled Australia, though they fortunately resisted this fate. The Malcolm family, described as 'the Croesus of Argyll', had brought spectacular colonial profits into Argyllshire and spent much of it on large building and improvement programmes in which were incorporated extremely unpopular clearances.[2]

At the very moment of the landlord's capitulation at Coigach there were much more notorious examples of clearances executed on both sides of the Highlands. These were brazened through, despite a great rage of abuse from the general public and the newspapers. The government certainly ignored the infamous events at Knoydart.

II. *Macdonnell of Glengarry and Knoydart*

The Knoydart clearances, executed in late 1853 in Glenelg on the west coast of Inverness-shire, took place in a blaze of publicity which influenced the course, but not the outcome, of the episode. The Knoydart people, like those in Lewis, were under landlord pressure to accept clearance on to emigration ships. According to one observer, their resolution not to co-operate was encouraged by the sympathetic publicity in the *Scotsman* and *The Times*. The Knoydart case belonged to the category of clearances marked by the extreme poverty of both the landlord and the people, and by the fact that the landlord offered the crofters relatively liberal conditions on which to depart the estate. The financial cost to him was equivalent to many years' rent.

Knoydart was the last remnant of the properties of the Macdonnells of Glengarry. At the end of the eighteenth century the population of the estate had been close to a thousand, even though Canada had already attracted away many of its people for several decades. There had been large-scale evictions in Knoydart as early as 1764 and 1786,[3] and by 1850 its population was still above 900. The financial difficulties of the estate had been acute for more than ten years before the new evictions.

The cause of the financial chaos, everyone agreed, was

proprietorial extravagance on the part of Macdonnell of Glengarry, fifteenth of that name. This was the most 'colourful' of Highland dynasties: Glengarry was said to have murdered his gamekeeper and committed several bloody assaults but celebrated his patriarchal charisma with grand Highland gatherings at Invergarry each year. The estate had extended more than fifty miles, from Loch Oich to the west coast of Knoydart. Despite great clearances on the estate the Glengarry apparently remained popular: the war-like Alister Ronaldson was the prototype for Fergus Mac-Ivor in *Waverley*. He had succeeded to a considerable inheritance but had squandered it. Glengarry may have been immortalised in the work of Sir Walter Scott, but Henry Cockburn was highly critical. He wrote that Macdonnell had been:

> a fine specimen of the chieftain. But none knew better than Scott that he was a paltry and odious fellow, with all the vices of a bad chieftain and none of the virtues of a good one; with the selfishness, cruelty, fraud, arrogant pretension and base meanness of the one, without the fidelity to superiors, and the generosity to vassals, the hospitality, or the courage of the other.[4]

Another evaluation of Macdonnell was equally scathing:

> His ambition was to be a Highland Chief of the olden time, so far as that could be attained under modern conditions. Glengarry moved about with a body of retainers, which constituted his 'tail'. He was eager for a leading place among his contemporaries. Though he possessed talent and many kindly qualities, his overbearing temper led him repeatedly into difficulties, and his careless expenditure far exceeded his income.[5]

Rambunctious to excess, he died after jumping on to rocks from a steamer in 1828.

When the squanderer died, there was a spectacular Highland funeral. The estate and its vast debts were inherited by Aeneas, sixteenth chief of Glengarry. He was then ten years old and his estate was under trust. The young Glengarry had been reared to lairdship and paraded in the full regalia; he was to be the very model of the chief. 'He was dressed in full Highland costume with eagles' pinions in his bonnet, covered with crepe.'[6] But in 1840 he was forced to sell off all his Highland properties, except for Knoydart, to Lord Ward. The young Glengarry, 'a respectable young man', according to Cockburn, emigrated to Australia in the hope of retrieving his finances. He returned a broken man in 1842 to his old home in Inverie, but died in June of that year. His own heir was also a minor, and the vestigial estate was now precariously balanced on the brink of bankruptcy; his mother, Mrs Josephine Macdonnell, acted as managing curator, while Messrs McKenzie and Baillie were retained as agents of the estate.[7]

Though none had starved, the people of the estate suffered both from the effects of the potato famine and from the migration of the herring out of Loch Nevis. Their most elementary subsistence was in doubt from year to year. The people of Knoydart were crofters and small tenants, together with squatters who paid no rent at all, and constituted, in the words of Sir John McNeill, 'a parasitical population'. The nominal rent of the estate was £250 per annum but little or no rent had been paid for several years; arrears of £1500 had accumulated by the start of 1853. In these circumstances, asserted the estate managers, there was a clear choice – either the property could be surrendered to the crofters from whom no economic rent could be extracted, or the people must be removed to make way for tenants who would pay the rent. Later it was alleged that the real motive for the eviction was to rid the estate of the burden of poor relief, though this was hotly denied.

III. Clearances and emigration

Heavily encumbered with debts, the Knoydart estate administrators moved to clear the people and pass the land over to sheep farmers. In the spring of 1853 the people were summonsed to be off the land by Whitsunday of that year. This action was entirely legal, and the proprietor had no further obligation beyond the proper delivery of notice. Nevertheless (perhaps for fear of public outcry) the landlord offered all the people free passages to Canada or Australia; he also forgave all arrears and there would be no confiscation of property. Four hundred people accepted these terms. The costs of the scheme were great: clothing, bedding and passages amounted to £1700, which the landlord borrowed under the Emigration Advances Act of 1853. Mrs Macdonnell was credited with great efforts for the comfort of the emigrants. But when the ship, the *Sillery*, arrived, only 332 of the people embarked. They disembarked in Canada on 7 September 1853, and the authorities reported:

> They are a fine, healthy body of emigrants. They received a free passage as far as Montreal, and were allowed each 10 lbs oatmeal on leaving the ship; and owing to the increasing demand for labourers of all description throughout the province, they cannot fail to do well.[8]

These Knoydart emigrants were, in this last respect, more fortunate than previous groups of migrants who happened to arrive (in Canada and Australia) at times when the local labour markets were already awash with excess labour. So far, the Knoydart clearance was a calm landlord success.

The *Sillery* did not convey all the people who had originally agreed to the terms of the removal. A handful of sick families were permitted to remain on the estate for the time being, but additionally:

> Some families . . . refused to embark, though not prevented by any [. . . specific . . .] cause, and continued to occupy the houses which they had been duly summonsed to vacate at Whitsunday.

Thus a small rump of unco-operative tenants remained, preventing the completion of the clearance plan. The estate moved to eliminate the last small remnants of the traditional population. It was, in effect, the final act in the long drama of the Glengarry exoduses which had begun many decades previously.

New legal summonses against these people were executed in August 1853. In this phase, the Sheriff's party pulled down the houses without resistance. Most of the people thus dispossessed gained refuge with friends, or in other cottages, but a number (between twenty and thirty) erected temporary shelters of blankets, and simply refused to shift. The officers then demolished these blanket dwellings, in a concerted effort to prise the squatters off the estate. But still they remained.

Soon distressing accounts of these events were circulated in the press, which, according to Sir John McNeill, had the effect of 'exciting public sympathy on their behalf, and public odium against the curators'. As for the people, 'the countenance and assistance they received very naturally encouraged them in their passive resistance to the law.' The curators of the estate renewed the earlier inducements to the people: they were offered free travel to Inverness, or Glasgow, or Fort William, or to any other place in Scotland, as well as free lodgings until the following April; they were also given full compensation for their crops. These terms were meant to persuade the people to get out without further bother, while guaranteeing that the landlord would not be charged with causing destitution among them. Few landlords in the rest of Britain felt the need to use such kid gloves when it came to a change of tenancy. Nevertheless the people once more rejected the offer.

In November 1853 the law was again pressed into action against the residual Knoydart folk. This time there were widespread allegations of culpable violence perpetrated by the evicting party. There were several versions of these controversial events and they show the distortions to which the record was always prey.

In his report, following enquires into these matters, Sir John McNeill, Chairman of the Board of Supervision for the Relief of the Poor in Scotland, discounted the stories of violence, but admitted that

> there is reason to believe that at least one premature birth occurred shortly after those proceedings; and there can be no doubt that the result was a considerable amount of suffering and much excitement.

Further controversy over the role of the Board of Supervision in the Knoydart events broadened into a general attack on the administration of poor relief in the Highlands. A local proprietor, Edward Ellice, Liberal MP for St Andrews, pursued the matter with great tenacity, claiming that the entire clearance at Knoydart had been motivated by a desire to avoid poor rates. He cited several specific examples of extreme suffering. Sir John McNeill reported that he was unable to find any substantiation of Ellice's claims, which he described as misinformed; he found further that the main reason for the Knoydart clearance was the desire of the landlord 'to recover possession of the land occupied by tenants who paid little or no rent, for the purpose of letting it to tenants who would pay rent'. He reported that the incoming sheep farmers had augmented the estate rental by £166 a year.[9]

Sir John McNeill's account of the Knoydart evictions is sometimes regarded as partial because his purpose was to defend the Board of Supervision's administration of the Poor Law. His words were in total contrast to those of many other commentators, of whom W.H. Murray serves as a recent example:

Josephine MacDonnell cleared the remaining humans to make way for sheep, her purpose being to enhance the value of her property before selling it to a Lowland ironmaster. Four hundred people were evicted by force from Airor, Doune, Sandaig, and Inverie. Their holdings were destroyed, and the people driven like cattle aboard a waiting transport supplied by the British government.[10]

IV. Corroboration

Contemporary newspaper reports, fortunately, provided an extensive check on the Knoydart controversy as it emerged in the last months of 1853. Though they contain inconsistencies – for instance, about the precise number of migrants and the level of arrears – the general picture emerges clearly. *The Times'* own correspondent reported that sixty people who had originally agreed to move actually refused to go, and they had then been given forty-eight hours' notice to quit. At that point the evicting party set to work:

The scene was now a truly painful one. So long as there was hope of being left with a covering over their heads the cottars were comparatively quiet, but now that they were homeless many of them became frantic with grief, and were driven to seek shelter in some of the neighbouring quarries, where some are now living, and others among the caves of the rocks with which this wild district of the Highlands abounds.

There was a real danger of starvation among these fugitive people since they had not been accepted on the Poor Roll. *The Times* observed that wool and sheep prices were very buoyant, but that the recent repeal of the Corn Laws had made the prospects for arable production virtually hopeless in such a marginal region. 'It is thus clear that the Highlands will all become sheep walks and shooting grounds before long', and future clearances were likely to be less liberal than those of Knoydart. The northern reporter asked, rhetorically, what was the moral responsibility of the Highland landowner, who gained by the change, to 'the chief sufferers by these transitions'? A letter to the editor remarked sharply, 'Sheep farmers are now becoming so valuable that it will pay our English sheep farmers to hire ships at any time, to pay for the removal of all who stand in their way.'[11]

In October 1853 the *Scotsman* also sent its reporter to Knoydart, where he found the evicted people huddled in flimsy shelters. The estate had meantime been converted into four large sheep farms and the former population of 606 (in 1847) had been reduced to sixteen families. The arrears had reached £2300 – partly because Glengarry had forgone all rents for the duration of the famine and thus allegedly encouraged the people into slack habits.[12] As economic conditions improved slightly, after the worst days of the famine, the people had offered to redeem some of their arrears, but the factors had refused to accept their money. There had been confusion about the destination of the people: in April Mrs Macdonnell had told them that they were to go to Australia, but in June they learned that Canada was to be their new home. At first it was not known that the offer applied equally to the cottars. The emigration removals had begun on 2 August, and within four days the people had been ferried to Isle Ornsay, whence the *Sillery* departed on 9 August – 'leaving the last miserable remnant of Clanranald to suffer eviction from their houses at the instance of the head of the clan'. It was on 22 August that the Knoydart managers began the ejection of these people. The *Scotsman*'s reporter was persuaded that these people had never agreed to emigrate. Five of the families were allowed to remain, for reasons of humanity, but the remaining sixteen families were expelled, and twelve houses were destroyed in the process. The people were exposed to bad weather.

The latest eviction continued over several days:

> On the third evening, when returning to Inverie, the factor's party came upon a small boat house erected on the shore, at Doune, which they had overlooked. In this the ejected families had huddled at night, for two nights, not daring to put up any artificial shelter. Fire was immediately applied to the roof, and the structure burned down. This completed the work of destruction, and eleven families were left absolutely without shelter – for unfortunately for them the coast of Knoydart has no caves in which protection from at least the rain might be found.

They then spent more than a month exposed to the weather, living under blanket constructions which were repeatedly overturned by the evictors on the specific orders of the manager. They were pursued relentlessly, and winter approached.[13]

Most of the subsequent controversy related to the fate of these people, rather more than sixty of them, who were being hounded about the Knoydart estate during the final months of 1853. The *Scotsman* examined several individual cases and produced vivid detail of the extreme wretchedness. The reporter castigated the proprietor for trying to shift them onto the charity of other landowners. He criticised the Parochial Board for its inactivity, and blamed the people themselves for their indolence. There had been no good reason for the clearance in the first instance because, he contended, the crofters could have produced better rents than the sheep farmers – but the estate management was inert, and the people had never been properly motivated.[14] It is evident from these reports that by the end of October 1853 many of the temporary dwellings of the Knoydart folk had been demolished four or five times. The agent would not permit them to erect tents for the winter. He announced:

> my clients commiserate as much as any one to the hardships to which the poor people of Knoydart have exposed themselves. They willingly agree not only to pay the expense of conveying the parties with their families to the county town of Inverness, or to any town where work is abundant, but also to supply them with the means of engaging suitable lodgings for the earlier months of the winter.

The *Northern Ensign* claimed that the people were too feeble to move seventy miles, and that there was little chance of employment as well as every danger of fever and cholera in Inverness. 'To offer to pay the expense of getting the people away from Knoydart, and landed in Inverness, is scarcely better than offering to pay for powder and balls if anyone should agree to shoot the victims!'[15] They would become beggars and paupers in the town.

The same newspaper, a powerful advocate of their cause, described one of the evicted men as 'a prize specimen of a Highlander', who had been presented to George IV in Edinburgh in 1823; he had passed a blameless life, and was now a widower of fifty-four with four children, reduced to living like an animal in a hovel.[16] At the end of November 1853 the local Catholic priest provided an acre of land for the erection of the tents which Donald Ross had brought from Glasgow.

In the midst of so many reports of the plight of the remnant of the Knoydart community, the *Scotsman* published an account from one of the migrants who had chosen to take the free passage to Canada a few months before. He testified to the pleasure of the journey, and his success since arriving:

> They are all very kind people in Canada, and at home one would not believe how well to do they are all in circumstances . . . Tell all the young men about Inverie that they are in the dark stopping there when they can get such good pay here, and all ready cash . . . I need not mention the prices of victuals . . . but a bottle of good whisky can be got for fivepence.[17]

In February 1854 the remaining Knoydart people were still in their tents; they had experienced extreme hardship during that winter: one man among them was said to have become deranged.[18] The final stage in the Knoydart story occurred in May 1854. The landlord now moved to evict those families who had been allowed to stay till spring 'for motives of charity'. A medical officer accompanied the party to ensure the health of those to be evicted. As the *Scotsman* pointed out, no one wanted these people because they would become a public burden wherever they went. It noted also that 'The gentlemen to whose extensive sheep walks are added the lands left vacant by the expatriation of last year must not give a house or shelter to any of the evicted people; a prohibition of this cruel nature is in their leases.'[19]

The final eviction at Knoydart prompted Edward Ellice MP to renew his attacks on the entire system of poor relief in the Highlands while the Board of Supervision produced counter evidence of the efforts made by the officials to relieve the Knoydart victims, even 'beyond what the Statutes required'.[20]

V. *Poverty and wealth*

Whatever the cause of poverty and human wretchedness in Knoydart during these years, and whatever the moral responsibility, there is no doubt that, in the wake of the clearances, there remained a group of pathetic human beings, living in appalling squalor, unattended by either landlord or Poor Law. Even the conservative *Inverness Courier* exclaimed that 'such scenes bring disgrace on the Highlands of Scotland'. In June 1854 it described the home of Kate MacPhee, aged fifty-four, who was living near the Manse of Inverie:

The place in which Kate lived was nine or ten feet long, five or six feet broad, and three feet in height. It was made up of branches of trees, brackens, and rags, and covered with a piece of canvas and an old Scotch blanket, fixed by cords and wooden pins. There was a sort of porch or entrance on the east side of the hovel, made of larchwood and divots. This door was barely sufficient to admit a full sized person, and then only by going on hands and feet and crawling in, which I had to do when I went in. As to the condition of the interior, a brood of young rats was found in Kate's bed when she was removed. Such was the wretched place in which this poor woman took her abode and lived throughout the whole of the late tempestuous winter.[21]

Ten months later the district still had thirty-eight paupers, almost all of them women – one of them more than a hundred years old, five in their nineties, three in their eighties, and fifteen in their seventies. Between them they had received a total of £96 in annual sustentation from the parochial funds. They represented the human wreckage left behind by the storm of famine and clearance; and by the greater longevity of women over men.[22]

A few years later the Knoydart estate was sold to James Baird (1802–76), who acquired a property now unencumbered by a pauperised tenantry. Baird was a hugely successful Lowland coal and ironmaster, leader of one of the great enterprises of Scotland's industrial revolution. His family bought landed estates to the value of £1 115 000 in the years 1853–63, including Knoydart for £90 000.[23] Many of the outgoing Glengarry family's effects were sold off at an auction at Invergarry – some cattle, a few goats, five ponies, some farming implements, 'several dozens of superior wine, a superior pleasure barge made of Glengarry oak, etc.' The local reporter noted that 'the young Chief of Glengarry, who appears to have little of the feudal ambition which was at once a source of pride and pain to his father, is now studying law in Edinburgh.' The last of the Glengarrys were farewelled from the native glens by the local gentlemen and small tenants, and the newspaper reported, surprisingly, that 'never was there a lady of Mrs Macdonnell's rank and station in the country, so respected and beloved by the tenantry, and all who had the honour of her acquaintance.' The agony of the clearances had served to pave the way for the easy entry of a Lowland entrepreneur seeking peace and sport away from the hurly-burly of southern industry.

When the county historian of Inverness, J. Cameron Lees, looked back over the events of Knoydart from the perspective of the 1890s, he was prepared to acknowledge that the clearances may have been to the ultimate benefit of the people themselves – they had been given the opportunity of exchanging Highland poverty for Canadian progress and prosperity. He maintained, however:

> That it was not to promote their comfort that they were sent away, but too often to satisfy the greed of those who disposed of them, and in not a few instances they were evicted from lands fertile enough to have sustained them in comparative comfort.[24]

Yet this last assumption ran counter to all the evidence of famine and deprivation in the 1840s. Although conditions in the Highlands improved significantly after 1852, the phrase 'comparative comfort' was rarely an apt term for the general state of the small tenants of the region.

As for the landlord, the post-clearance rent increases were not especially lucrative, but there were considerable capital gains which affected the value of all Highland properties in the middle decades of the century. For instance the lands which the eccentric and erratic Lord Ward had bought in Glengarry in 1840 for £90 000 were resold in 1860 for £120 000 – to Edward Ellice, who had campaigned so vigorously on behalf of the people of Knoydart in 1853–5.[25] The sale was much welcomed in the glen. Lord Ward had made little improvement, and had regarded his Highland estate chiefly as a shooting ground and a place of seasonal residence. Ellice himself was a comparative newcomer. He was the only son of an English family which had settled in Aberdeenshire; the family's money had been made mainly in the Hudson's Bay Company, and in land trading in North America. The family had bought Glenquoich, had lived lavishly, and entertained more than a thousand guests a year. Of Edward Ellice it was said in an obituary:

> He loved the Highlands, and at Invergarry on Loch Oich built a house of extraordinary comfort in a situation which combined all the beauties of mountain, water and woods. He did all in his power to improve the dwellings of his tenantry, and by plantations, fencing and roadmaking did much for their comfort. He knew personally everyone who lived on his estates, and had great influence with them.[26]

VI. 'The slaughter at Greenyards': Spring 1854

The concentration of major clearances in 1853–4 at Sollas, Suishnish, Coigach and Knoydart entailed such large dislocations of people that they could not have passed unnoticed. The scale and intensity of publicity about the Highland Clearances of 1853–4 was unequalled and owed much to the vigour of the journalists in the north.

As a climax to these events came the events at Greenyards in Strathcarron, Easter Ross (about five miles from Bonar Bridge), in the spring of 1854 – the most dramatic of all the clearances. The people who created such a sensation at Greenyards were encouraged by the indignation provoked by the recent Knoydart episode, as well as the widely celebrated success of the Coigach folk from which the Greenyards people drew confidence and courage. But, obversely, the defeat of the law at Coigach, and the humiliation heaped upon both the landlord and the police, caused the authorities to redouble their determination to reassert the full rule of the law. In the outcome, Greenyards was the last great confrontation and the last great clearance before 'the Crofters' War' of the 1880s.

Most subsequent accounts of the Greenyards affair derive from the eloquent but melodramatic descriptions which Donald Ross later republished as a pamphlet entitled 'The Massacre of the Rosses'. Ross was eyewitness to some of the episodes; his transparent purpose was to rouse public opinion against the landlords of the Highlands. Ross's anger led him into hyperbole which naturally places his credibility at risk. There are, however, two other sources to set beside his version of the events at Greenyards in 1854.

The *Inverness Courier*, a sober but relatively independent newspaper of the day, was unlikely to exaggerate the turmoil at Greenyards. It observed that the proprietor of Greenyards had given notice to the people of their removal, which would be executed in late March and early April 1854. The evictor was Major Robertson of Kindeace, who had achieved notoriety in 1845 for the Glencalvie evictions (see Chapter 2). The opposition to the eviction was greater than had been anticipated. The *Courier* reported that Sheriff Taylor and his party of about thirty-five men travelled in the night from Tain and arrived at Greenyards at dawn. They had been expected – a crowd of about 300 (two-thirds of them women) assembled from the surrounding district, 'all apparently prepared to resist the execution of the law'. The people aligned themselves in the formation common in such episodes:

> The women stood in front armed with stones, and the men occupied the background, all or nearly all furnished with sticks.

The Sheriff addressed the people to persuade them of the futility of any resistance. Some of the women tried to grab him, and in the process assaulted him. Cummings, Superintendent of the Ross-shire police, also attempted to reason with the people but without success. At that point, said the *Courier*, the Sheriff was 'reluctantly obliged to employ force'. The police were led into the heart of the crowd; there was a short, sharp skirmish and they dispersed. The Sheriff then served the summonses on four tenants. It was during this incident that violence occurred:

> The women, as they bore the brunt of the battle, were the principal sufferers. A large number of them – fifteen or sixteen, we believe – were seriously hurt, and of these several are under medical treatment; one woman, we believe, still lies in a precarious condition. The policemen appear to have used their batons with great force, but they escaped themselves almost unhurt. They tried to apprehend some of the ringleaders, but the men had fled and all they caught were some of the wounded women. They were imprisoned in Tain but released on bail next day.[27]

These newspaper reports of the Greenyards events created a sensation in Scotland. They were greatly refuelled by the passionate and detailed accounts in Donald Ross's letters to the press, although his florid style caused many contemporaries to be sceptical. He wrote an open letter to the Lord Advocate, chief law officer in Scotland, in which he demanded an enquiry into 'the slaughter at Greenyards'. He said that the eviction concerned twenty-two families who were the residue of the much greater population which had been cleared in the name of the octogenarian landlord, the notorious Major Robertson of Kindeace. The people were sub-tenants of a tacksman named Munro. The people's record was stainless; nor were they a penny in arrears. Some of the menfolk of Greenyards were currently serving in the 93rd Regiment at Sebastopol in the Crimean War. This community was under notice of removal to make way for sheep. It was a replay, in almost every detail, of the clearances perpetrated in the time of the Napoleonic Wars.

Ross elaborated his allegation in vivid terms, relating that there had been high tension on the estate for some time and there was already a record of resistance. The people of Greenyards had been aware of a likely summons: on a previous occasion the law officer who had attempted to deliver the notice had been stopped, searched and had his papers burned before his eyes. This had been a standard tactic in Highland resistance since the turn of the century. But the law officer had not been hurt, nor further intimidated. Subsequently there had been a bizarre incident in which a group of drunken gangers had impersonated law officers and feigned the identity of a removal party as an elaborate prank. During the confrontation a pistol had been drawn by one of the gangers, but he had been persuaded to desist. When 'the jest' was discovered the men were despatched out of the district – but again without injury or humiliation – even though they later claimed that they had been stripped naked and carried shoulder high out of the property. This incident, said Ross, had helped to compound the tension among, as well as against, the police, whose purpose was to quieten the district. Ross then claimed that the police had filled themselves with ale, porter and whisky before they reached Greenyards on the morning of 31 March, and that 'they brought with them, to near Greenyards, large baskets full of alcoholic liquors, of which they drank copiously before they made their savage onslaught on the poor females'.[28]

In Ross's account of the events of 31 March he said that the police party was met at a pass leading to Greenyards by about sixty-five women, a dozen men, and a lot of boys and girls who were spectators. The Sheriff instructed the people to get out of the way – in English, even though he knew Gaelic perfectly well. He did not read the Riot Act. The people did not move immediately and the police were ordered to move in – 'with the full force of their batons on the skulls of the women', who were knocked to the ground and then further beaten while in that position. Ross continued:

> Such was the brutality with which this tragedy was carried through, that more than twenty females were carried off the field in blankets and litters; and the appearance they presented, with their heads cut and bruised, their limbs mangled, and their clothes clotted with blood, was such as would horrify any savage.

Four or five of the wounded, claimed Ross, were in danger of their lives, and two were past all recovery when Ross saw them a month later. The women had held no weapons or staves, nor had they made any move. In typically graphic terms Ross wrote:

> Such indeed was the sad havoc made on these females on the banks of the Carron . . . that pools of blood were on the ground – that the grass and earth were dyed red with it – that the dogs of the district came and licked up the blood.

Ross had seen the bloodied clothes of the women in which:

> there are also pieces, or patches of the skin, which the police with their batons stript off the heads and shoulders of the women when they were beating them.

After the conflict four of the wounded women were captured and, despite their bloody state, were handcuffed together and taken to jail in Tain. They were released on bail the following day. Meanwhile the victorious police returned to the tacksman's house to drink more whisky.[29]

VII. *The official account*

Ross's account was received with some incredulity in the Scottish press but a third version of events has survived. The law officers were nervous of the legal repercussions of their involvement in the episode and they preserved a running commentary on the events as they unfolded. Their purpose was utterly at odds with the motives of Donald Ross. There was, indeed, a danger that the Greenyards affair would be raised in the House of Commons, and the legal officers involved in the action were careful to prepare full and detailed reports to the Lord Advocate. One letter, full of the immediacy of the events, was written to the Sheriff of Ross and Cromarty (who was 'happy to report that the expedition has proved successful') by his substitute, Taylor, within a couple of hours of the actual fracas.

Taylor penned his report from Ardgay Inn, at 9 a.m. He said that the eviction party had rendezvoused at 5 a.m. and proceeded to within two miles of Greenyards by carriages. They then marched quickly in order to surprise the people, 'but we soon heard shots from different quarters, which we knew were fired as signals of our approach'. They observed many people converging on Greenyards. On the arrival of the police party, the people were already assembled:

> They raised quite a clamour of voices, all vociferating at once. I tried to obtain silence, told them who we were, and required them to allow us to pass and to disperse quietly; but my voice was quite drowned, and the crowd made towards us in a menacing way, when the police were ordered to clear the road, and then began a regular skirmish, in which the women used their sticks and were assisted by a number of the men. But the police likewise used their batons vigorously, and seeing and feeling that we were in earnest, the mob soon gave way and began to make their escape in all directions. We had thus the way open, and proceeded without further molestation to the cottages, and had the citations duly served.

The police tried in vain to capture some of the men, but caught only five of the women. One of the women was badly hurt and a doctor was sent for, by express. The others were not so badly hurt. 'I think the people have had such a lesson today as will effectually prevent a recurrence of the lawless deforcement of the officers of the law in this quarter.' Taylor estimated that the crowd numbered 300; he believed that they had been secretly forewarned of the police plans – 'and consequently they assembled in force last night and had been watching throughout the night for us.'[30]

Sheriff Mackenzie outlined the background, saying that there had been a series of outrages (thereby partially confirming Ross's account). Three weeks before the fracas at Greenyards the premises of a new tenant had been set afire and 'forty head of cattle besides horses were destroyed'. An officer had been sent to Greenyards to execute a summons of removing on four subtenants. The people had anticipated the visit and fifty or sixty had collected, and 'stripped him naked, seized and burned his papers, and finally marched him out of the district. A police officer who happened to go to the place at the time was similarly maltreated.'[31] All this was fully reported and a precognition had been taken. Major Robertson said that it would be pusillanimous to give way to reckless violence;

he called for the law to be fully enforced. Taylor had pointed out that a small force would be useless:

> It is, I think, high time to put an effectual stop to these lawless deforcements – for which this County has now an enviable notoriety. And I shall regret if energetic steps be not taken for that purpose in this instance, which appears to have nothing in it in the way of hardship to the people to enlist public sympathy.

In accord with these opinions a plan was mounted to implement the eviction and also 'to apprehend the ringleaders of the previous deforcement'. Taylor learned that the people of the strath kept a watch day and night, with never less than forty at the ready. An excise officer who had fallen into their hands had been able to extricate himself only by showing his pistol. Taylor's plan had been designed to surprise the people and so avoid a large confrontation. However the *Inverness Advertiser* had thwarted this ploy by publishing a report that the police party was being readied; the newspaper also reminded the public that 'the parish of Kincardine was famous for its resistance to officers of the law'. (This was a reference to the events of the 1790s, 1820s and 1845.) Sheriff Mackenzie described the author of the article as 'this Free Church paper writer' and said that it was an incitement to rebellion.

Having outlined the origins of the resistance, Mackenzie gave his own version of the conflict. He contended that the women had been armed with sticks and stones, and the men with cudgels. They had been signalled to the spot at Greenyards by gunshots, and some were reinforcements who had come from Sutherlandshire. Taylor had asked them to disperse, but they refused. The ensuing resistance was routed in a few minutes. Mackenzie described Taylor as 'a very *humane* and *judicious man* . . . he has planned and conducted this unpleasant expedition with judgement and energy'. The medical officer had been sent for immediately and he reported on six cases of Injury: 'Two women who were engaged in the scuffle with the police have been badly hurt . . . [and they] were in a precarious state from wounds on the head'; another dozen were slightly injured. Taylor had greatly regretted the injuries, but there was no doubt that the people had provoked the violence.

Mackenzie concluded by saying that the whole affair was too much like the current troubles in Ireland.[32]

Sheriff Mackenzie, in further letters to the Lord Advocate, contended that public sympathy for the people of Greenyards was essentially misguided. Specifically, he adverted to the question of the women who had participated in the violence:

As Sir Robert Peel said of Ireland, 'my chief difficulty' on Ross-shire has been '*the women*'. It was the women as you are aware who at Coigach, aided and abetted by the men, *twice* defeated Sheriff Cameron and the *posse comitatus* of the County. It was the women, who, in the Invergordon riots, when the Military were called in, attacked the soldiers with staves and other missiles, and compelled the officer in command to charge them with the bayonet. It was only after this charge and after some of the women had been wounded with the bayonet that the mob was dispersed. In the present instance it was the women, who, according to custom, maltreated the officers sent to execute the summonses by stripping them naked and burning their papers; and who violently obstructed the police in the execution of their duty, so as to leave them no alternative but to repel force by force, or allow themselves to be defeated as their predecessors were at Coigach.

Mackenzie argued that if the police had not acted decisively against the Greenyards people, they would have been overwhelmed. In an important justificatory remark, Mackenzie said that he had given Taylor

peremptory instructions . . . to act with vigour because on a former occasion your Lordship had an impression (in which I was disposed to concur) that they had not used their batons with proper spirit and energy when attacked by the people.

He concluded rhetorically:

Besides what apology can be made for the whole inhabitants of a country covering an area of *15 miles* rising in insurrection to prevent a landlord exercising his legal rights to serve summonses of removal on four small crofters from premises occupied by them? I believe two of these crofters were not intended to be removed, but only to be shifted to a different part of the same property.[33]

Sheriff substitute Taylor, a fortnight later, provided a broader perspective on 'the almost systematic' opposition to the law that had developed in the county. He recollected similar resistance in 1840, in Coigach in 1853, and in other cases. The Greenyards affair was 'an extensive combination' and the people had clearly expressed their resolution to resist all summonses. This, he said, was fully demonstrated by the assembly of 300 people at six o'clock in the morning. Many had travelled eight or ten miles for the purpose, and they had been in a state of continuous preparedness for four weeks. They had shown a pistol on a previous occasion. All of this showed the seriousness of the resistance. Taylor said that the police had acted with great restraint and, although he deeply regretted the injuries that had occurred, he was 'satisfied that if the Police had not used their batons to force a passage, in the manner they did, our party would have been deforced and maltreated'. They would have been stripped naked by the women; and, without decisive action, it would have confirmed their idea that women have an immunity from attack (for which reason they are always put in the front of the mob) and thus encouraging the refractory spirit among them till a military force would become necessary – probably ending fatally.[34]

The account of the Greenyards eviction provided by the impassioned pen of Donald Ross differed in several important respects from the newspaper and official reports. Ross implicitly denied that there had been a systematic resistance to the law; he contended that the people had been unarmed and had behaved in an orderly manner. He gave a much smaller estimate of the size of the crowd that confronted the police; and, most importantly, he alleged that the police had acted with extreme brutality towards the womenfolk.

Nevertheless, beyond these specific disagreements, there was a considerable unanimity between the accounts. The basic facts of the case were not challenged: a body of baton-swinging police had indeed ploughed into a crowd of women, and they had inflicted severe, almost fatal, wounds upon them. The police sustained no injury. The confrontation had obviously been much premeditated by both sides: the Lord Advocate, the Sheriff, the proprietor, the newspaper and the people all expected a bloody conflict. It was undoubtedly a trial of strength between the peasantry of Ross-shire and its police force.

In the aftermath four of the people captured at Greenyards were sentenced at the Circuit Court in Inverness 'to a long confinement and hard labour in prison'. One year later the clearance at Greenyards was completed, to the accompaniment once more of allegations of cruelty, but without resistance. The *Northern Ensign* reported the final act:

A few days ago the Greenyard evictions were repeated; and what had been *left* unfinished by the *heritors* and tacksmen of these lands, of the revolting tragedy of last spring, has been accomplished.

A civil force had been brought in from Tain. The furniture of the evictees was put out into the nearby fields; the fire in the hearth was extinguished and the inmates were ejected, 'like a band of felons'. One bedridden woman was placed, in her bed, in the open air, 'exposed to the piercing cold in intense frost and snow storm' until she was rescued by a neighbour from across the Carron.[35]

Notes

1 Evan Macleod Barron (ed.), *A Highland Editor: Selected Writings of James Barron of the Inverness Courier* (Inverness, 1927), p. 50.

2 See Macinnes, 'From Clanship', op cit. p. 29, *Clanship*, op cit. pp. 192–4, and Eric Richards, 'Highland emigrants to South Australia in the 1850s', *Northern Scotland*, vol. 5 (1982), pp. 1–30.

3 Fraser-Mackintosh, *Letters*, pp. 311–2, Cockburn, op. cit., p. 126, Rixson, *Knoydart*, pp. 199–125.

4 Cockburn, *Journal*, p. 109.

5 Barron, *Northern Highlands*, vol. III, p. xxxviii.

6 Mitchell, op. cit., I, pp. 73–6.

7 See Eric Richards, 'The Highland passage to colonial Australia', *Scotlands* (1995) pp. 28–44.

8 Papers relative to the emigration to the North American colonies, PP, XLVI (1854), p. 79.

9 Ninth Annual Report of the Board of Supervision for Relief of the Poor in Scotland, PP, 1854–5, XXIV (1854–57), Appendix A, No.1 (Report of Sir John McNeill).

10 W.H. Murray, *The Companion Guide to the West Highlands of Scotland* (London, 1968), p. 250.

11 *The Times*, 20 and 27 September 1853. These reports were reprinted with approval in the *Northern Ensign*, 29 September 1853.

12 The *Northern Ensign*, 27 October 1853, alleged that the people had understood Glengarry to have waived their arrears during the famine.

13 *Scotsman*, 17 September, 22 October 1853; *Northern Ensign*, 8 September 1853.

14 *Scotsman*, 26 October 1853.

15 *Northern Ensign*, 10, 24 November, 8 December 1853.

16 Ibid., 20 and 27 October, 8 December 1853.

17 *Scotsman*, 20 October 1853.

18 *Northern Ensign*, 2 February 1854.

19 *Scotsman*, 27 May 1854; *Northern Ensign*, 15 June 1854.

20 SRO, H.H. 23/5/(2253); *Northern Ensign*, 16 March 1854.

21 *Inverness Courier*, 15 June 1854.

22 *Northern Ensign*, 8 March 1855; *Scotsman*, 12 August 1854.

23 *Dictionary of Scottish Business Biography, 1860–1960*, ed. A. Slaven and S. Checkland, I (1986), pp. 20–4.

24 Cameron Lees, *A History of the County of Inverness* (Edinburgh, 1897), pp. 200–2, 339.

25 Alexander Mackenzie, *History of The Macdonalds and The Lords of the Isles* (Inverness, 1888), pp. 360–61; Cameron, 'Scottish emigration to Upper Canada', op. cit., p. 388 et seq.

26 *Inverness Courier*, November 1860; *Inverness Advertiser*, April 1856; *Historical Pamphlets of Inverness-Shire*, passim; entry relating to Edward Ellice, *Dictionary of National Biography*, vol. VI, pp. 665–6. See also the thoughtful remarks on the district in Rixson, op. cit., chapters 8–10.

27 *Inverness Courier*, reprinted in *Scotsman*, 8 April 1854.

28 Ibid., 11 and 25 May 1854.

29 *Northern Ensign*, 4 May 1854.

30 SRO, Lord Advocate's Papers MS/117, Taylor to Mackenzie, 31 March 1854.

31 Ibid., Mackenzie to Lord Advocate, 4 April 1854.

32 Ibid., Mackenzie to Lord Advocate, 4 March, 8 March [this should read 'April'] 1854.

33 SRO, Lord Advocate's Papers, AD56/309/3a, Mackenzie to Lord Advocate, 9 April 1854.

34 Ibid., Taylor to Lord Advocate, 12 April 1854.

35 *Northern Ensign*, 15 February 1855.

17

Nervous Landlords, 1855–86

I. The landlords' fear

THE HIGH-PITCHED PUBLICITY given to the burst of great clearances around the famine years in the mid-nineteenth century focused attention sharply on the Highlands, the plight of its people and the behaviour of its landlords. Twenty years later the controversy turned political with a vengeance. For the landlords the greatest threat arose when questions were posed about the moral and legal bases of proprietorial oppression. This inevitably created a debate about popular land rights. The public shudder of revulsion from the clearances caused the democratic press to question the basis of the legal system that permitted such acts.

Thus in 1853, in the wake of the Knoydart evictions, the *Northern Ensign* thundered:

The man who can do a barbarous and inhuman act, and who then jumps behind that wretched subterfuge, 'legal rights', is a coward of the most consummate meanness. The civil law, which, when enforced, violates the natural rights of man as well as the dictates of humanity, is in my opinion not to be boasted of. It is a principal duty of the civil law to protect the natural rights of man. 'The right to live,' as was well observed by Lord Jeffrey, '*lies deeper than* the *right to property itself.*' I know well that the 'law' by which Highland lairds effect these sweeping and cruel clearances has been for a long time on the statute book. The act which warrants forcible ejections is dated 1591, cap 217. It was *foisted* upon Scotland when feudal barons and heritors 'ruled the roost' in the Scottish Parliament. The country was at that time overrun with beggars, squatters and sorners; yet, after a lapse of 250 years, this old law is still in force, and no steps are taken to repeal it.[1]

Spokesmen for the Highlanders demanded the abolition of land laws which permitted landlords to evict tenants with virtually no institutional restraint and there were urgent voices demanding a parliamentary inquiry into the condition of the north. It was 'The Land Question' in Highland garb, the local version of the challenge made by every peasantry in Europe from Donegal to Corsica, from Jutland to Galicia. In practice the crofters did not yet rally collectively to this call. They settled into two decades of quietude, broken only by sporadic individual evictions which raised merely a few local ripples of protest.

Landlords had always feared a parliamentary visitation, and rightly so in the ultimate outcome. But government was not enthusiastic about questioning the sacred territory of proprietorial rights. Nevertheless, in the three decades before the Napier Commission into Crofting, appointed in 1883, there was a significant shift in the age-old contest between the landowners of the Scottish Highlands and the occupiers of the land. Thus, whereas in 1850 the popular cry was, essentially, that the landlords should be stopped in their work of eviction, by 1880 the initiative had changed hands. Thenceforward the crofters and their leaders took the battle to the landlords and sought to wrest control of the land from their masters. The conflict became openly and vociferously politicised into a battle to recover 'lost rights', to repossess ancestral territory. Instead of landlords clearing the people, by the 1880s the crofters were invading their old lands – in the phrase of the time, they were 'land-raiding'. The crofters, with some outside assistance, created a movement of considerable political sophistication, and laid siege to Highland landlordism. Between 1855 and 1880 all the rules of the contest for the land had changed.

At all stages in the emergence of a crofter movement there was an Irish parallel. But, in the early 1850s, the Highland debate was only a quiet echo of the Irish furore. It was even calmer through the rest of that decade and for another twenty years: subsidised emigration channelled some of the heat and energy to distant places.[2] The return of relatively good times in the mid-1850s, even for the crofters, reduced passions in the north. There were two decades of comparative prosperity for most strata of Highland society. The sheep farmers fared exceptionally well, but even the crofting population experienced a mild prosperity which encouraged expectations of security and stability. Seasonal migration brought a vital supply of income to the lowest echelons of the region's population.

Cattle prices rose several-fold and this was the key element for crofters in this comparatively comfortable plateau.[3] In many though not all places population pressure eased after the middle of the century, and harvests were relatively generous, with occasional localised exceptions. Just as important was the low level of crofters' rents. Evidence drawn from several estates shows that small rents rose very little (if at all) and generally lagged behind the increase of cash income. While this did not guarantee prosperity for the crofters – whose lives remained extraordinarily pinched by general British standards of the day – it was a large advance on the conditions which applied in the days of the destitution.

II. *The decline of clearances*

The most powerful consideration in lowering the level of conflict in the Highlands during these years was the decline of clearances. After the hysteria of Greenyards in 1854–5 there were no more mass evictions in the Highlands. The rancour and public abuse associated with the events of 1849–55 had demonstrated to landlords the folly of wholesale eviction. Better economic conditions reduced pressure on the Poor Law administration and reduced some of the imperative for clearances. The fear of a national conscience, increasingly sensitive to distant social cruelty, was part of this change of attitude: mass eviction forced through by the arm and fist of the law came to be regarded as entirely too crass. Landlords restrained their natural inclination to shift their people, holus-bolus, off their estates. They learned patience and, whether humane or otherwise, generally chose to encourage emigration rather than force the people from their lands. Thereafter most clearances that came to the public attention were small-scale affairs,

usually involving one or two families rather than entire communities. When the crofting community eventually roused itself to
unprecedented agitation against the landlords in the 1880s, it was
stimulated not by renewed clearances, but by a positive urge to
recover lost rights and by the encouragement of a sympathetic press
and public opinion.

The actual rate of eviction in the Highlands between 1855 and
1883 has never been calculated and there is no *prima facie* case for
believing that it was any greater than in the rest of Britain or in
Ireland. The crofter was not much more vulnerable to eviction than
the ordinary English agricultural labourer in his tied cottage. For
both the omnipresent possibility of eviction remained as the
governing element in landlord–tenant relations. It was a time of
sporadic clearances, of mainly invisible pressure on the people, to
ease them out of the region.

III. Riddell and the new élites

The dilemma of many Highland landlords in mid-century was
nicely captured in the case of Sir James Riddell, who conformed to
the more sensitive model of his class. The Riddells owned estates at
Ardnamurchan and Sunart in Argyllshire and had conducted
clearances in the first half of the century.[4] But the Riddell estates
had not been fully cleared, the population remained large and there
was still scope for the extension of sheep farms. The famine of
1846–9 had ravaged the district and Riddell sought governmental
assistance for the relief of his people. He spent large amounts on
improvements, but by 1848 he had accumulated a total debt of
about £50 000. His factors urged him to evict the small tenants
who had run up arrears during these years, but Riddell appears to
have resisted the temptation.[5] The estates were placed in the hands
of trustees in an attempt to extricate the family from its difficulties.

In April 1848 Thomas Goldie Dickson prepared a report for
Riddell's trustees, dealing specifically with the question of arrears
among the small tenantry, and the advisability of clearances. Since
1848, the tenants had accumulated rent arrears of £5674; in a

Domesday-like survey of the lands, Dickson instituted an enquiry into the circumstances of each tenant. There were about 400 small tenants arranged in the traditional pattern under the sway of several large tacksmen. Dickson judged that the arrears of many tenants were irrecoverable, so that it had become 'necessary with the view of turning their possessions to profitable account, that they be dispossessed and removed to smaller crofts'. Many of them were in debt well beyond the value of their cattle, their only exchangeable asset. Dickson thought that the people could be removed from the estate without any further provision being made for their resettlement; they would be able to look after themselves. He was anxious, however, to 'avoid when the removals take place any risk being run of parties being left without the means of procuring shelter for themselves and their families'. He also discovered that neither the landlord nor the existing tenants could afford to stock the lands with sheep, and that they would have to seek a large capitalist sheep farmer for the enterprise. Dickson believed that the old small-tenant system had become anachronistic. In a revealing passage, he wrote:

> The proper working of the system of small Tenant Farms depends so much upon a proper feeling subsisting between the Proprietor and the Tenant. A feeling on the part of the Proprietor of anxious concern for the welfare of his Tenantry evinced by acts of kindness and consideration, and on the part of the Tenant of respect, confidence and gratitude that when an Estate falls under Trust management, there being no room for the exercise of these feelings, the position of matters is entirely altered and the working of the system becomes necessarily defective.

Dickson believed that removals were justified, so long as alternative employment was reasonably accessible to the people displaced. This was a principle with which few landowners anywhere in Britain would have disagreed. On examining the local opportunities for work in the region of Ardnamurchan, Dickson found that employment was available in wood-cutting, bark preparation and at the lead mines at Strontian; in addition there was seasonal work to be had at the dye-works of Glasgow. One of the obstacles to removals as advocated by Dickson was the 'aversion on the part of Sir James Riddell to compulsory measures'.[6] In the past this had operated as a restraint on the trustees, and had been the root cause of the arrears. The outcome of Dickson's report is unknown, but in 1855 the Riddell estates were sold to John James Dalgleish.[7]

The Riddell sales were part of a remarkable acceleration of land transfer in the Highlands. Between the 1820s and the 1880s two thirds of the Highlands changed hands, including the Clanranald estates of the Macdonalds, Campbell of Islay, the estate of Knoydart, Lewis, Kintail, Glenshiel, Barra, Skye, Glenelg, Reay, Morvern, Badenoch, Lochaber and many more. Increasingly ownership ended up in Lowland, English or even American hands, a new dissociated élite in a region of traditional family allegiance. It was a social revolution.[8]

The circulation of élites was greater in the Highlands than elsewhere in Britain. Often, as in the case of Riddell, the sales were forced on the old owners when debts reached beyond the capacity of estate income to cope. As T.M. Devine says, 'Only a combination of stable or increasing levels of income, lower annual costs and sound estate management could have saved the Highland landed class.' He quotes Malcolm Gray who remarked that 'the first breath of falling rents was sufficient to sweep them on to the market.'[9] The paradox, of course, was the continuing rise in external demand for Highland estates at a time when incomes were sluggish or worse. The high valuation placed on Highland estates expressed the peculiar attraction which the Highlands exerted upon the Victorians, led by the Queen herself. The magic of the Highlands was proclaimed by the social Darwinian, Herbert Spencer, and poetized by Tennyson himself. It was powerfully facilitated by the extension of railways and steamships to the Highlands. Thus, though incomes were low, capital values rose strongly and good pickings were available to canny investors in the Highlands. And, in any case, Highland estates were much cheaper than in the south. All this simply sharpened the edge of local anger against the élite, home grown or otherwise.

IV. *Carnegie and others*

One of the new owners was Alexander George Pirie (1836–1904) who soon chose to embark on clearances in Wester Ross in an effort to satisfy his sporting instincts. Pirie was an immensely successful paper manufacturer near Aberdeen who bought the Leckmelm estate in the 1879. He resided on his sporting estate for twenty years, removed tenantry and introduced cricket to the district, the ultimate symbol of cultural imperialism from the south. Pirie's lordly evicting behaviour, as early as August 1880, brought the Highlands to Parliamentary attention and precipitated renewed political agitation.[10]

Another rich but less controversial newcomer, in the following decade, was Andrew Carnegie. The Lowland-born United States steelmaster was the greatest entepreneur of the age. He bought much property in the Highlands and certainly believed that his was more in tune with local customs. He acquired Cluny Castle in 1888 and spent a decade of summers there, somewhat to the irritation of his American clients and investors. It was said that Carnegie was 'as good a Highlander and as good a clansman as the rest. A lusty piper . . . circumnavigated the house in the morning, stopping under each window.' Carnegie later also bought Skibo Castle in Sutherland, which he described as his 'Heaven on Earth', where he spent five months each year. He was 'home at last', he exclaimed.[11]

Another proprietor with every reason to be sensitive to public criticism was the Duke of Sutherland. The memory of the great removals of 1810–21 was invoked with undiminished outrage whenever clearances were discussed. In 1855 the Sutherland factors removed a small number of individual families who had occupied crofts without the approval of the estate. They were squatters. The removals were heatedly denounced in the newspapers, much to the discomfort of the Duke of Sutherland, who had little stomach for public debate.[12] In response to his demand for detailed information, he was told that a sub-tenant named Angus Sutherland had, in defiance of the estate rules about sub-division and accommodation of married children, lived on the croft which was let in the name of his mother-in-law, until he had quarrelled with her, at which point he and his family were evicted by her into a snowstorm. They chose simply to squat on the far end of the croft. When the ground officer told Sutherland to get out, he refused. 'It then became necessary to eject them by legal means, which was done.' According to George Loch, the duke's Commissioner, 'the roof was taken off the hut, but by great mismanagement it was otherwise left entire – they immediately resumed their residence in the adjoining cottage.' Subsequently the removal was fully executed, and Loch emphasised to the Duke the indispensability of a policy which 'prevented the growth of a squatting and pauper population . . . [and] the evils social and moral that must ever accompany such a state of things.'

The Sutherland estate officials believed that they were no longer able to pursue a rational course in cases such as that of Angus Sutherland without provoking 'a fresh outcry . . . by the [*Northern*] *Ensign*'. They realised now that even the smallest removals must be implemented with the greatest circumspection. On the other hand they considered it imperative that the rights of the landlord be 'vindicated' in these circumstances. Sometimes they were led a merry dance. For instance, again in 1855, the Sutherland estate agents were accused of evicting the wife of a squatter by carrying her 'out in her blankets and depositing her on the ground outside'. The ground officer explained that there had been a 'trick' and 'that while he was detained outside the cottage she got into bed for the purpose'. Loch thought that although it was 'by no means improbable that such was the fact – it is however unfortunate that such an occurrence took place'.[13] The estate officials believed that cases were invariably sensationalised by the newspapers.

By 1860 the atmosphere of public opinion was entirely hostile to clearances and the vigilance of the northern newspapers undoubt-edly helped to curb the estate owners. Few landlords were prepared to risk the deluge of vilification that fell upon them even if they were to evict a single cottar. These feelings unquestionably inhibited the Sutherland estate. In 1864, for example, the infamous factor of the Scourie district, Evander MacIver, recommended to the Duke of Sutherland that the township of Nedd be cleared. There were excellent economic and managerial reasons for so doing. But George Loch placed the matter in its true context:

I need not suggest to your Grace how serious and formidable a proposal this is – and that it would require to be justified by the strongest possible reasons – in these days a measure deliberately undertaken as 'a clearance' would attract the most unfriendly criticism – and it would be impossible so to conduct it as not to encounter some difficulty and opposition which would be immediately taken up by the public voice from one end of the country to the other – it would be difficult anywhere, but in Sutherland almost impossible. I have no doubt that the people might be made happier and more comfortable elsewhere – but that would not serve very much to help in carrying it through. It may be very right to make some partial change in the occupation of the township of Nedd, but I should apprehend great discomfort to ensue in any attempt to effect a 'clearance'.[14]

This was a realistic measure of the spirit of the age. Indeed, for the entire period 1862–81, in the large district of Tongue, in Sutherland, there were only forty-nine cases where summonses of removal were taken out against small tenants, and in no single instance was an eviction actually executed.[15] So far as the adjustment and rationalisation of the crofting population was concerned, the estate was now hamstrung. On the island of Skye in the period 1840–1883 there were 1740 decrees of removing pronounced of which only a small proportion were actually executed; but as J.P. Day pointed out, 'the person summoned had to pay the costs, about 10 shillings, and was made to realise the insecurity of tenure.'[16]

The fact that some landlords no longer felt themselves free to evict whenever they wished was small comfort to those already dispossessed as well as the landless strata of the Highland population. The voice of the cottar and the squatter is heard in a petition which Angus Sutherland wrote to the Duke of Sutherland in 1855. He described himself as a fisherman and cottar from Armadale, a married man with two infant children, and 'of good moral character'. He declared that he had

occupied a room at Armadale built by himself without authority for some months before Whitsunday last when he was removed from it and this room unroofed, since which time the petitioner's wife and family have been forced to live in an open barn having been unable to procure any other shelter, and the petitioner has been employed in the Herring Fishing at Wick . . . as the weather is now getting broken the winter season fast approaching and the Petitioners whose ancestors have been tenants on the Sutherland and Reay Estates for centuries back, is unable to procure any place of shelter, he humbly prays that it may please your Grace with your usual generosity to the Poor and helpless to order some place at Armadale or any other part of your Grace's Reay estate to be procured to protect the Petitioner, his wife and helpless infants from perishing from exposure to the weather, and the Petitioner as in duty bound will ever pray.[17]

In response to this plea, though it was against the estate's most basic philosophy, Sutherland and his family were provided with accommodation to see them through the coming winter, on condition that they departed in the following April.[18]

V. Shetland and Mull

After 1855 the transformation of the Scottish Highlands continued in less dramatic fashion. It was shaped primarily by market forces, particularly by the prosperous days of sheep farming which continued through the middle decades of the century and until the late 1860s. After that, adverse price trends and seasons produced agricultural depression which was more severe and more prolonged than in the rest of Britain. The Highland economy was again required to adjust to these secular trends and to the continuous growth in demand for sporting facilities which, of course, maintained the direction of the long-run structural transformation. This meant fewer people in the glens and the further devotion of landed resources to uses determined outwith the region.

The continuing adjustment of land use and occupation was in no sense confined to the main upland mass of the Highlands. Even the peripheral low-lying parts of the region – Easter Ross, Caithness and the northern isles – were also subject to radical agrarian change which entailed the movement of population. In Caithness, by 1850, agriculture had been reorganised for both grazing and arable production. Large capitalist farms emerged in which efficient tenants raised wheat and oats almost entirely for the inter-regional trade with the south. They employed a class of proletarians who were part agricultural labourer and part fisherman, with only a tenuous claim on the land itself. In the less cultivable areas of Caithness, sheep farmers took control of great tracts for grazing. The consequence, in the long run, was the dissociation of the bulk of the population from the ownership and occupation of the land. The common people became a landless labour force, and the new agriculture became outstandingly efficient in its use of land, labour and capital. But the social consequences even in this most favoured part of the region were, arguably, much the same as in other parts.[19] The once corn-clad Strath of Berriedale was converted to sheep, and a correspondent from Halkirk in 1853 spoke of the 'ill-advised and reckless proprietors . . . [who listened] to the subtle suggestions of designing and avaricious land monopolizing capitalists'.[20] But at least the capitalist arable farmers and the local fishing trade created more jobs for the people of Caithness than did sheep farming.

Far to the north, the Shetland Islands were similarly transformed by the mid-century, and there were also cases of sudden clearances. In 1809 Arthur Edmondston had accurately predicted that commercial sheep farming was inevitable and that it would bring no benefit to the small tenantry.[21] From the 1840s there was an increasingly commercial and rational approach to landlord–tenant relations in Shetland: fishing was no longer made a condition for tenancy, and when crofts were vacated they were swallowed into sheep farms. The process accelerated, and landlords served notices to quit. As a historian of the islands observed in 1879, eviction was generally the first step towards progressive improvement, and a more recent writer explains that

> The preliminary policy of clearances met with little opposition from the tenants; for the people were accustomed to move at frequent intervals and few crofts had been held by one family for more than a generation or two. It was when the lairds laid claim to the common grazings that the people objected, and in a few places resisted fiercely.

The valley of Veensgarth, Tingwall, was cleared in the 1850s when twenty-one families were removed in favour of sheep. Unst was the scene of similar events in 1867 and no resistance was offered.[22] Witnesses before the Napier Commission made reference to other clearances in the previous thirty years – in North Yell, for instance, it was said that whole villages had been erased for sheep pastures. As for the people, it was remarked, 'They all removed; some went to other countries and some removed to other farms', to be replaced by a solitary shepherd.[23] The persuasive work of emigration agents had helped to syphon off a large part of the population. More dramatic than most were the evictions at Queendale in 1874 where, according to a contemporary historian, 'the houses were stripped and in some cases burned as soon as the tenants were out. Twenty-seven families were evicted at Martinmas and many went immediately to Australia and New Zealand.'[24]

Among the Western Isles, Mull had witnessed all manner of clearances. James Forsyth cleared Dervaig in 1857, and Treshnish was cleared in 1862, but there had been particular events at Calgary half a century earlier, at Mishnish in 1842, and F.W. Clarke was a vigorous evictor in the years of the famine.[25] None of these had reached the attention of the Scottish newspapers. Of Tobermory, on Mull, it was remarked to the Napier Commission:

> Many years ago [the town] became a harbour of refuge for many that were evicted from different places, including Ireland, leaving it to the present day a seat for propagating paupers ... Volumes could be written in connection with the clearances of a character that would not reflect much credit on those who were the sole cause of them.[26]

Such volumes have still to be written.

VI. Lesser clearances

After 1855 clearances were usually part of the ongoing and gradual erosion of the population. But from time to time individual evictions caused an eruption of anger against particular landlords. For instance, in August 1859 there were pathetic accounts of the eviction of a poor tailor and his family from Applecross by the

Duchess of Leeds. The scene was reminiscent of the Suishnish episode half a decade before:

> The poor tailor they made short work of. They found him quietly sitting down to his breakfast, when they seized him and pitched him outside the door, sending his humble breakfast after him. They next turned on his wife, who was lying sick in bed. They dragged her from her bed screaming, and sent her outside, bruising and discolouring her arm. Her infant child, who was sucking at her breast, was then taken out and laid upon the ground. The whole effects were thrown out after him, and the door locked. The people stood by horror-struck by such cruel treatment, and could only express their sympathy for this afflicted family by raising a small subscription on their behalf.

The people were warned that if any shelter were given to the family, those involved would also be evicted.[27]

Most small clearances passed unnoticed. Local historians are thrown back on the evidence of oral traditions and of the empty landscapes. In the Hebrides, Islay has no written documentation, even though it is almost certain that people were evicted. In North Gigha 'there is a very definite oral tradition of the removal of eighteen families in one day.'[28] On the mainland, in the west, the Gairloch district was spared the worst of the clearances but, according to Ian Fraser, 'it was by no means uncommon for tenants to be turned out' for sheep stealing, poaching and like misdemeanours. In this respect Highland lairds behaved in the same way as their southern counterparts.[29] There was a small clearance at Oronsay in Morvern ordered by Lady Gordon in 1868, but the main part of the population had been cleared during the previous fifty years.[30] By contrast, on the Matheson estate on Lewis, in 1872, the people of several districts petitioned the landlord to be removed and assisted to emigrate, creating a special category of voluntary clearances.[31]

Though the population of the Highlands was in general decline after 1860 it is not possible to separate the causes. Spontaneous and subsidised emigration operated to the same effect as eviction, and there were various shades of pressure exerted by landlords which, though falling short of outright clearance, acted as an effective expulsive force. In Jura the process had been in train since the beginning of the century. Its most recent historian insists, 'It must be understood that . . . here and there, one by one farmers' tenancies have quietly not been renewed, and the ground turned over to the owner's sheep and deer. The trend continues.'[32] More identifiable and devastating were the clearances pushed through on estates in Orkney, by alien landowners, especially the blustering General Burroughs.[33] He was yet another proprietor who had brought a familial fortune from East India service to the Highlands and islands. Speaking before the Napier Commission in 1884, Burroughs described his sheep-farming experiments and the way in which he had taken over the old grazing land. He expostulated:

> I think they ['the people'] have as much right to my common as I have to their clothes; the land is mine, and the coats and hats are theirs, and I cannot see how they can claim the pasture. It never did belong to them.

Burroughs had developed firm views on the crofter question and told the Commissioners that

> my own experience is that tenants can very well take care of themselves; in fact, instead of making Acts of Parliament to protect tenants, it would be much more to the point to make Acts of Parliament to protect landlords.

General Burroughs would not assure the Commission that his crofters would face no retribution as a result of their evidence to the inquiry. It was little wonder that they spoke of 'landlord-terror hanging on them'.[34] Another who refused to give an assurance of indemnity to delegates before Lord Napier in 1883 was an absentee proprietrix of Islay, Mrs Baker. She too taunted the Commissioners: 'I hope your delegates are not losing their brave spirits, and beginning to show the white feather.'[35]

Rannoch, in Perthshire, provides a further example for the period between the famine and the Napier Commission. During that time the population halved, partly as a consequence of voluntary emigration, and partly because of individual ejections. There were no outstanding clearances, but the landlord, Sir Alistair MacDonald of Dalchosnie, was alleged to have made the position of his tenants 'so hot . . . that they had to leave'.[36] Similarly the island of Raasay was visited by famine and clearances in the period 1847–53, and thereafter the fate of the remaining people appears to have depended primarily upon the personalities of each of the successive proprietors who came to own their lands. George Haygarth Rainey, for example, personally resisted all factorial advice to remove the people despite the financial sacrifice that such an attitude required. A later owner, a romantic Londoner named Armitage, lived in a cloud of absentee beneficence and liked to think of the island as 'our little kingdom'. His successor, an industrial sportsman from the Potteries, turned most of the land over to deer, pheasants and rabbits.[37] Sir Archibald Geikie had first visited Raasay in the 1850s, just after some of the crofters had been removed and, half a century later, he recollected that scene:

> Many of the cottages still retained their roofs, and in one of the deserted houses I found on a shelf a copy of the Bible wanting the boards and some of the outer pages. When I revisited the place a few days ago, only ruined walls and strips of brighter herbage showed where the crofts had been.[38]

VII. Deer and a different bleating

Public wrath against sheep clearances was inflamed anew when, especially after 1860, much of the Highlands was converted into deer forests. This appeared to compound the original crime for decidedly frivolous reasons. The sporting possibilities of the Highlands had been pioneered before 1814 by English and Irish shooters as they began their annual assaults on red deer, ptarmigan, black game and grouse.[39] In 1846 Henry Cockburn had exclaimed about

> the autumnal influx of sporting tenants . . . Almost every moor has its English tenant. On the whole, these birds of passage are useful. They are kind to the people, they increase rents, they spend money, and they diffuse a knowledge of, and a taste for, this country. The only misfortune, that though some of them try to imitate Celticism, on the whole, the general tendency is to accelerate the obliteration of everything peculiarly Highland.[40]

The influx was not new except in scale, as we have seen. It has been calculated that twenty-eight deer forests were formed by 1839, sixteen in the 1840s, ten in the 1850s and eighteen between 1855 and 1860.[41] Deer forests soon began, in aggregate, to account for large tracts of the region.

In 1844 William Howitt had described the ludicrous situation that developed in tiny villages in the west Highlands when a deluge of sport-crazed 'Southrons' descended – 'Into one miserable village, or one poor solitary inn, pour, day after day, the summer through, from seventy to a hundred people.'[42] Some clearances (for example, the Coigach fiasco in 1852–3) were connected with deer forests. Glen Tanar was cleared in 1855–8 in favour of deer, dispersing families to other parts of the estate.[43] It was indeed during this phase of the Highland revolution that sheep farmers were cleared to make way for the free run of deer, and this introduced a new type of bleating into the north of Scotland.[44]

The transition came mainly after 1860, by which time railways had made the Highlands much more accessible. The development was favoured by two trends – one was the increasing fashionability of expensive sport among the aristocracy and plutocracy of the new industrial nation; the other was the sharp decline in the profitability of sheep farming in the 1870s. Sheep (then and since) were blamed for the destruction of the forests and the devastation of the landscape, though recent opinion suggests that 'The impact of sheep farming on the Highland environment is uncertain.'[45] The improvement of sporting rents had already been demonstrated: the rental value of Glenurquhart, as a consequence of deer shooting, doubled between 1836 and 1872; Glenmoriston was worth £100 a year in 1835 and possibly £3000 in 1872; on some estates the rent increase was of the order of twentyfold. The collapse of wool prices after 1873 (under the impact of foreign competition) increased the relative importance of the sportsmen, who paid rent worth £33 690 in Ross-shire alone.[46] By 1914 more than three and a half million acres were devoted to deer forests in the Highland counties.[47]

In many places sheep were cleared from estates to make way for the deer. On the Chisholm estates, for instance, much fine grazing in Glencannich, Sleasgarve, Carnagullan and Millardoch was taken over for sport. There was concern for the fate of the evicted shepherds: at Glenaffric, a sheep farm tenanted by Lord Tweedmouth was cleared for deer and left four shepherds entirely redundant. Public feeling about deer forests was sufficiently passionate to give credence to some wild flights of the imagination. Thus, as J.P. Day wrote, despite the evidence to the contrary (and the considered opinion of the Napier Commission), 'the idea that the homes of hundreds of crofters had been pulled down and people turned adrift in order to establish deer forests became a somewhat popular delusion.' In later years Lloyd George waxed eloquent on deer forests, though he had small understanding of the subject.[48]

Deer did not, in reality, cause clearances in a manner at all comparable to the scale of the sheep evictions. The deer simply exacerbated the land hunger of the region and symbolised, in the most dramatic way, the existence of the two nations that inhabited the Highlands. There were, on the one hand, the sporting magnates, the 'Nimrods', who massacred animals in the strenuous pursuit of leisure and prestige; and, on the other, the crofters and cottars who eked out their lives on the fringe of the land mass, unable to gain access to the pastoral lands because of the greater profitability of capitalist sheep farming and the new sports industry, neither of which had much use for crofters. In more recent times a neo-mercantilist doctrine has asserted that 'vast tracts of land were effectively removed from the process of production' though the rent yields suggest otherwise.[49]

Many landlords in the Highlands, by design or by their own indolence, continued to invest too much local authority in the hands of their factors. The management class worked under distinct conditions and were required to squeeze profits out of large and small tenants alike. In 1874 small tenants were removed from the estate of Sir James Matheson. The factor confessed that he had not consulted Matheson because it was 'too small a matter to trouble Sir James about'.[50] Ultimately, of course, the landlord carried the can.

Notes

1 *Northern Ensign*, 24 November 1853.

2 Emigration may have acted as a safety valve to social protest, though it is difficult to establish the claim, see 'The Failure of Radical Reform in Scotland in the late Eighteenth Century', in Devine, *Conflict and Stability*, p. 61.

3 Hunter, *Crofting Community*, pp. 107–8; Napier Commission, Evidence, Appendix A, pp. 68–72.

4 Napier Commission, Evidence, pp. 2282 et seq.

5 SRO, GD1/395/26, Correspondence on Memorial relative to a Distall of Ardnamurchan etc. by Sir James M. Riddell Bart. November 1848, Report on the State of Affairs of Sir James M. Riddell 1848.

6 SRO AF/49/6.

7 Napier Commission, Evidence, p. 2282.

8 See Devine, *Clanship*, appendix.

9 Op.cit., pp. 118–9.

10 *Dictionary of Scottish Business Biography, 1860–1960* ed. A. Slaven and S. Checkland, 2 (Aberdeen, 1990), p. 202, Willie Orr, *Deer Forests, Landlords and Crofters* (Edinburgh, 1982), pp. 37–43, 60–1.

11 Joseph Frazier Wall, *Andrew Carnegie* (New York, 1970), pp. 942–3.

12 See Richards, *Patrick Sellar*, op. cit., Chapter 16.

13 SCRO, D593/N/4/2/4 Mr Loch's Report concerning removals in 1855 and 1856.

14 SCRO, D593/P/24/2/1, George Loch to Duke of Sutherland, 16 February 1864.

15 SCRO, D593/N/4/2/4, Note of Summonses.

16 Day, *Public Administration*, p. 187. See Napier Commission, Evidence, p. 633.

17 SCRO, D593/N/4/2/4, Petition of Angus Sutherland (and that of his wife Dolina Sutherland).

18 SCRO, D593/N/4/2/4, Loch to Duke of Sutherland, 17 October 1855.

19 See Richards, *Scottish Food Riots*.

20 *Northern Ensign*, 28 September 1854; *New Statistical Account*, vol. XV (Halkirk).

21 Arthur Edmondston, *A View of the Ancient and Present State of the Zetland Islanders* (2 vols., Edinburgh, 1809), vol. I, pp. 219–20.

22 *Northern Ensign*, 12 January, 15 February 1855; James R. Nicolson, *Shetland* (Newton Abbott, 1972), pp. 74–5.

23 Napier Commision, Evidence, pp. 1285, 1302.

24 R. Cowie, quoted in Nicolson, *Shetland*, p. 75.

25 P.A. McNab, *The Isle of Mull* (Newton Abbott, 1970), passim.

26 Napier Commision, Evidence, pp. 2279.

27 *Northern Ensign*, 25 August 1859.

28 John Mercer, *Hebridean Islands* (London, 1974).

29 Ian Fraser, review of Osgood Mackenzie, *A Hundred Years In The Highlands* (London,1972), in *SS*, vol. 17 (1973).

30 Gaskell, *Morvern Transformed*, p. 111.

31 Macdonald, *Lewis*, p. 162.

32 Mercer, *Hebridean Island*, p. 20.

33 See Miller, *Orkney*, pp. 82, 126; W.P.L. Thomson, *The Little General and the Raasay Crofters* (Edinburgh, 1981).

34 Napier Commission, Evidence, pp. 1557–82.

35 Ibid., p. 3109.

36 Mackenzie, *Highland Clearances*, pp. 242–5.

37 Richard Sharpe, *Raasay : A Study in Island History* (London, 1977), pp. 67–72.

38 Geikie, *Scottish Reminiscences*, p. 227.

39 Sir John Sinclair, *General Report on the Agricultural State and Political Circumstances of Scotland* (Edinburgh, 1814), pp. 115–6.

40 Cockburn *Journeys*, p. 195.

41 See Orr, op cit., pp. 6–8 and Appendix V.

42 William Howitt, *The Rural Life of England* (Shannon, 1971 edn.), p. 37.

43 Watson and Allan, op. cit., p. 31. See also Orr, op. cit., pp. 120–1.

44 See Orr, op. cit., pp. 120–2.

45 See the papers in T.C. Smout (ed.), *Scotland Since Pre-History* (1993) especially those by Mather and Smith. The impact of sheep may have been less decisive than that of the larger human population in some parts. See R.A. Dodgshon, 'Budgeting for survival: nutrient flow and traditional Highlands farming', in S. Foster and T.C. Smout (eds), *The History of Soils and Field Systems* (1994).

46 D.G.F. Macdonald, *Cattle, Sheep and Deer* (London, 1872), pp. 705 et seq.

47 Watson, 'Sheep industry', p. 16.

48 Ibid., p. 203; see also Mitchell, *Reminiscences*, vol. II, p. 109.

49 Orr, op. cit., p. 149.

50 Robert Matheson, *The Survival of the Unfittest* (Edinburgh, 2000), p. 7.

18

The Crofters' First Triumph

I. Anarchy and triumph

The landlords are going, Ho ro,
We shall have the land, Ho ro Morag.[1]

In the early 1880s, with a sudden urgency, the Crofter question at last reached boiling point. Looking back over that period of Highland turmoil, an official report observed:

> From 1882 down to 1887 the Highlands and Islands were in a state of unrest – in many places there was open lawlessness. Rents were withheld, lands were seized, and a reign of terror prevailed. To cope with the situation the Police Force was largely augmented – in some cases doubled. Troopships with marines cruised about the Hebrides in order to support the Civil Authorities in their endeavour to maintain law and order.[2]

In 1886, Reginald Macleod, a spokesman for Highland landlords, summarised the current state of affairs in the north, and the conflict which finally drew sustained national attention and legislation to the condition of the crofters:

> The Island of Skye is in a state of anarchy. The Queen's writ does not run, debts are not paid, rates are fearfully in arrears, the poor law and educational system are in danger of collapse, landowners are on the road to ruin, credit is at an end, all improvements have ceased, and there is no demand for the labour of the people.

Macleod believed that there was a total contempt for law and a neglect of contract in the relations between landlord and tenants. Arrears could not be recovered because there was no adequate power to enforce payment. Any officer attempting to discharge his duties was 'at once deforced'. The authorities looked on 'in imbecile inaction': 'the government of agitation is paramount.' The government, moreover, had sponsored a Crofters Bill which 'passed-by all the teachings of political economy [and] . . . deprives the landowner of rights which he has bought with full sanction of the state.'[3]

Within a few years the Highlanders had been roused to extraordinary action against their landlords, and had successfully overturned many of the sacred principles and assumptions of Highland landownership.

The 'Crofters' War', as the agitation of the 1880s became known, was a great triumph of popular protest. As one of its historians has remarked, it 'produced a revolution in land tenure and social condition in the Highlands and led to the creation of the first independent "labour" party in the British parliament, the Crofters' Party.' It was a remarkable achievement, the more so because the crofters were renowned for their alleged 'congenital passivity', and because the region had been comfortably ignored for so long.[4]

The success of the crofter agitation in the 1880s effectively marked the end of the clearances because the consequent legislation bound the hands of the landlords in a manner which, only a few years before, had seemed unthinkable. The authority of the State, very late in the day, was exerted to inhibit a landlord policy which had dominated the Highlands for the previous century. The Crofters Act of 1886 was a decisive and unambiguous piece of class legislation on behalf of the common people: it was specifically designed to prevent clearances. It was also meant to solve the 'Highland problem'.

II. Revolting crofters

The eruption of crofter agitation in the 1880s is not easy to explain. There were disjointed and sporadic outbreaks of agitation in Wester Ross and Lewis in the 1870s, but the first concerted effort began in Skye in 1882, when the people asserted their 'historical right' to graze stock on land held by sheep farmers from Lord Macdonald.[5]

The Highlands had been relatively prosperous and politically calm for most of the twenty-five years since the famine. All previous agitation had been politically unsophisticated, poorly co-ordinated and highly localised. The events of the 1880s were on a totally different plane from anything attempted in the past. There were a number of contributory influences at work. Land reformers took up the championship of the crofting population, thus widening the political significance of the dispute. The methods of Parnell's Irish Nationalist Party and the Irish Land League provided a working model. There had always been a fear that the Irish trouble would infect the Highland question. Links were forged in the 1870s, but as early as 1866 there were rumours of Fenianism in Argyllshire, and in March of that year the local militia advised that there might be 'an attempt upon the store of arms . . . made by some Irish Fenians in the town of Campbeltown . . . where there is always a considerable number of Irishmen'.[6]

But the Irish influence was more effective as a 'demonstration effect' transmitted, in particular, by John Murdoch,[7] a Scot who had lived in Ireland and knew Parnell and Davitt personally. In 1873 he founded the Inverness newspaper, *The Highlander*, which printed strenuous diatribes against landlordism. The spread of literacy after the Scottish Education Act of 1872 probably increased general political awareness in the north, widened the democratic spirit, and helped give more shape to the previously inchoate sense of grievance in the crofting community. Several southern newspapers were vocal in support of the crofters, whose cause was also assisted by the favourable attitude to land reform among some sections of the Liberal Party in Scotland. An even more persuasive factor was the development of the Victorian conscience, which was markedly more responsive than ever before to accounts of poverty and oppression in the remote Highlands and Islands.[8]

The government could gain no popularity by springing to the aid of landlords, who were by now notorious for their record of eviction. Within Scotland the level of awareness was raised by the growth of Celtic societies, especially in Glasgow, and by the radical and romantic support from second-generation Highlanders in the south. The literary anger (and leadership) of John Stuart Blackie and Alexander Mackenzie also created an atmosphere profoundly sympathetic to the aspirations of crofters. Indeed much of the leadership and stimulus derived from outside the Highlands. It is likely that all these external elements encouraged a more actively resistant spirit among the crofters.

The sudden deterioration of economic conditions in the north at the beginning of the 1880s may have helped to concentrate the anger of the people against the rent policies of some Highland landlords. The winter of 1882–3 was the bleakest since the famine of 1846–9: the potato crop was a failure, the grain crop was lost in October gales, the coastal fishing was very bad and many boats were lost in storms. The income earned in seasonal employment in the Lowlands was half the average return. The agitation, however, continued through the good harvests of the mid-1880s. Important also were a number of Land League connections which were established, especially in Glasgow, and these groups promoted notions of peasant proprietorship, separate political representation for the crofters and a 'no-rent' campaign.

The crofter agitation was a direct challenge to landlordism in the Highlands, but did not erupt into open conflict until a series of relatively small provocations led to physical confrontation in 1882. Pirie's Leckmelm evictions of 1879 in Wester Ross[9] had helped to generate tension, but the 'Land War', as it came to be called, was not primarily a response to evictions; indeed there had been no wholesale clearances for many years. The image of the 'alien, absentee, rack-renting predators who evicted their defenceless tenants at will' no more applied to Highland landlords in this period than, apparently, to their Irish counterparts.[10] Highland discontent, in this period, was directed towards the restoration of old grazing rights and the preservation of existing tenures. It was a campaign specifically designed to turn back the clock, to recover the lost past. In 1882 there emerged a more active form of obstruction of landlords.[11]

The tactics and strength of crofter resistance changed once they began to refuse to pay rent, a tactic first employed on the Braes estate of Lord Macdonald in Skye. Here the tenants protested about their deprivation of certain grazing rights some seventeen years before, and refused to pay their rents until the land was restored to them. Macdonald responded with a summons of eviction. This, however, was dealt with in the time-honoured fashion: on 7 April 1882 the Sheriff Officer was met by a body of crofters, and his papers were burnt before his eyes. Ten days later the law returned, bolstered by fifty men from the Glasgow Police Force. They faced a large crowd of people at the Braes of Benlee: 'men, women and children rushed forward in all stages of attire, most of the females with their hair down and streaming lovely in the breeze.' Eventually, in the 'Battle of the Braes' the police succeeded in subduing the people and prisoners were taken.[12]

This skirmish was, however, merely a prelude to widespread insubordination sustained in the western Highlands over the following eight years. The prisoners taken at Benlee were tried at Inverness and fined by the Sheriff, but after sympathisers paid the fine the people continued both to run their stock on the land at Benlee and to withhold their rents. Another attempt to remove them later in the same year was equally unavailing. A similar and even more widely publicised sequence of resistance was played out at Glendale at the end of 1882. The new pattern of crofter agitation that emerged from these events assumed two main forms. One was the political campaign which channelled energy into parliamentary representation, pamphleteering, protests and fund raising. The other, at the literal grassroots, was the action of the crofters who refused to pay rents, who 'invaded' or 'raided' old lands and resisted the law in many ways. Both methods attracted national publicity and the story was reported fully in such newspapers as the *Illustrated London News* and the *Graphic*.[13]

III. Running the gauntlet

The entire atmosphere of landlord–tenant relations changed in these years.[14] Events on the Sutherland estate illustrate the alteration in the times. By 1880 the estate agents experienced the greatest difficulty in controlling the crofter population. They frequently allowed crofters to remain in arrears, or to run foul of estate regulations, rather than risk a noisy public outrage. Any small incident could swell into an uncontrollable commotion. In August 1882, for instance, the Sheriff Officer of the county tried to carry out a small eviction at Muie, but was prevented by a crowd of men and women. An agent reported: 'There was plenty of bad language and some rotten eggs and slops made free use of . . . but the officer appears to have beat a retreat before any *violent deforcement* took place.' When police officers were called in to supervise the eviction, they found themselves running the gauntlet of abuse:

> Before the ejectment had been completed there were upwards of sixty people present, many of them carrying heavy sticks. Although there was no attempt to interfere with or prevent the officers carrying out the warrant of ejectment there was a great deal of exciting talk chiefly directed against Ormiston, the incoming tenant, who it was declared would never be allowed to occupy the place. A number of women made themselves very conspicuous.

The crowd broke into the house and occupied it. The police feared that a riot would erupt if the new tenant tried to enter. And in this, as in other cases, the Sutherland estate administrators simply capitulated. The action of the people of Muie was within the classic pattern set in the previous century – the main change was in the confidence and persistence of the revolt, its alliance with a rent strike, and the change in the receptivity not only of the public but also of the government. The episode was significant because it demonstrated that some landlords had already become unnerved before the passing of the Crofters Act and that the contest for the land was already running strongly in favour of the common people. As for the Muie people, it was only four years later that they 'invaded' the adjacent sheep farm of Blairich and took possession of the grazing for their own use. Eventually brought to court, they defended their action with these words: 'We were always under the impression that the land belonged to ourselves.'[15]

Crofter resistance, especially the vigorous action on Skye in 1882 and 1883, caused the government to strengthen the law in the north (even to the point of dispatching a gunboat and troops), and to set in motion a Royal Commission into the condition of the crofters and cottars in the Highlands and Islands, under the chairmanship of Lord Napier and Ettrick. The government had been reluctant to take this step, and was forced into it by the pressure of civil disobedience and public opinion. Its members were two moderate landlords, two crofter spokesmen, and two Gaelic scholars.[16] The Commission began its tour of the region at Braes on 20 May 1883 and concluded at Tarbert on 20 December 1883. It eventually produced a massive report which constitutes the greatest single document on nineteenth-century Highland society, economy and history. It is a remarkable work of collective oral testimony, with all the strength and weakness of that form of evidence.

Despite the hopes of the government, the establishment of the Napier Commission did not diminish agitation, resistance and rent-striking in the north. The election of five crofter members into a delicately balanced Parliament in 1885 increased the political dimensions of the Highland problem; the intervention of Henry George and Michael Davitt served to complicate and confuse further the aims of the land reform groups. At least three different groups of land reformers were at work outside the Highlands, and it cannot be said that the movement was, in general, well co-ordinated.[17] The support for the crofters lacked unity of tactics and philosophy, and it was easy for the opponents of reform to brand the entire movement as 'extremist'. In July 1885, one critic denounced the agitation as 'the work of a few individuals influenced by ambition and vanity, acting under the guidance of crafty revolutionists in London, Ireland and America', who brought to the north the danger of 'rank communism'. He invoked the spectre of revolution and war:

I venture to ask the crofter sympathisers to pause for a little and consider whether it is wise to encourage an excitable race in dreams which cannot be realised, unless, indeed, as the agitators say, a social revolution and the horrors of civil war are at hand.[18]

IV. Napier, 1884

The Napier Report, published in 1884, was a detailed and thorough exposé of the problems of the Highland economy. It identified the basic elements which caused poverty and discontent – notably the smallness of the holdings, insecurity of tenure, lack of compensation for improvements by the tenants, high rents, the poor infrastructure of the economy, population congestion and the failure of attempts to widen the base of employment in the region. The commission acknowledged the central conflict in tenurial relations between landlords and crofters:

> The opinion was often expressed before us that the small tenantry of the Highlands have an inherited inalienable title to security of tenure in their possessions while rent and service are duly rendered, [which] is an impression indigenous to the country though it has never been sanctioned by legal recognition, and has long been repudiated by the actions of the proprietors.[19]

The report drew the exact analogy between the crofter's life and 'the handloom of the cottage, the sailing craft along the shore, the yeoman's freehold' which were either gone, or were doomed to disappear. To rescue the crofter from similar extinction the Report recommended

> a complex system of interference on behalf of a class in the community which is not numerous, which does not contribute a preponderant share to the aggregate sum of national wealth, and which does, after all that has been said, possess, in ordinary times, conditions of welfare and happiness unknown to some orders of the people, for instance, to the poorer sort of rural day labourers in England, or to those who depend on casual employment in the cities.

The Commissioners justified such special treatment on several grounds: on the peculiar value of a fishing population as a reserve for the navy (a classic Adam Smithian defence of government intervention), on the importance of giving working people a stake in the land, on the danger of famine, and on the necessity of reducing the 'collisions between proprietary rights and popular demands'. But their main justification was couched in these terms:

To suffer the crofting class to be obliterated, or to leave them in their present depressed circumstances, if by any justifiable continuance their condition can be improved, would be to cast away the agencies and opportunities for a social experiment connected with the land of no common interest.[20]

The 'social experiment' recommended by the Napier Commission[21] involved a consideration only of the crofter population, that is tenants whose holdings were worth more than £6 and less than £30 per annum. There were about 40 000 families in the region, but, according to a sample of four parishes analysed by the commissioners, a quarter of them were 'without land, and without regular access to local wages, most of them, it may be assumed, scattered amongst the poorest sort of occupiers, to whom they are a heavy burden'. This class (mainly cottars) was the most tragic casualty of land hunger in the Highlands, the victims of economic and demographic transformation in the region. The Napier Commissioners defined them out of existence and recommended their emigration; as J.P. Day puts it, 'the Commissioners wished to obliterate' that class. A century later Allan Macinnes declared that the Crofters' Holdings Act of 1886 should be lamented not celebrated because it gave privilege to the peasant class at the expense of the Gaelic society as a whole and, into the bargain, created congested districts which became 'a ready reservoir of cannon fodder for British Imperial service'.[22]

The central recommendation in the Napier Report was the recognition, improvement and enlargement of the Highland 'township', the communal core of the crofting mode of agriculture. The recommendations entailed also provision for the independent valuation of rent, compensation for improvement and a framework in which changing patterns of production could be introduced by occupiers and landlords. The Report was reluctant to offer perpetual security of tenure but advocated that the state should assist the crofter to buy his or her own holding. In all, the Napier Report recommended striking alterations in the organisation of life in the Highlands. It was, however, only the beginning of the political debate for a Crofters Act which, two years later, showed a curious and somewhat tenuous relationship to the original recommendations.

V. Politics and the crofters

The publication of the Napier Report, amid continuing crofter and land-reform agitation, simply added further fuel to the blazing controversy in Scotland. The government was reluctant to take legislative action but, given other priorities, acted with surprising promptness on the issue. Two factors helped the crofters. Although Gladstone was alarmed about the drift towards socialism by way of 'exceptional expedients' of government intervention, he recognised the essence of the crofter case. In January 1885 he wrote to Sir William Harcourt: 'The crofters' title to demand legislation rested on "the historical fact" that they had enjoyed rights of which they had been surreptitiously deprived to the injury of the community.' Gladstone believed that the common Highlanders had suffered a terrible wrong in the clearances, by the 'the withdrawal of the common grazing to convert them into sheep farms', and he was clearly moved to right 'the great grievance'.[23] This was an important measure of the success of the crofters' advocates who had sustained the historical argument against, for example, the Duke of Argyll who believed that the crofters' ancestors had never possessed land in any way, and contended that the entire crofter case was based on an historical fiction.[24]

Both Gladstone and Chamberlain were extremely sympathetic to the crofters' cause and reflected most public opinion on the question. But the government was loath to become involved in any further extension of state paternalism, or any further invasion of the sacred territory of private contracts. In reality, the key political element in formulating the Crofters Bill was the strategic placement of the five crofter members in the balance of strength in the Parliament of 1885.

In some ways the Crofters Act of 1886 was the logical culmination of the agitation which had begun in a small way in the western islands, had grown to national attention and finally emerged as a significant political pressure in Parliament itself. In H.J. Hanham's view the entire episode was inflamed by the maladroit response of the legal and political authorities. They allowed the crofter question to get out of hand. Referring to the original agitation in Skye, Hanham remarks that nothing usually came of such stands. It required the publicity machinery of the British press, alerted to the land problem by the campaign of the Land League in Ireland and the over-elaborate reaction of Sheriff Ivory to the stand of the Braes crofters, to make a movement out of a very minor land dispute. And the press would have been able to make nothing of the incident had not the importation of the Glasgow police drawn attention to the affair.[25]

This view tends to sell short the tenacity, unanimity and stamina of the crofter movement in these years. There had been identical confrontations between police, factors and the people in the previous decades. In earlier episodes the authorities had behaved in a manner no less elephantine, yet the resistance had failed to cohere into a social and political movement. In the 1880s there was more iron in the souls of the crofters, their leaders were much more dexterous and knowledgeable and, most of all, public opinion was immeasurably more responsive.[26]

VI. The Act

The Crofters' Holdings (Scotland) Act of 1886[27] was the malformed offspring of these diverse influences. It undoubtedly breached landlord rights of property, and intruded an elaborate governmental machinery between landlord and tenant. Clearances were now outlawed. For the statutory crofter (not cottars, nor farmers who paid more rent than £30 per year) it gave extraordinary security of tenure and a mechanism (the Land Court), by which their rents and arrears could be arbitrated against the quasi-medieval notion of 'fairness'. The Act recognised also the conception of the 'township' as a communal arrangement of tenurial rights. It provided compensation for unexhausted improvements to the land. It prevented the dismemberment of the crofting community by clamping strict controls on the sale of crofting land. All these conditions represented unambiguous gains for the crofters at the expense of the landlords. The Crofters Act was a great victory for the common people. The gilt upon the victory was reduced somewhat by the suggestion that the landlords were at that time less averse to concession because the decline of wool prices made any sacrifice to the crofters less painful.[28]

Despite the legislative triumph, the Act is more usually judged by its omissions than by its positive virtues. Much of the crofting community was dissatisfied with the provisions of the legislation; the Land War continued for several years after the passage of the Act. The legislation signally failed also to stem the exodus of the people from the Highlands and Islands. Moreover the cottar and squatting populations remained as great a problem as ever; the fishing industry stagnated; the crofters refused to purchase their holdings; and the average size of holding did not grow towards the optimum specification. Landowners, pinched by low rents and high rates, were worse off than ever and could find no buyers for their estates, not even the State. For these reasons, the old subsistence economy continued to decay and the region remained a rural slum far into the twentieth century.[29]

The most fundamental criticism of the legislation of 1886 (and its successors) concerned, therefore, its failure to establish the conditions of economic progress for the crofters. It provided no long-run answers to the problem of poverty and congestion in the Highlands. There was no adequate provision for the enlargement of holdings or for a system which allowed the more energetic and efficient crofter to expand his or her acreage by taking up the crofts of their less successful neighbours. It created only a poor mechanism for the land transfer by which a more economically efficient size of holding might emerge, appropriate to the technology and market conditions of the late nineteenth and early twentieth centuries.

A logical evolution of landholding was prevented by the legislation of 1886, even though the Napier Commission had recommended a more flexible approach. It was ironic that a region which had experienced the most turbulent effects of the free exercise of market forces for an entire century should be denied some of the positive benefits of such competitive forces. It was the cost of giving security to the crofters and of preserving the quasi-communal system of landholding.

The crofters, despite the Napier Commission's hesitation on the question, were given absolute security. The effect was to 'freeze' the structure of the economy and so prevent development. It was a measure of the victory achieved by the crofters in the Land War; and it was the retribution (diminished in reality by the decline in the value of sheep grazings) imposed by a democratic government on a landowning class which was judged to have misused its traditional authority in a peasant community over the previous fifty years. It was the final price the landlords paid for the clearances. As Bruce Lenman has written:

> In the last analysis the provision of the crofting legislation that a crofter could make his tenancy heritable, or assignable to another, destroyed the reality of his landlord's ownership of the croft.[30]

But the consequences of this triumph were highly questionable: as Ian Grimble put it, the legislation 'created a system as rigid and obstructive to progress as the old runrig system of the eighteenth century. It has frustrated every attempt to solve the Highland problem during this [the twentieth] century.'[31] As Ewan Cameron has said, the legislation created 'a static structure of landholdings, with only limited opportunity for the relief of congestion'. It provided the crofters with very little more land, it perpetuated small crofts and offered little scope for modernisation, yielding 'a near absolute incapacity for change.' According to Cameron it was, therefore, 'a pyrrhic victory'.[32] By creating tenancies which were virtually perpetual, the Crofters Act exerted a profoundly conservative force upon the community. David Turnock, the geographer, summarised the general verdict:

> In short, the effect of the legislation was to fossilise the crofting landscape as it happened to appear in 1886. Change is now frustrated by the high degree of security which crofters enjoy as well as the essentially communal nature of the system, which allows a conservative minority to obstruct the progressive majority.[33]

While the legislation of 1886 failed to meet the development needs of the crofting community, it was nevertheless effective in dealing with the popular demand to prevent landlords evicting the people. The Highland peasantry were accorded extraordinary security of tenure and the landlords lost their discretionary power: it was a vindication of the peasant mentality. But it did not solve the Highland problem, and it did not reconcile the contest for land between landlord and crofter.

Thirty years before, in 1851, Sir John McNeill had identified the central dilemma of the crofter economy: 'The inhabitants of these distressed districts have neither capital enough to cultivate the extent of the land necessary to maintain them if it could be provided, nor have they land enough were the capital supplied to them.'[34] Neither the Crofters Act of 1886, nor later legislation, was able to conquer this critical paradox which characterised the plight of the people in the Highlands in the years of the Crofter Commission, just as it had before Culloden.

It would be a mistake to believe that the crofter legislation of 1886 (and the subsequent Acts of the next three decades) brought much sunshine into the relations between the owners and occupiers of the Highlands. The wings of the landlords were clipped, but controversy and conflict continued, albeit in a different social and legal framework, now defined by the Crofter Commission. Clearances were a thing of the past, but landlord oppression and popular indignation repeatedly broke the peace of the north. For, though the new legislation granted unprecedented security to the crofters, there were still circumstances, notably in connection with arrears of arbitrated rent, in which they could be evicted. Even after the passage of the Act, individual evictions caused occasional explosions of anger.

VII. Recidivism

In October 1886 there was a classic case of eviction in Strathglass which aroused all the old indignation. Evidence before the Crown Agent in Edinburgh demonstrated, in miniature, many of the features of earlier clearances, including the recourse to fire. The eviction was executed at the insistence of Chisholm of Chisholm against Peter Shaw, a ploughman, who lived in a house on a croft at Rimivraid with his wife, who had taken over the nineteen-year lease from her dead father in 1880. The Shaws were £142 in arrears of rent, and had become bankrupt. As a consequence their farm was 'displenished' under law, and Shaw committed himself to vacate the farm by August 1886. Chisholm had offered Shaw a house in Inverness, but Shaw rejected the offer. In fact the Shaws did not shift and Chisholm asked for their legal ejection. Three adults, including the Shaws, were evicted. The weather had been overcast. The task had taken two hours and, at the end, it had begun to rain very heavily. Furniture and blankets removed from the house were drenched. The Shaws, though literally penniless, eventually gained asylum with a Cannich innkeeper. The officer stated that

> in order to prevent the Shaws returning he must burn the house, and he accordingly set the dwelling houses and other buildings on fire. After a time the fire took effect, and the dwelling-house, the barn and stable were consumed except the bare walls.

The officer had had no authority for burning the houses and Chisholm raised an action against him for damages. The Procurator Fiscal observed that the episode had created much unpleasant feeling in the locality. Peter Shaw claimed that the officer had threatened

> that he would throw myself into the fire if I did not be quiet . . . When the officer saw that the house was burning he and his assistants went into the barn and began to drink whisky. He shouted to his men saying that when he got a job from the chief of a clan, [such] as the Chisholm of Chisholm, he would go into it manfully, and that was the way to do it – pointing to the fire.

Chisholm blamed the law officer, Macdonald, for exceeding his authority. The Lord Advocate ordered 'a severe reprimand' for the errant officer and the landlord was distanced from the effects of his own policy.[35]

The Crofter Commission eventually provided a means of appeal for such people as Peter Shaw, and was able to adjudicate fair rents and the settlement of arrears. This worked well in general but did not guarantee harmony, or prevent stories of the continuing abuse of proprietorial power. In 1897, for example, William Carson, a

Catholic priest, reported from Lochmaddy that the laird, Sir John Orde, had behaved with outrageous tyranny towards his tenantry and that 'the workhouse was filled with victims that he had evicted from their homes simply for being a little in arrears with their rent'. The melodrama at Lochmaddy was compounded by unconfirmed allegations that Orde had forced some of the people to drink contaminated water, and had thereby caused their deaths, saying 'Let them die, they're much better dead than alive.'[36]

VIII. The demand for land

The impact of the Napier Commission and the Crofters Act was to alter the basis of landlord–tenant relations. The legislation, naturally, was not nearly as radical as many in the north had demanded, and it did not herald a golden age. Still, it did place relations on a different footing and represented a genuine discontinuity in government policy. It was a retreat from the dogmas of *laissez faire* and an early shift towards governmental responsibility for regional development. The Act had been, for the radical wing of the crofter movement, 'far short of what Highland people were entitled to expect'.[37] Yet, though 'the restoration of the land of the Highlands' to the people was not accomplished, unprecedented inroads into landlord authority were achieved.[38] It is difficult to measure precisely the net value of the changes for the people, but three years after the passing of the legislation, one of the leaders of the crofters, Dr Macdonald MP, gave the question careful calculation. Speaking in Gaelic at a gathering at Loch Carron, he observed that the Crofters Act had already done some good:

> It had transferred about £100 000 of money from the pockets of the landlords to those of the crofters, rents had been reduced at least 30 per cent, and a large proportion of the outstanding arrears had been cancelled.

The administration of the Act perpetuated some inequities, he said, but the main task facing the crofters was to extend the gains that they had already achieved. Emigration, he insisted, was inappropriate until 'the land now under sheep and deer [is] occupied by tenants from the congested townships'. Macdonald had great faith that Gladstone would eventually break up the Highland estates 'and the people . . . would have their own again.' To this end, Macdonald 'exhorted the people to attend to organisation and to agitate.'[39] For several years, the crofter agitation continued to frighten the landlords. The most dramatic episode in the period was the famous 'raids' carried out on the Matheson property in the mid-winter of 1887–8, which caused the authorities to dispatch 500 marines to the Lewis.

The bare statistics of the operations of the Crofter Commission provide a rough gauge of the effects of the 1886 legislation. In the twenty-six years to 1912, the Commission heard 22 111 applications for fair rents, and in response reduced old rents of £89 503 to £67 496, and cancelled arrears of £124 826. These figures understated the force of the legislation because landlords, in anticipation of the intervention, began reducing their rents before the Commission reached them. In its provision for the compulsory enlargement of holdings the Act achieved, in the same period (1886–1912), a transfer of 73 341 acres from the landlords to the crofters, though the benefits were generally somewhat marginal: the value of grazing land had been much reduced by the fall of stock prices in the 1870s.[40]

On the other side the reaction was predictable. Defensive positions were taken up by the landlord class, and there was a tacit redefinition of their obligations towards the people. The vestiges of the old deference society and the remnants of clan loyalty were washed away in the deluge of the 1880s. Among landlords there was a silent withdrawal of discretionary support for the small tenants and a quiet rejection of the old moral obligation that was associated with landownership. This constituted a collective abnegation of the old responsibilities which had always provided some legitimation to Highland landlordism; it signalled the end of all pretence that Highland society rested upon unique social foundations by which it was differentiated from the rest of Britain.

This qualitative change, intangible and difficult to chart, was expressed in small transactions between landlord and tenant. In

1889, for instance, the Duke of Sutherland chose no longer to respond in the accustomed way to the requests of his small tenants for building materials with which to improve their houses. The State had interposed itself between landlord and tenant, and the Duke, as a consequence, would no longer bestow largesse upon his people, for, as his Commissioner put the point:

> Now that the Crofter Act has so greatly altered the legal relations between tenant and landlord bestowing fixity of tenure and by means of the Commission, greatly lowering the rents, it has been found more difficult to continue the system of help which prevailed in the selection of cases – the poorest of course having preference.[41]

The Crofters Act of 1886 was the belated response to the accumulated anger of the crofter community. It was a recognition of the social and economic consequences of regional retardation. The Act altered the complexion of relations in the Highlands but it afforded no solution to the deep-seated problems of undevelopment and rural congestion in the region. Indeed it tended to reinforce some of the structural difficulties, and to bind the people more firmly than ever to a land which yielded a low level of subsistence. It thereby diminished the possibilities of economic growth and adjustment. The great Highland estates were not broken up and divided among the crofters.

Nevertheless the legislation brought to an end many of the frictions that surrounded tenurial arrangements in the Highlands; it curbed landlord power and set relations on a predictable course. Paradoxically the Act was an institutional expression of the oldest characteristic of Highland society: that is, the land hunger which had dominated the mind of the Highlander since at least 1745.

The Crofters Act changed the rules regarding the occupation of the Highlands, but the sense of wrong, and the contest for the land itself, remained unresolved. For landlords and tenantry in the Highlands the control of the land was rarely a straightforward question of economic maximisation. Conflict simmered for decades and occasionally erupted into land raids, in the following hundred years. The emotional commitment to a communal conception of 'the land for the people' persisted longer and more passionately in the Highlands than elsewhere in Britain. Before the close of the twentieth century the recurrent campaign for the community ownership of extensive estates achieved a spectacular local success in Assynt in Sutherland. This, together with a number of other cases, offered a remarkable expression of the power of posterity and the reassertion of a collective ideology, to turn against the tide of modern individualism and the dictates of the market.[42]

Notes

1 New words for an old Gaelic song, quoted in 'Home truths on the Crofter agitation', *Blackwood's Edinburgh Magazine* (1885).

2 Final Report of the Crofters Commission 1913, p. xxvi, quoted in Day, *Public Administration*, p. 187.

3 Reginald Macleod, 'The Crofters: How to benefit them', *Blackwood's Edinburgh Magazine*, vol. 139 (1886), pp. 559–63.

4 Hanham, 'Highland discontent', passim.

5 Ewen A. Cameron, *Land for the People? The British Government and the Scottish Highlands, 1880–1925* (1996), p. 17.

6 SRO, Lord Advocate's Papers, AD56/309, Duke of Argyll to Crown Agent, 13 March 1866. On Murdoch see James Hunter (ed.) *For the People's Cause: from the writings of John Murdoch* (Edinburgh, 1986).

7 See Hanham, 'Highland discontent', p. 35.

8 James G. Kellas, 'The Crofters' War 1882–1888', *History Today*, vol. 12 (1962), pp. 281–8.

9 See Chapter 17.

10 See review of W.E. Vaughan, *Landlords and Tenants in Mid-Victorian Ireland* (Oxford. 1994), by Catherine F. Shannon in *AHR* (December 1997), p. 1490.

11 See C.F. Gordon Cumming, *In the Hebrides* (London, 1883), pp. 135 et seq; Day, *Public Administration*, p. 119.

12 See James G. Kellas, 'The Crofters' War 1882–1888', *History Today*, vol. 12 (1962), pp. 281–8; Hanham, 'Highland discontent', passim; Day, *Public Administration*, passim. See also I.M.M. Macphail, 'The Skye military expedition of 1884–85', *Transactions of the Gaelic Society Of Inverness*, vol. XLVIII (1972–4), pp. 62–94; I.M.M. Macphail, 'The Napier Commission', *TGSI*, vol. XLVIII (1972–4), pp. 435–72; idem., 'Prelude to the Crofters' War', *TGSI*, vol. XLIX (1974–7), pp. 159–88.

13 Day, *Public Administration*, p. 187.

14 J.P.D. Dunbabin, *Rural Discontent in Nineteenth Century Britain*

(London, 1974), Chapters IX, XII.

15 SCRO, D593/K/Peacock to Kemball, 9 February, 4 August 1882; Tranquar to Kemball, 9 August 1882.

16 Hanham, 'Highland discontent', p. 59; 'The report of the Crofters' Commission', *Saturday Review*, 3 May 1884, p. 560.

17 Dunbabin, *Rural Discontent*, passim.

18 'An old Highlander', 'Home truths on the Crofter agitation', *Blackwood's Edinburgh Magazine* vol. 138 (1885), pp. 98–100.

19 Napier Commission, quoted in Grant, *Everyday Life*, p. 8.

20 Napier Commission, Report, pp. 108–11.

21 The clearest account is in Day, *Public Administration*, pp. 187–92; see also Devine, *Clanship*, p. 220.

22 Allan Macinnes, 'Crofters' Holdings Act of 1886: A hundred year sentence?' in *Radical Scotland* no. 25 (1987) and subsequent responses.

23 Quoted in Ewan A. Cameron, 'The Scottish Highlands as a special policy area, 1886 to 1964,' *Rural History* 8 (1997), p. 196.

24 See M. Barker, *Gladstone And Radicalism* (Hassocks, 1975), p. 14; J.S. Blackie, 'The Highland Crofters', *Nineteenth Century*, vol. XIII (1883); Duke of Argyll, 'On the economic condition of the Highlands of Scotland', *Nineteenth Century*, vol. XIII (1883); *Saturday Review*, 10, 30 December 1882, 3 May, 15, 21 November 1884, 13 March 1886. See also Lord Napier's own defence during the controversy, 'The Highland Crofters. A vindication of the report of the Crofters' Commission', *Nineteenth Century*, vol. XVII (1885), pp. 437–63.

25 Hanham, 'Highland discontent', p. 65. Cf. J.A. Cameron, 'Storm clouds in the Highlands', *Nineteenth Century*, vol. XVI (1884), p. 380.

26 Eric Richards, 'How tame were the Highlanders?' pp. 46–8.

27 The provisions of the Act are outlined in Day, *Public Administration*, p. 191.

28 Cf. J. Neeson, review in *Historical Journal*, vol. XLI (1998), p. 278.

29 For the most balanced view of the effects of the legislation see Day, *Public Administration*, pp. 395–9.

30 Bruce Lenman, *An Economic History of Modern Scotland 1660–1976* (London, 1977), pp. 199–200.

31 Ian Grimble, 'Unsceptred Isle', in D.C. Thomson and Ian Grimble (eds.), *The Future of the Highlands* (London, 1968).

32 Cameron, op. cit., pp. 39, 304.

33 D. Turnock, *Patterns of Highland Development* (London, 1970), pp. 64–7.

34 Quoted in Day, *Public Administration*, p. 202.

35 SRO, HH/1/823, Eviction at Strathglass.

36 Ibid., Carson, 'Diary', p. 98.

37 *Scottish Highlander*, 19 August 1886.

38 Ibid., 5 April 1889.

39 Ibid., 26 September 1889.

40 Day, *Public Administration*, p. 192.

41 SCRO, D593/K/1/7/23, Wright to Mackay, 11 December 1889.

42 See the account of the dramatic campaign in Assynt by John MasAskill, *We Have Won the Land* (Stornoway, 1999). A fine evocation of the realties of modern crofting is Alisdair Maclean, *Night Falls on Ardnamurchan: The Twilight of a Crofting Family* (1984).

19

The Highland Clearances: Answers and Questions

THE HIGHLAND CLEARANCES STRETCHED across more than a hundred years. Many of the events in that history have been described in the previous chapters. What answers can this narrative now suggest to the series of questions posed at the very start (in the Preface)?

I. Rural flights

Were the Clearances a uniquely Highland experience? In reality most modern societies have passed through rural re-construction and turmoil. A notable instance of this is the Canadian novelist, Margaret Atwood, who regards herself as the product of a modern rural exodus. She told an audience in her home town that she had been born in Ottawa in 1939 and declared:

> I would not have been there at all if it hadn't been for the Great Depression: my parents were economic refugees from Nova Scotia – here is your historical force.[1]

The Atwoods' experience was not uncommon, especially among rural people during the Depression. Indeed most families in modern western societies, in historical memory, have been detached from the land and have become urban. In 1999 it was reported that there were at least 7000 abandoned villages in Spain.[2] Families and individuals have moved off the land, sometimes under pressure from landlords, or banks, or prices, or competition or adversity. More often rural people have migrated in response to the magnetic pull of the towns. It is virtually an historical cliché to say that this is a universal force in modern times. Highland crofting communities were running down throughout the twentieth century.

But rural exoduses are not all the same. The clearing of the Highlands was more cataclysmic than in most places. A Highland Clearance was 'an enforced simultaneous eviction of all families living in a given area such as an entire glen'.[3] This was not unique to the Highlands, nor was it the only form of Highland transformation. But it was common enough to colour the entire experience of Highland history. The suddenness, and the almost total erasure of a highly distinctive society, distinguishes the Highland Clearances from the customary movement of other rural peoples from the land.

British history reveals several variants of the rural exodus. The disappearance of the small landholder in England, extending throughout the nineteenth century and into the twentieth, was usually more gradual than in the Highlands. It was less dramatic than the mass evictions in the north of Scotland and parts of Ireland. But, even in England, the ultimate outcome was much the same: the number of smallholders eventually shrank and the great commercial farmers triumphed; the agricultural system was transformed. Moreover, at the base of rural life, the condition of the agricultural labourer in England, like that of his Highland counterpart, improved barely at all before 1851.[4]

Agrarian adjustments continued across Great Britain in the nineteenth century. It was part of the general reduction of the agricultural population which affected virtually every region: agricultural cottages were demolished everywhere, and the destruction was not confined to any particular variety of farming community; and in urban areas the demolition of slums was carried out with enthusiasm in the name of benevolence and to the shrill protests of the evicted. Even the philanthropic Octavia Hill and Lord Shaftesbury evicted people when they thought the change would improve the moral climate. In Ireland eviction was strongly correlated with economic conditions in agriculture. Everywhere the displacement of population was the mark of a society and economy in the throes of rapid structural change. One expression of such a transformation was the Highland Clearances; another was the removal of an estimated 76 000 in different parts of Britain to make way for the railways in the period 1853–1901.[5]

Was the vehement Highland reaction to the Clearances exceptional? One of the abiding characteristics of the remnants of Highland society has been its sustained anger against the Clearances. The story has been re-told with the accumulated bitterness of posterity in the oral record of the Highlands. It is preserved also in remarkable density in the many volumes of the Crofter Commission of 1886 and that of 1892.

Rural societies, ruptured by the demands of modernisation, frequently generate a rich and angry literature of denunciation.[6] The sense of loss of the old society in many countries is a universal theme in their plays, novels and poetry, myth and melodrama.[7] There were moments of high drama in the story of the Clearances, of individual suffering and collective resistance. The entire experience was shocking at the time, and more shocking to a later age. There is in the Highlands a widespread sense of indignation undimmed by either time or distance from the original events and it would be extraordinary if enduring anger had not been generated.[8]

Anger against rural transformation is common in some of the best known historical controversies which have been focussed precisely on the politics and social consequences of rural upheavals when the people were disengaged from the land. The list is long and lengthening: the 'storms over the gentry' in seventeenth-century England, and the 'Enclosures' in the eighteenth, spring to mind. So do the debates about rural reorganisation in Stalin's Russia, about the dislocation of Aboriginal economies by white settlement in colonial Australia and in the Americas, about the introduction of sugar production into the Philippines, and about the razing of villages in Ceausescu's Romania.[9] They all, like the Clearances, aroused the deepest passions.

Did the Clearances constitute 'genocide'? The latterday use of the term in the context of the Highland Clearances is widespread and questionable. But even a contemporary, Sir Edward Pine Coffin, spoke of the 'extermination of the people'.[10] Genocide, however, requires mass deaths and a clear element of intention on the part of a superintending force. In reality, few if any died during the Clearances in a way which could be directly attributed to the effects of eviction. There were people who evidently wanted to marginalise the Highlanders, and the modern phrase 'ethnic cleansing' echoes in the advocacy of some of the extreme elements in the Highlands (notably in the views of Patrick Sellar). But most landlords and their ideologues wanted no more than the reduction of the population of the region to sustainable levels. If labels are required, then 'economic displacement' and 'population control' are more apt to the purposes of the clearers.

Were the Highlands a viable and contented society before the Clearances? For posterity it is clear that the pre-clearance communities in the Highlands and Islands, their culture and ways of economic life, have shared the same neglect as those of other agrarian peoples in the British Isles. Like the English cottagers of the pre-industrial world, they have (in E.P. Thompson's resonant phrase) 'eluded the attention of historians since they were neither [profit-oriented] agriculturists nor emergent proletarians, and were of no importance to anyone except themselves'.[11]

It is, nevertheless, evident that the old Highland society was not democratic in spirit; the paternalism of the old ruling class in the Highlands was commonly combined with brutal arbitrariness. All the historical evidence demonstrates that grinding poverty in the Highlands pre-dated the Clearances and continued after the landlords were curbed. Even in the late twentieth century, it remained a relatively poor region with a narrow economic base. Until the late 1990s all efforts to promote employment in the Highlands and Islands have produced poor results. No agency private or public had been able to sustain closer settlement in the Highlands. If new growth can now be consolidated it will reverse all the historical trends of the past 150 years.[12]

How did the Clearances affect the population of the Highlands? The population of the Highlands continued to rise until 1851 and then declined unevenly until it was reduced in most places. Migration had been much greater from the relatively favoured quarters of the south and east of the region; permanent migration was lowest in the most isolated and poorest parts, in the north-west; this district retained its population most persistently and suffered the most sensational poverty and congestion.[13] The general path of population change in the Highlands was not significantly different from that of other agricultural, and especially pastoral, regions in the rest of the British Isles. As two recent historians have remarked of the Highlands:

> even the most generous could not accept that the social and economic structure should remain intact and unchanged when it was so patently unable to provide the bare necessaries of life in many places for a rising population.[14]

Emigration from the Highlands pre-dated the Clearances and much of the later emigration was not directly associated with the Clearances. People would have left the Highlands in any case; the Clearances were a complicating and an accelerating factor.

Did the Highlands face special disadvantages? We know that regions on the peripheries of industrialisation always suffer the centrifugal effects of economic growth. In the Highlands these forces were released during the period of the Clearances and limited the range of manoeuvre for all parties in the region. Highland landlords were as various as those elsewhere, as benevolent and as avaricious as the rest of their class. Highland landlords were less constrained by the law than their counterparts in the rest of Britain. At the same time Highland lairds were caught in the grip of economic and geographical conditions which limited their policy options more than most of their counterparts.

The phrase, 'the Highland Clearances', does not account for the sheer diversity of agricultural change in the Highlands, especially from east to west. The record shows clearly enough that there were identifiable Clearances in the Highlands as early as the 1660s.[15] The expansion of cattle production before 1770 created pressure for larger farms. Demands of improvement widened and deepened, being part of the response of the Highland economy to the requirements and opportunities of national and local economic growth. The turmoil of agrarian change in the Highlands was greater and more sudden than elsewhere in the British Isles, accelerating dramatically in the 1790s under the impact of the sheep. Geographical isolation and relatively poor resources had sustained a resolutely peasant structure longer than in most other parts. Consequently the region was less prepared for change than, say, the West Midlands of England or Lanarkshire. When it came it was more devastating. Moreover, since this economy was unable (despite many aborted efforts) to industrialise or diversify along the lines emerging in the industrial south, the indigenous people had far fewer alternatives once diverted from their old activities.

II. The clearance model and its variants

Was there a particular model of clearance? In the outcome there were many types of removal. The most dramatic and infamous of these was the mass eviction of whole communities at short notice, often marked by manhandling and the destruction of houses and providing no alternative accommodation or employment for the people involved. Sometimes these policies, as we have seen, were executed by estate officials, reinforced by legal officers and a *posse* of police, and were the cause of great hardship among the people. In another category were many instances of large-scale removal in which the landlord (often in a hurry and at large additional expense) offered the people alternative accommodation on the same estate.

Did Highland landlords try to diminish the consequences of the Clearances? Some proprietors, especially before 1820, created employment, raised new enterprises and villages, invested in local infrastructure and subsidised migration. Mostly they failed, demonstrating the intractability of 'the Highland problem' and the long record of failure of capital investment in virtually all enterprises except sheep and deer forests.[16]

Were the Clearances a completely negative and uniform phenomenon? Until the mid-nineteenth century contemporaries referred to the changes in the Highlands as the 'Improvements'. They included a panoply of innovations in crops, technology, tenure, manufactories and new villages. Shifting the people about was termed 'removal'. The process involved agrarian changes on a broad scale. Sometimes it required the relocation, sometimes the outright expulsion of the existing population; this then released entire districts for large-scale production, both arable and pastoral.[17]

Why did the re-construction of the economy cause such revulsion? The landlord-initiated re-settlement schemes usually involved the creation of crofts on the fringe of estates and on the most marginal land. These necessarily required the people to make great adjustments in both status and means of livelihood. Most crofting was created on the assumption that the people would take up fishing or kelp-working, or else find other productive ways of dividing their labour. Some of these Clearances were also forced through by legal process and in clear defiance of the wishes of the people. Rarely, if ever, were the common people consulted about their future: they were simply given their marching orders. Only the more dramatic episodes were recorded. But more prevalent were smaller-scale and longer-drawn-out Clearances which punctuated the life of the region, especially in the years 1800 to 1840. Most seem to have involved relocation rather than outright eviction. Evictions of individuals (not normally termed Clearances) sometimes caused great commotion and brought the entire community up in arms.

How much violence was employed? As the previous chapters have shown, in some of the more dramatic clearances (e.g. at Greenyards and Glencalvie) considerable physical force was applied. Whenever the people to be evicted resisted their fate, there were scenes of physical combat. There were many episodes of direct confrontation and several pitched battles in which injuries were incurred on both sides. In some of the most infamous cases, as in Sutherland in 1813–4, houses were demolished or set afire in order to prevent their re-occupation by the evicted tenantry. All this was part and parcel of the process of forced eviction in the Highlands and there is clear evidence of atrocious behaviour by some of the evicting officers. Sometimes the evicting parties were connected with emigration agencies who had contracted the people to depart on waiting ships. When some refused, at the last moment, estate officials tried to force them to fulfil their promises.

Rough-handling and episodic resistance were bound to occur in circumstances of sudden agricultural re-organisation and eviction. As the people were obviously being moved against their wishes some coercion was inevitable. Some landowners were patient, some not. Often the work was done by factors or incoming farmers. Patrick Sellar in Sutherland in 1814 was both; he was extremely impatient and used methods of eviction which few then or since could justify. Summary eviction, at the best of times, was a harsh way to deal with people whose main crime was their poverty and their inability to pay economic rents.

The history of the Clearances was, therefore, punctuated by many ugly encounters, but how much resistance was generated? The level of violence was less than in similar events in contemporary Ireland. There were no assassinations, and very few reprisals were either threatened or recorded. It is still widely thought that, having been broken by the impact of Culloden and government policy in the aftermath, the Highlanders withdrew into a pathetic stoicism and met their fate without resistance or even volition: they were cowed into submission to the will of the landlords, led by their ministers who preached co-operation and passivity.

In reality there was considerable resistance, passive and active, to the Clearances. Highland resistance was in the mould of pre-industrial collective behaviour and sometimes occurred in a large and relatively sophisticated form, most notably in the campaign against Patrick Sellar. Moreover the ministers were by no means uniformly complicit in the evictions and some provided support to the victims of the events. Equally evident, as we have seen in many episodes, Highland women were especially prominent in the sporadic resistance to the Clearances, often leading the affray and confronting the law officers and the police. The participation of women in many episodes emphasises the communal character of protest during the Clearances.[18] Highland resistance was, indeed, comparable with rural protests in other parts of the British Isles during other phases of rural transformation. Nevertheless the fact remains that the resistance was, at best, only partially successful. Few Clearances were actually stopped and most of the agrarian transformation proceeded, checked only in part by the fear of adverse publicity.

Did the Highlanders resist as much as an historian would expect? The strength of popular resistance in the Highlands has to be judged against the realistic possibilities of success in local conditions. Looking beyond the Highlands, it becomes clear that few peasant societies of this sort have been able to stop agrarian transformation in its tracks, whatever resistance was offered by the people. The great transformation of agriculture in the Scottish lowlands passed with 'relative tranquillity'.[19] The victims of English Enclosures were likewise known only for their grumbling passivity, though as Jeanette M. Neeson has emphasised, there was a 'visceral hostility that the term "grumbling", so effectively obscures'.[20] She argues that 'Resistance is no guide to the extent of hostility to enclosure. The sense of loss, the sense of *robbery* could last forever as the bitter inheritance of the rural poor'.[21] Neeson maintains that enclosure was a turning point in the social history of many English villages because it struck at the roots of the peasant economy and its class relations. What was true of English villages applied with greater force in Highland townships because the impact was more severe and because the historical preparation time was so much shorter than in England.

What were the expulsive forces in the Highlands? The removal party was not the only form of coercion in the Highlands. There were also more generalised pressures which worked to lever the people out of their old communities. Wherever the agricultural sector responded to national needs, market mechanisms were set in motion which promoted changes in land use. Eventually the pressures were transmitted to the least efficient elements in the community, helping to dislodge them in favour of producers who promised and delivered higher yields to the land and its capital. In the Highlands the pressure took the form of the inexorable upward movement of rents from about 1760 to 1815, which effectively pushed out those least able to pay, and was mainly fuelled by the competition of incoming sheep farmers. Sometimes the pressure came to a sharp focus – when, for instance, a tacksman's lease ended and newcomers (often from the south) entered the arena and bid up the rent beyond the capability or willingness of the current occupiers to pay. This was the common precipitant of a clearance.[22]

More usual was the gradual attrition of the local population, of people choosing to walk off the land rather than accept the more stringent conditions of landholding. *In extremis* some of the poorest elements of the crofting population begged their landlords for assistance to emigrate. Whatever the particular propellant, these people became part of the general mobility patterns of agrarian change, moving to local villages or adjacent estates, perhaps as a prelude to a move to the coast or to the south or even abroad.

Did the Clearances produce a particular economic structure in the Highlands? The effect on population movement was not necessarily radically different from that in several other rural areas in the British Isles during industrialisation.[23] But in the long run the Highland economy came to be segregated into two distinct sectors – the large farms (both pastoral and arable) and the crofts. The rents of the two sectors tended to diverge. For instance, real rents in the period 1845–80 rose much faster for the large tenants and sporting lessees than for the small tenantry; the crofters' relative contribution to total income fell throughout the century. The position of the small tenants was also weakened by the widespread refusal of Highland landlords to permit sub-division. This meant, of course, that families could not provide separately for their growing number of children as they reached adulthood. In extreme cases some landlords forbade children to remain on a croft once they married. Partly this was motivated by an effort to staunch the rapid growth of what was seen as a redundant population; undoubtedly it operated as a further expulsive force on the crofting community.

How did landlords justify the Clearances? Some proprietors argued that the Clearances were necessary because the people were too numerous and were forcing the entire region to the brink of famine; depopulation was imperative for their own good. This, however, was a reversal of the more common logic of the situation. The poverty of the people and their general inability to pay economic rents simply rendered alternative uses of the land the more attractive. Moreover there were managerial benefits from a cleared estate: it was easier and cheaper to extract rents from a few dozen capitalist tenants than from a dense population of hundreds of lotters.

What did the people in general feel about the great changes? Perhaps the nearest we can get to an answer is provided by the Celtic scholar, Donald E. Meek, who has explored furthest into the heart of the popular reaction to the removals. Drawing on the heritage of the Gaelic poets in the century after 1760, Meek has re-constructed vital parts of the mental world which had been thrown into turmoil by the invasion of the sheep economy and the concurrent tensions in the Highlands. The response of the poets was 'confused', but there can be no mistaking the revulsion and the popular resentment against the economic pressures which faced the people even before the sheep invaded the north. A poem of about 1770, originating in Islay, berated landlords for the accumulating rent increases. But the poet also celebrated the escape route offered by a beckoning Gaelic Arcadia in North Carolina. Three decades later other poets were attacking the shepherds and their sheep which they associated with the loss of traditional loyalties in the old community. In Glenshiel the decline of social cohesion and old values was registered by the poet Ailean Dall MacDougall who satirised the 'filthy' ways of the shepherds, their disgustingly smeared sheep, and 'the yelling dogs of lowlanders'. In the 1820s, McLachlan of Rahoy, familiar with Ardnamurchan, Morvern and Mull, initiated a cycle of poems against the shepherds:

> I see nothing there now but a ragged shepherd
> and his fingers blacker than a crow's pinion.

A sense of disgust and revulsion, as well as incomprehension, dominated the poetic indictment which, not surprisingly, carried a racial edge:

> The ill-will of Lowlanders has scattered
> those who have left us and will never return.

It was defined as a conflict between the *Gaidheal* and the *Gall* – that is, 'between the indigenous person and the economically motivated incomer'. Emigration, however, was perceived as 'a merciful deliverance from a collapsed world order', a liberation from the terror of eviction and the behaviour of oppressive landlords. There had been an unforgivable betrayal. The anger and the despair of the community were captured in these poems.[24]

III. The landlords

How should landlords, especially those in the Highlands, be judged?
They were regarded as the custodians of the land and possessed
customary responsibility for the welfare of the people and the
efficient conduct of the local economy. They could be expected to
supply leadership, stewardship and a rational use of the resources
within a framework set by a tradition which had clearly shifted its
foundations. They may also have been charged with responsibility
to the nation at large. In the modern era their traditional roles and
their new agenda were often at odds and at times this put them in a
quandary.

Landlords held the levers of power in the Highlands and they
made decisions on behalf of the region. They could not insulate the
region from the outside world; they had to balance the requirements of economic development against the forces of inertia and
the minimisation of dislocation. The old peasant economy was
unable to respond effectively to the demands of the market.
Improvers pointed this out at great length and proclaimed
Improvement as a national duty. Landlords observed their costs and
living expenses rise decade after decade and were fully conscious of
the attractions of the southern model. The fact that small
producers, either collectively or individually, were unable to match
the rents offered by capitalist farmers meant that their days were
numbered. Many of the newcomers (in both sheep and arable
farming) were from the south, though there were many
Highlanders among them too. The great attraction of the
Highlands was the relatively cheap and under-exploited land to
which more productive modern agricultural methods could be
applied. Expertise, capital and a willingness to pay higher rents
were the entry costs which most local small tenantry could not
match. The essential story is told in the farm advertisements
published in the northern newspapers from 1780 onwards.
Highland proprietors, in this respect, simply followed national
trends and were not much different from landlords elsewhere.
When wool prices fell after 1815 rents fell more slowly and the
pressure on marginal producers was redoubled. Many landlords

had committed themselves financially on the expectations generated in the period of inflation and now felt greater urgency in extracting income, with fewer concessions to their tenantry.

What did contemporary economic advisers recommend? Improvement propagandists encouraged landlords to increase their scale of operations and the introduction of tenants with good reserves of capital. The old peasant agriculture was not only palpably less competitive, it was equally a waste of the region's resources and could not even provide the people themselves with a decent secure livelihood. The ultimate cause of the Highland Clearances was located in the extraordinary increase in the nation's demands for food and raw materials, which in turn generated internal pressures, over many decades, for a structural transformation of the northern economy. By 1820 the Highlands clearly contributed to the transformation which enabled the country as a whole to feed itself and prosper. Eventually even the Highlands participated in improved living standards, though this was contingent also on the reduction of the population of the region.

The landlords therefore were, in a sense, functionally the intermediaries in this structural change. But they reacted to it in many ways. Some followed the trend (and their own financial interest) without much restraint. Others followed the general dictates of the economy with great hesitation, often precipitated into radical change by some local circumstances such as an impending bankruptcy, or a change in ownership, or a subsistence crisis among the crofters on an estate. Some landlords tried to compromise, balancing the introduction of capitalist agriculture with the retention and redeployment of the old population within their estates. This compromise was the main origin of crofting in the nineteenth-century Highlands.[25] Other landowners delayed the change as long as possible, often attempting to extract as much rent increase from the old occupiers as they could. Some of them permitted sub-division to a dangerous extent. A few landlords were successfully blocked by popular resistance (or the threat of it) and were unable to restructure their estate economies. A few landowners tried to revitalise small-scale holdings by organising them into new and efficient systems of agriculture, but the results were very poor for landlords and people alike.[26] Some landowners and ideologues argued straightforwardly that there was no future for small producers in the Highlands and that mass migration was the only solution. But many landowners clung to the view that the Highlands could be developed in a way which would solve the problem of poverty for them and for the people.

Did Highland landlords lack enterprise and capital? From about 1760 onwards, through the years of the Clearances, external capital flowed into the Highlands as never before. Much of this capital had been generated in the Lowlands, in England and in the colonies, some brought home by expatriates returning with the booty of empire. Capital went into estate purchases, land improvements, industrial and commercial enterprise, famine relief, and the building of mock castles and other follies. At minimum, the capital imports created short term employment effects in many parts of the Highlands. But the return on capital was almost certainly very low by contemporary standards. Much of the imported capital simply haemorrhaged in the Highlands. It is also clear that some of the most successful entrepreneurs of the age were drawn north to the Highlands. They included men full of zeal, urgent to crack the problem of the Highlands, prepared to plough their commercial and industrial wealth into the region. But the return on their investments was almost always derisory. The dividends of empire and industry were thus often wasted in the Highlands. It was indeed a loss to the national economy to be set beside any gains to be tallied.

The history of the Clearances is, therefore, only a partial record of the landlord response to the opportunities and pressures which were generated in the Highland economy in the period 1760 to 1880. Evictions were undoubtedly a dominant characteristic of this behaviour, but it would be a travesty to say that this was the only form of landlord activity in this period. The record of the many efforts to reconstruct local economies in the Highlands in order to generate new employment and cushion the decline of old industries, and to ward off the worst consequences of over-population, congestion and famine; the expenditures devoted to subsidised emigration; the extraordinary patience of many landlords with uneconomic rents – all this, and more, should be set beside the story of the Clearances. There were among the Highland proprietors sensitive and humane landlords who bankrupted themselves in vain efforts to hold back the implacable pressures of economic and demographic change. Several fortunes derived from places outside the Highlands were sunk into the region in unavailing attempts to establish the economic foundation of a more secure way of life. The story of these recurrent failures is instructive in the sense that they provide a measure of the difficulties which confronted and broke even the best motivated, most prosperous, and most humane of landlords.

With or without sheep and deer, it was always extremely difficult to modernise or shift the economy of the old society. At Gairloch in 1845 an ambitious attempt was made to re-construct the local economy. More than 370 cottars and small tenants of the MacKenzies of Gairloch and Conan (influenced by similar experiments in Sussex and Belgium) were shifted into a new pattern of settlement; new crofts were created and one fifth of the settlers were brought in from beyond the estate. Eventually the landlord was forced to admit failure for himself and the people. This was indeed an example of positive clearance – and not associated with the introduction of sheep – designed to renovate the estates specifically to retain the population. Whatever the motivation, however, the Gairloch experiment was not a success and was greeted with predictable rejection by the local small tenantry.[27]

Were Highland landlords especially oppressive? Some clearly were, as the previous chapters have demonstrated. But most Highland landlords, like those elsewhere, generally accepted the conditions that they faced. These were no wiser than other landlords: they consumed their rentals, they sought the best tenants they could get, they subsidised large numbers of unproductive relatives, and they cleared small tenants off their lands. The timing, the manner, and the consequences of these evictions varied widely from landlord to landlord, and from district to district. In the long run – by cataclysmic clearances, or gradual erosion, or voluntary emigration – the result was the same, and the expulsive forces were triumphant. In the long run, the transformation of the economy and the dissolution of this peasant society were, arguably, irresistible.

What was the value of good intentions? Much of the drama and tragedy of the Highlands is told in the negotiations between financially-racked landlords and their creditors, agents and trustees. Even those proprietors most loyal to the traditional values of the Highlands eventually either fell bankrupt, or reluctantly followed the path of the improvers. The story of David Stewart of Garth, the champion of the old Highlands and proclaimer of all the virtues of landlord paternalism, was the most pathetic. His estates finally collapsed under the weight of family debt and annuities and sinking rents. He found himself trying to bolster his Highland estates from the profits of his West Indian slave plantations. He ended up urging his own sub-tenants to emigrate – in effect, to clear themselves off his estate so that he could raise his rents. Similarly the last of the Glengarrys sold off his West Highland estate and tried to re-create his clan in New South Wales, ending as a broken reed, all dreams destroyed. The best of intentions were never enough amid the more populous and improvement-driven world of the mid-century Highlands.[28]

IV. A people adrift

How do we measure the consequences of the Clearances? This is one of the most difficult tasks in modern Scottish history. But the medical historian Robert Matheson has recently asserted that 'The Clearances dispossessed a people, expelled them to wholly inadequate sites and condemned them to misery and disease'. He roundly blames the Clearances for all the social problems of the post-clearance Highlands: destitution, pauperism, malnutrition, ill-health and disease. 'After the clearances, subsistence was threatened, immunity weakened and overcrowding made more severe. Thus contamination was much more often fatal.' This is the severest of modern indictments yet it depends on a very optimistic assessment of the pre-clearance conditions of the Highlands. It equally relies on the idea that conditions of Highland poverty were caused by landlord policy rather than any of the other circumstances affecting levels of welfare in the Highlands. Most of all, Matheson's 'causal pathology' depends on an implicit hypothesis, namely that the Highlanders would have been healthy and prosperous but for the removal policies. This, of course, is the crux of the matter, and remains unresolved by modern historians.[29]

The impact of the Clearances as such is difficult to disentangle from the effects of other simultaneous changes in the fabric of the Highlands. De-industrialisation and rapid population growth were both great influences on levels of social welfare. So too were the effects of emigration agents and greater employment opportunities outside the region, both activating an outward flow of Highlanders. Concurrent with the coercive effect of the Clearances were streams of 'voluntary' migrants both seasonal and permanent. In the 1850s young emigrants left the Highlands for North America and Australasia in a spirit of adventure, escape and liberation: their experience can be set beside the pathetic human remnants of famine and eviction who required special nursing and feeding before they could be readied for their oceanic voyages.[30] Yet poverty, disease and famine all pre-dated the Clearances.

What was the precise number of Highlanders directly cleared off the land in the various categories of coercion? This is not known but must have entailed several tens of thousands. Aside from the Clearances, it is likely that the generally inhospitable economic conditions, much worsened by rapid population growth, induced or persuaded many more people to take their own paths out of the Highlands. When living standards improved more rapidly in the south, after the 1840s, the outflow accelerated.

Why is the population question so perplexing? Population growth was virtually universal by the 1770s and continued in many places until the 1860s, but within the broad trend were differences which bedevil a clear understanding of the Clearances. In the east of the Highlands (for example in Easter Ross), agricultural change required major shifts among the local population and a consolidation of farms. But, compared with the rest of the region, the proportion of arable land was high, the level of farm investment and labour intensity much greater, and the development of local villages and fishing much more vigorous. Yet in this relatively rich district, with good alternative employment opportunities, the level of population growth was low. Population here did not accumulate and out-migration was copious. By contrast, in Wester Ross, where sheep farming was far more dominant and where fishing and kelping failed very badly, and where subsistence was palpably more precarious, population accumulated very rapidly (and did not decline until 1870). In some parts of the west the population trebled between 1770 and 1850.

Can the landlords be blamed? It is often said that the landlords were responsible for the demographic crisis in the west because they deliberately promoted close settlement at the time of expanding kelp and fishing enterprise. There is truth in this, but the argument ceases to apply after 1815, when population continued to increase despite the clear reversal of landlord policy.[31]

Thus population congestion was greatest in the poorest and most remote districts, in the areas where the effects of the Clearances were most delayed and where the tenacity of the people to cling on to the land which rewarded them so poorly was greatest. Out-migration, and absolute population decline, occurred precisely during the generation in which crofter living standards rose demonstrably, that is from 1860 to 1890. It is also well established that other rural regions in the British Isles lost their people at a faster rate than the Highlands, even though these societies never faced Clearances.

In the case of Barra, the expansion of the population after clearance seemed to give little comfort to those who saw the solution of the Highland problem in terms of emigration. Between 1841 and 1851 the population of the island fell from 2363 to 1873. But by 1881 it had risen again to 2161, and by 1911 it reached a record level of 2620. The experience of North Uist was much the same. On the other hand many parts followed a downward curve much earlier: both South Uist and Lochbroom declined continuously after the mid-century.

Although there were several episodes in which people were cleared and directly embarked for overseas, it has yet to be demonstrated that, in general, the Clearances accelerated either migration or emigration. Landlord policy may have strengthened the crofters' determination to cling on to their homeland. J.M.

Bumsted, following earlier work of Margaret Adam, has argued that the earlier emigrations were acts of choice rather than coercion.[32] It is obvious that, despite much movement from the west coast, emigration was inadequate to prevent extraordinary population growth.

The demographic history of the Highlands after 1840 shows that the problem of explanation was more complex than Malthus or the emigration enthusiasts had believed. In practice the clearing landlords of the 1850s had little more systematic knowledge of likely population trends than their predecessors who had pursued reverse policies only fifty years before. For the most part the Highland Clearances constituted the crudest type of social engineering, and were, in the event, a blunt instrument wielded by landlords with only the most rudimentary understanding of the repercussions of their actions.

V. Famine in Highland history

Why did the Highlands suffer famine in 1840s? The West Highlands and Islands of Scotland were the last region of mainland Britain to escape from the grip of recurrent famine. Famine had affected the Highlands from time immemorial. Even the east, as late as 1817, was still subject to severe harvest shortfall, but by 1830 the eastern Highland grain lands were regular surplus producers (even in 1847/48). But in the west, famine continued to descend on the people, especially in 1835–6 and 1847–9, also in lesser known crises in each decade until the end of the century. The great difference between the nineteenth-century famines and those of earlier times was that few if any of the population starved to death. Relief measures were better mobilised and the isolation of the region was decisively reduced.[33] In 1847–8 death rates may even have fallen during the great subsistence crisis. Nevertheless there was great suffering and distress in the west coast communities and, indeed, fear and turbulence in the east coast villages.[34]

That a large population in mainland Britain should continue victim to recurrent harvest failure in the heyday of Victorian economic development stirred the national conscience and darkened the reputation of the landlords who presided over the region. The role of the Clearances is often regarded as central in these episodes and it is indisputable that famine accelerated evictions on some estates. It is equally true that the introduction of sheep farming could only have intensified congestion along the coasts. The Clearances were a critical element in the set of circumstances which caused a large growing population of peasants to live on the margin of a poorly endowed region with little chance of ancillary employment or a productive division of their labour. Indeed, more remarkable than the persistence of famine was the sheer survival of so many people in such difficult circumstances: it was a tribute to the food value (per pound, per acre, and per man-hour) of the potato, and also to the observable fortitude and communal resilience of the people themselves. In a special sense the West Highland economy was a resounding success in that it kept alive a huge increase of its population without the benefit of diversification, industrialisation or (in the main) emigration. But the vulnerability of the Highlands to famine in the 1840s was a consequence of the perpetuation of pre-industrial conditions; in essence the dangerously increasing population was caught in an economy in which the demand for labour was declining.

VI. Winners

Who were the beneficiaries of the great changes in the Highlands? Some of the original landowners benefited from much higher rents and were able to survive into the new commercial era. But there was a great rate of turnover in landownership and many owners sold out and left the Highlands. The return on land ownership in the Highlands has never been calculated but seems to have been lower than elsewhere in Britain. The sheep farmers made good profits and some became wealthy despite the high risks they shouldered. Even so the sheep farmers as a class did not emerge as a great plutocracy noted for their conspicuous consumption; nor was the sheep farming industry the basis for illustrious pastoral dynasties. The offspring of the sheep farmers found little future within the Highlands and they migrated as much as the small tenantries.

The winners are less easily identified than the victims. Patrick Sellar, who had more than an axe to grind, rejoiced in the fact that his own grandfather had been ousted from the inland districts of Banff and forced to begin a new life of personal improvement. It is not known whether his forbear would have agreed with this view, though Sellar made the same proto-Smilesian claim on behalf of Sir William Grant (1753–1832), Master of the Rolls (1801–17). Grant's father had also been a very small farmer catapulted from Elchies in Banff into the wider world.[35] But Highlanders on the whole did not thank their landlords for clearing them from their lands.

The reduced population of the region eventually, after the passage of perhaps five generations, experienced better living standards. But the most effective method of increasing average levels of welfare was, in a powerful paradox, to reduce the population. The true benefits of the Highland Clearances were, in reality, widely diffused in the form of cheaper commodities to the rest of the British economy: the clothes of the people, the food they ate, their employment in the industries of the south. In the great parallel debate on the land question in Ireland, as W.E. Vaughan points out, contemporary advocates of freedom of contract invoked a wider concept of 'the public good'. They made a stark implicit calculation: 'if large-scale sheep farming could reduce the price of woollen socks even by a small fraction of a farthing, sweeping changes in rural society might be justified'.[36] The imperative of economic development had indeed required the appropriation of the Highlands to serve the needs of the national economy, and the excision of a culture. But was the reduction in the price of wool by 'a penny a pound' worth so much turmoil?

Do we know enough about the Highland Clearances? The story of course contains abundant fuel for indignation, but the focus has become blurred partly because of the confusion of criteria employed in the ongoing debates.[37] For instance, a realistic view of the events requires a systematic comparison of the fate of those Highlanders cleared with those who remained in the undisturbed districts of the region. This has not yet been tackled. Moreover the histories of several large estates are still uninvestigated.[38] Similarly darkness shrouds the exact state of economic and social life in the Highlands before the Clearances and this undermines our evaluations of subsequent changes. The critics of Highlands landlords still generally fail to give substance to their denunciations by specifying plausible alternatives for the region in the age of the clearances.[39] It remains clear that, despite the spectrum of solutions applied at different times and places, the economic problems of the Highlands have hardly yet been solved[40] and the notion that the problems of the present can still be blamed on the Clearances becomes increasingly implausible as time passes.

VII. Losers

Do we need to revise the story of the Highland Clearances? When all the qualifications have been made, it remains beyond dispute that large but unknown numbers of Highlanders were cleared from their ancestral homes. A peasant society and a distinctive culture were, in many places, razed from the face of the land. The Highlands of Scotland were transformed as much as any colony in the Empire in that age, fully incorporated into the role of supplying the metropolitan economy, and routed by the forces of change. The benefits which accrued from this great upheaval did not flow in the direction of the people who inhabited the region. The central historical question is not what happened, but why the Highlands underwent this appalling experience, and why this tragedy was not ameliorated or tempered by a nation which had become the richest and most dynamic the world had seen.

Moreover, despite the great sympathy widely felt for the fate of the Highlanders in general, little consideration was accorded the lowest strata of Highland society, most prominently the cottars and the squatters who lived on the margins of a marginal society. These anonymous sub-peasantry were the most serious losers in the transformation. The problem of the landless in the Highlands is still capable of arousing angry dispute, even amongst the most sympathetic observers of the cleared Highlands.[41]

The contemporary documentation of the Highland Clearances, subjected to the normal tests of historical evidence, therefore broadly vindicates the popular version of the story. The iron fist of landlord power in the Highlands was employed with little restraint in many cases. There was probably an unspecifiable number of accelerated deaths among the victims of the evictions. The poverty of the people was often desperate. Fire and hatchets were used to carry through many clearances. On occasion the people were coerced on to emigrant ships and despatched to barely-understood destinations. The forces of the law and the military were borrowed to implement cruel evictions. The government refused to intercede on behalf of the common people.

Highland landlords behaved as variously as other landlords under such conditions. The forces of conservatism belonging to the old vested interests obstructed rural change in the Highlands. Newcomers to the Highlands displayed both ignorance and incomprehension of the vestiges of the old society which they appropriated. The Clearances were resisted intermittently and on a scale and with an intensity which was not unusual in such a society undergoing transformation. The level of leadership was poor but the involvement of women was striking and recurrent in a clearly established pattern. But the extent of violence and bloodshed was small by historical standards. The role of posterity has been to exaggerate and polarise the account and to diminish the underlying economic dilemma of everyone in the region. The exceptionalism of the Highlands has been over-rated at the expense of the significance of the Clearances as a well-documented exemplar of the perils facing a poor society located on the edge of industrialisation.

Notes

1 Margaret Atwood, 'In Search of *Alias Grace*', *American Historical Review*, 103 (1998) p. 1504.

2 See *Guardian Weekly*, 25 Nov. 1999.

3 See Adam Watson and Elizabeth Allan, 'Depopulation by clearances and non-enforced emigration in the North East Highlands', *Northern Scotland* (1990), p. 31.

4 See W.R. Wordie, 'The Chronology of English Enclosure, 1500–1914,' *Ec H R* XXXVI 1983. Most works on the history of English agriculture do not contain the word 'eviction' in their indexes.

5 See Enid Gauldie, *Cruel Habitations* (London, 1974), pp. 33, 56, 87.

6 A small selection of the Highland literature includes Neil M. Gunn, *Butcher's Broom* (1934), *The Silver Darlings* (1941); Iain Crichton-Smith, *Consider the Lilies* (1970); David Foster, *Moonlite* (1981); John McGrath, *The Cheviot; the Stag and the Black Black Oil* (1974); the Grampian Television series *The Blood is Strong* with accompanying booklet by Angus Peter Campbell (1988), and John Prebble, *The Highland Clearances* (1963). Another genre is the travelogue in the form of a quest for the descendants of the people who emigrated from the Highlands: see Craig, op. cit., James Hunter, *A Dance Called America* (1994), and the works of Derek Cooper, for example, *The Road to Mingulay* (1985).

7 See, for instance, Rosalind Mitchison, 'The Highland Clearances', *Scottish Social and Economic History* no. 1 (1981), pp. 1–24.

8 See especially the remarkable work of Donald E. Meek from original Gaelic sources, op. cit., passim.

9 Similar parallels are drawn by David Craig, *On the Crofters' Trail*, (1990; 1997 edition), pp. 7–8.

10 Quoted in Devine, *Clanship*, p. 60.

11 E.P. Thompson, *Customs in Common*, p. 178, as quoted by Roger Wells in *Journal of Peasant Studies*, 21 (1994), p. 204.

12 See James Hunter, 'Balance of Power', *Scotsman*, 11 Nov. 1999.

13 See Cameron, op. cit., p. 2.

14 See R.H. Campbell and T.M. Devine, 'The Rural Experience', in *People and Society in Scotland II 1830–1914* edited by W. Hamish Fraser and R.J. Morris, p. 50.

15 See R.H. Macdonald, 'Estate of Chisholm', *Transactions of the Gaelic Society of Inverness*, vol. LIV (1984–6), p. 88.

16 See A.J. Youngson, *After the Forty-Five* (Edinburgh, 1973); Philip Gaskell, *Morvern Transformed* (Cambridge, 1968); Nigel Nicolson, *Lord of the Isles* (1968); Eric Richards, *Leviathan of Wealth* (1973).

17 See the studies reported by J.B. Caird, 'The Creation of Crofts and New Settlements. Patterns in the Highlands and Islands of Scotland', *Scottish Geographical Magazine*, vol. 103, no. 2 (1987), pp. 67–75.

18 See especially Alexander B. Mearns, 'The Minister and the Bailiff: A study of Presbyterian clergy in the Northern Highlands during the clearances', *Scottish Church History Society, Records*, XXIV; and

especially the vigorous paper by David M. Paton, 'Brought to a wilderness: the Rev. David Mackenzie of Farr and the Sutherland Clearances', *Northern Scotland*, op. cit.

19 T.M. Devine, *Exploring the Scottish Past* (Edinburgh, 1995), Chap. 13. See also John Stawhorn, *The History of Irvine* (Edinburgh, 1985), pp. 71, 84.

20 J.M. Neeson, *Commoners*, op. cit., p. 280.

21 Ibid., p. 291.

22 Frequently an incoming tenant would make his occupancy dependent on the removal of the people. There were many cases in which the rent of the land was clearly greater if the people were evicted altogether.

23 See, for instance, R.H. Campbell, 'Inter-County Migration in Scotland and the Experience of the South-West in the Nineteenth Century', *Scottish Economic and Social History*, vol. 4 (1984), pp. 55–63.

24 I am most grateful to Professor Meek for allowing me to quote from his unpublished lecture, 'Concepts of the Clearances in Contemporary Gaelic Verse' (1999).

25 See J.B. Caird, op. cit. See also Adam Collier, *The Crofting Problem* (Cambridge, 1953), and James Hunter, *The Making of the Crofting Community* (Edinburgh, 1976).

26 See *Pigeon Holes of Memory. The Life and Times of Dr John Mackenzie* (1803–1886), edited by Christina Byam Shaw (Palo Alto, 1988).

27 See James B. Caird, 'The Creation of Crofts', pp. 67–75.

28 On the promotion of 'Highlandism' see J.E. Cookson, 'The Napoleonic Wars, Military Scotland and Tory Highlandism in the Early Nineteenth Century' *SHR*, LXXVII (1999), pp. 60–75.

29 Matheson, op. cit., pp. vii, ix, 5, 121, 167, 179.

30 See Richards, *Scotlands*, op. cit., passim.

31 A convenient review of population and migration trends in the different parts of the Highlands is found in Charles W.J. Withers, 'Highland – Lowland migration and the making of the Crofting Community, 1755–1891', *Scottish Geographical Magazine*, vol. 103, no. 2 (1987).

32 J.M. Bumsted *The People's Clearance 1770–1815* (Edinburgh 1982). See also the work of Bernard Bailyn, *Voyagers to the West* (New York, 1986); T.M. Devine, 'Highland migration to Lowland Scotland 1760–1860', *Scottish Historical Review*, vol. 54 (1975); and Don Watson, *Caledonia Australis* (Sydney, 1984).

33 See Devine, *The Great Highland Famine* (1989) and Eric Richards,

'Poverty and survival in nineteenth century Coigach', in J. Baldwin (ed.), *Peoples and Settlement in North-West Ross* (Edinburgh, 1994).

34 See Eric Richards, *The Last Scottish Food Riots* (1981).

35 See Richards, *Patrick Sellar*, Chap. 2.

36 W.E. Vaughan, *Landlords and Tenants in Ireland, 1848–1904* (Oxford, 1994), p.10.

37 See for instance Stuart R. Sutherland, 'Ethics and economics in the Sutherland Clearances', *Northern Scotland*, vol. 2, no. 1 (1974–5).

38 But see Leah Leneman, *Living in Atholl, 1685–1785* (Edinburgh, 1986), Eric Richards and Monica Clough, *Cromartie: Highland Life 1650–1914* (Aberdeen, 1989), and I.F. Grant, *Everyday Life on an old Highland Farm* (London, 1924).

39 R.H. Campbell's Introduction to 1980 edition of Gaskell, op. cit.

40 See Michael Pacione, 'Rural problems and *Planning for Real* in Skye and Lochalsh', *Scottish Geographical Magazine*, 112 (1996) pp. 20–8.

41 See Allan I. Macinnes, 'The Crofters' Holdings Act of 1886: A Hundred Year Sentence?' *Radical Scotland*, no. 25 (Feb/March 1987).

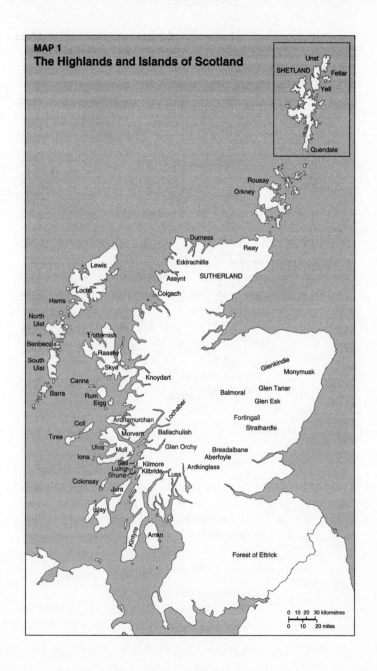

MAP 1
The Highlands and Islands of Scotland

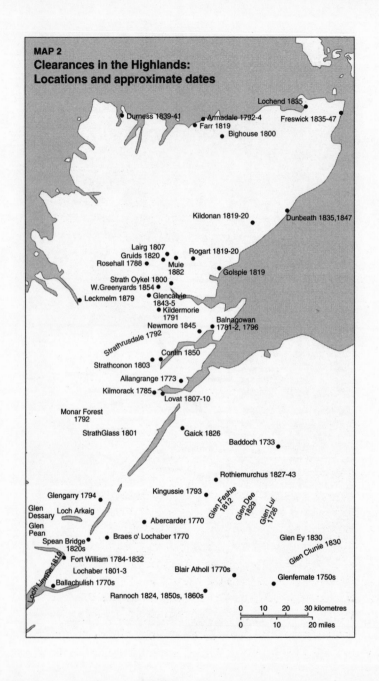

MAP 2
Clearances in the Highlands: Locations and approximate dates

Lochend 1835
Durness 1839-41
Armadale 1792-4
Freswick 1835-47
Farr 1819
Bighouse 1800

Kildonan 1819-20
Dunbeath 1835, 1847

Lairg 1807
Rogart 1819-20
Gruids 1820
Rosehall 1788
Muie 1882
Golspie 1819
Strath Oykel 1800
W.Greenyards 1854
Leckmelm 1879
Glencalvie 1843-5
Kildermorie 1791
Balnagowan 1781-2, 1796
Newmore 1845
Strathrusdale 1792
Contin 1850
Strathconon 1803
Allangrange 1773
Kilmorack 1785
Lovat 1807-10
Monar Forest 1792
StrathGlass 1801
Gaick 1826
Baddoch 1733
Rothiemurchus 1827-43
Glengarry 1794
Kingussie 1793
Glen Feshie 1812
Glen Dee 1829
Glen Lui 1726
Glen Dessary
Loch Arkaig
Abercarder 1770
Glen Pean
Braes o' Lochaber 1770
Spean Bridge 1820s
Glen Ey 1830
Glen Clunie 1830
Fort William 1784-1832
Lochaber 1801-3
Blair Atholl 1770s
Glenfernate 1750s
Ballachulish 1770s
Loch Linnhe 1816
Rannoch 1824, 1850s, 1860s

0   10   20   30 kilometres
0   10   20 miles

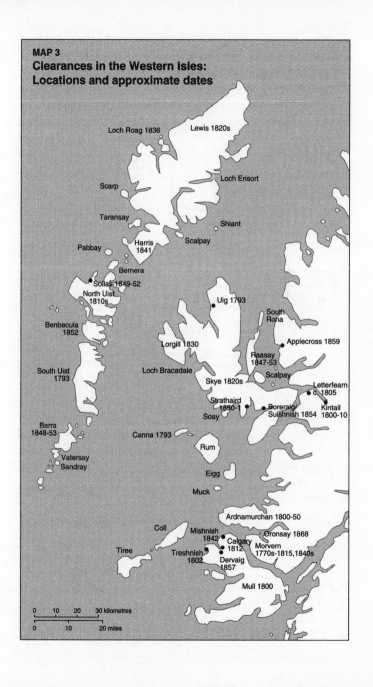

MAP 3
**Clearances in the Western Isles:
Locations and approximate dates**

Loch Roag 1836
Lewis 1820s
Loch Erisort
Scarp
Taransay
Shiant
Pabbay
Harris 1841
Scalpay
Bernera
Sollas 1849-52
North Uist 1810s
Uig 1793
South Rona
Benbecula 1852
Lorgill 1830
Applecross 1859
Raasay 1847-53
South Uist 1793
Loch Bracadale
Scalpay
Skye 1820s
Letterfearn c. 1805
Strathaird 1850-1
Boreraig Suishnish 1854
Kintail 1800-10
Soay
Barra 1848-53
Canna 1793
Vatersay
Sandray
Rum
Eigg
Muck
Ardnamurchan 1800-50
Coll
Mishnish 1842
Oronsay 1868
Calgary 1812
Tiree
Treshnish 1802
Morvern 1770s-1815, 1840s
Dervaig 1857
Mull 1800

0   10   20   30 kilometres
0   10   20 miles

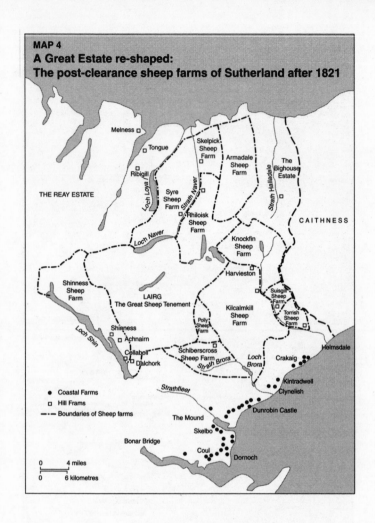

MAP 4

A Great Estate re-shaped:
The post-clearance sheep farms of Sutherland after 1821

Melness

Tongue

Skelpick Sheep Farm

Armadale Sheep Farm

The Bighouse Estate

Ribigill

THE REAY ESTATE

Syre Sheep Farm

Loch Loyal

Strath Naver

Rhiloisk Sheep Farm

Strath Halladale

CAITHNESS

Loch Naver

Knockfin Sheep Farm

Harvieston

Shinness Sheep Farm

LAIRG
The Great Sheep Tenement

Kilcalmkill Sheep Farm

Suisgill Sheep Farm

Torrish Sheep Farm

Loch Shin

Shinness

Achnairn

Polly Sheep Farm

Cellaboll

Dalchork

Schiberscross Sheep Farm

Strath Brora

Loch Brora

Crakaig

Helmsdale

Kintradwell

Strathfleet

Clynelish

The Mound

Dunrobin Castle

Skelbo

Bonar Bridge

Coul

Dornoch

● Coastal Farms
□ Hill Frams
–·–·– Boundaries of Sheep farms

0   4 miles

0   6 kilometres

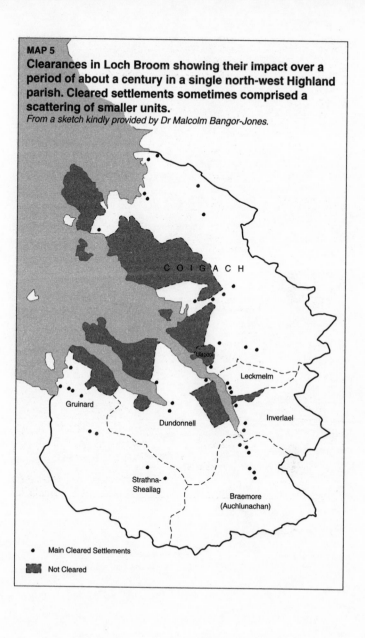

MAP 5

Clearances in Loch Broom showing their impact over a period of about a century in a single north-west Highland parish. Cleared settlements sometimes comprised a scattering of smaller units.
From a sketch kindly provided by Dr Malcolm Bangor-Jones.

COIGACH

Ullapool

Leckmelm

Gruinard

Dundonnell

Inverlael

Strathna-Sheallag

Braemore
(Auchlunachan)

• Main Cleared Settlements

▓ Not Cleared

Bibliography

The following books have useful bibliographies:

Gray, M. *The Highland Economy 1750–1850* (Edinburgh, 1957).
Hunter, J. *The Making of the Crofting Community* (Edinburgh, 2000).
Richards, E. *The Leviathan of Wealth* (London, 1973).
Symon, J.A. *Scottish Farming, Past And Present* (Edinburgh, 1959).
Turnock, D. *Patterns Of Highland Development* (London, 1970).

Abbott, E. and Campbell, L. *The Life and Letters of Benjamin Jowett* (1897).
Adam, M.I. 'The causes of the Highland emigrations of 1783–1803', *Scottish Historical Review*, vol. 17 (1920).
————'The eighteenth century Highland landlords and the poverty problem', *Scottish Historical Review*, vol. 19 (1922).
————'The Highland emigration of 1770', *Scottish Historical Review*, vol. 16 (1919).
Adam, R.J. (ed.) *John Home's Survey of Assynt* (Scottish History Society, Edinburgh, 1960).
————(ed.) *Papers on Sutherland Estate Management* (Scottish History Society, 2 vols., Edinburgh, 1972).
Adams, J.Q. *Writings of John Quincy Adams*, ed. W. C. Ford (New York, 1968).
'Agricola'. 'On the improvement of the Highlands', *The Weekly Magazine of Edinburgh Amusement*, vol. 25 (1774).
Alison, W.P. *Letter to Sir John McNeill on Highland Destitution* (Edinburgh, 1851).
Alister, R. *Barriers to the National Prosperity Of Scotland* (Edinburgh, 1853).

Alister, R. *The Extermination of the Scottish Peasantry* (Edinburgh, 1853).

'Amicus' *Eight Letters on the Subject of the Earl of Selkirk's Pamphlet on Highland Emigration as they Lately Appeared under the Signature of Amicus in One of the Edinburgh Newspapers* (Edinburgh, 1803).

Anderson, G. and P. *Guide to the Highlands and Islands of Scotland* (Edinburgh, 3rd edn., 1851).

Anderson, J. *An Account of the Present State of the Hebrides* (Edinburgh, 1825).

Anderson, J. *General View of the Agriculture of the County of Aberdeen* (Edinburgh, 1794).

Anderson, J. *Prize Essay on the State of Society and Knowledge in the Highlands of Scotland* (Edinburgh, 1825).

Anon. *Emigration from the Highlands and Islands of Scotland to Australia* (London, 1852).

——*Hints for the Use of Highland Tenants and Cottagers, by a Proprietor* (Inverness, 1838).

——'Landed tenures in the Highlands', *Westminster Review*, vol. 34 (1868).

——*Notes and Sketches Illustrative of Northern Rural Life in the Eighteenth Century* (Edinburgh, 1877).

——*Observations on the Causes and Remedies of Destitution in the Highlands of Scotland* (Glasgow, 1838).

——*On the Neglect of Scotland and her Interests by the Imperial Parliament* (Edinburgh, 1878).

Argyll, Duke of (George Douglas Campbell). *Autobiography and Memoirs*, edited by the Dowager Duchess of Argyll (2 vols., London, 1906).

——'A corrected picture of the Highlands', *Nineteenth Century*, vol. 16 (November 1884).

——'On the economic condition of the Highlands of Scotland', *Journal of the Statistical Society of London*, vol. 26 (1883).

——*Scotland as it was and as it is* (2 vols., Edinburgh, 1887).

Armstrong, W.A. 'The influence of demographic factors on the position of the agricultural labourer in England and Wales, c.1750–1914', *Agricultural History Review*, vol. 29 (1981).

Ashton, T.S. *The Industrial Revolution* (London, 1968 edn.).

Atwood, M. 'In search of *Alias Grace*: on writing Canadian historical fiction', *American Historical Review* 103 (1998), pp. 1503–1516.

Bailyn, B. '1776. A year of challenge – a world transformed', *Journal of Law and Economics*, vol. 15 (1976).

——*Voyagers to the West*. (New York, 1986).

——'The challenge of modern historiography', *American Historical Review*, vol. 87 (1982).

Bain, R. *History of the Ancient Province of Ross* (Dingwall, 1899).

Baker, A.R.H. and Butlin, R.A. (eds.) *Studies of Field Systems in the British Isles* (London, 1973).

Baldwin, J. (ed.) *Peoples and Settlement in North-West Ross* (Edinburgh, 1994).

Balfour, R.A.C.S. 'Emigration from the Highlands and Western Isles of Scotland to Australia during the nineteenth century', unpublished M.Litt. thesis, University of Edinburgh, 1973.

Bangor-Jones, M. *Assynt Clearances* (Dundee, 1998).

Barker, M. *Gladstone And Radicalism* (Hassocks, 1975).

Barron, E.M. (ed.) *A Highland Editor. Selected Writings of James Barron of the Inverness Courier* (Inverness, 1927).

Barron, J. *The Northern Highlands in the Nineteenth Century* (3 vols., Inverness, 1907–13).

Barzun, J, and Graff, H.F. *The Modern Researcher* (San Diego, 1985).

Basu, P. *Narratives in a Landscape: Monuments of the Sutherland Clearances*. M.Sc. thesis, University College (London, 1997).

Bayne, P. *The Life and Letters of Hugh Miller* (2 vols., London, 1871).

Beames, M. 'Rural conflict in pre-famine Ireland', *Past and Present*, no. 81 (1978).

Bear, W.E. 'Obstruction to land tenure reform', *Contemporary Review*, vol. 48 (1885).

Belsches, R. *General View of the Agriculture of Stirlingshire* (Edinburgh, 1796).

Beresford, M. *The Lost Villages of England* (London, 1954).

Bischoff, J. *A Comprehensive History of the Woollen and Worsted Manufactures* (2 vols., London, 1842).

Black, R.D.C. 'The classical view of Ireland's economy' in A.W. Coats (ed.), *The Classical Economists and Economic Policy* (London, 1971).

———*Economic Thought and The Irish Question 1817–1870* (Cambridge, 1960).

———'The Irish experience in relation to the theory and practice of economic development' in A.J. Youngson (ed.), *Economic Development in the Long Run* (London, 1972).

Black, R.I.M. 'An emigrant's letter in Arran Gaelic, 1834', *Scottish Studies* 31 (1992–3) 62–87.

Blackie, J.S. *Altavona* (Edinburgh, 1882).

———'The Highland crofters', *Nineteenth Century*, vol. 13 (1883).

———*The Scottish Highlanders and the Land Laws* (London, 1885).

———*Scottish Song* (Edinburgh, 1889).

Blair, D.B. 'On the early settlement of the lower provinces by the Scottish Gael: their various situations and present prospects', *Transactions of the Celtic Society of Montreal* (1884–7).

Botfield, B. *Journal of a Tour through the Highlands* (Norton Hall, 1830).

Boyd, W.K. *Some Eighteenth Century Tracts Concerning North Carolina* (Raleigh, 1927).

Breen, H. *St Lucia* (London, 1844).

Brenner, R. 'The agrarian roots of European Capitalism', *Past and Present*, no. 70 (1976).

Bristow, E. 'The liberty and property defence league and individualism', *Historical Journal*, vol. 18 (1975).

Broady, M. *Marginal Regions* (Oxford, 1973).

Brock, W.R. *Scotus Americanus* (Edinburgh, 1982).

Broeker, G. *Rural Disorder and Police Reform in Ireland 1812–1836* (London, 1970).

Broeze, F.J.A. 'Private enterprise and the peopling of Australasia, 1831–1850', *Economic History Review*, vol. 35 (1982).

Brooking, T. *Lands for the People* (Dunedin 1996).

Brown, C. *The Social History of Religion in Scotland since 1730* (1987).

Browne, J.A. *History of the Highlands and of the Highland Clans* (4 vols., Glasgow, 1838).

Bruce, J. *Letters on the Present Condition of the Highlands and Islands of Scotland* (Edinburgh, 1847).

Bruce, S. 'Social change and collective behaviour: the revival in Eighteenth Century Ross-shire', *British Journal of Sociology*, vol. 34 (1983).

Bryden, J. 'Core-Periphery Problems – the Scottish Case' in Dudley Seers, Bernard Schatter and Marja-Lilsa Kiljunen (eds.), *Underdeveloped Europe*, (London, 1979).

Buchanan, J.L. *Travels in The Western Hebrides* (London, 1793).

Bulloch, J.M. *The Gordons of Cluny* (Buckie, 1911).

Bumsted, J.M. *The People's Clearance: Highland Emigration to British North America 1770–1815* (Edinburgh, 1982).

———'Settlement by chance: Lord Selkirk and Prince Edward Island', *Canadian Historical Review*, vol. 59 (1978).

Burns, Sir A. *History of the British West Indies* (1965).

Burton, J.H. 'Celtic clearings', *Edinburgh Review*, vol. 86 (1847).

Cain, P.J. and Hopkins, A.G. *British Imperialism, 1688–1914* (1993).

Caird, J.B. 'The North West Highlands and the Hebrides' in Jean Mitchell (ed.), *Great Britain. Geographical Essays* (Cambridge, 1967).

———'The creation of crofts and new settlement patterns in the Highlands and Islands of Scotland', *Scottish Geographical Magazine*, 103 (1987) 67–75.

———(ed.) *Park: a Geographical Study of a Lewis District* (Nottingham, 1958).

Cameron, E.A. *Land for the People? The British government and the Scottish Highlands, 1880–1925* (East Linton, 1996).

———'The Scottish Highlands as a special policy area, 1886 to 1964', *Rural History*, 8 (1997).

Cameron, J.A. 'Storm clouds in the Highlands', *Nineteenth Century*, vol. XVII (1884).

Cameron, J.M. 'A study of the factors that assisted and directed Scottish emigration to Upper Canada, 1815–1855', unpublished Ph.D. thesis, University of Glasgow, 1970.

————'The changing role of the Highland landlords relative to Scottish emigration during the first half of the nineteenth century' in *Proceedings of the Fourth and Fifth Colloquia on Scottish Studies* (Guelph, 1971).

Cameron, T. *The Old and the New Highlands and Hebrides, from the Days of the Great Clearances to the Pentland Act of 1912* (Kirkcaldy, 1912).

Campbell, A. *The Romance of the Highlands* (Aberdeen, 1927).

Campbell, D. and R.A. Maclean. *Beyond the Atlantic Roar: a Study of the Nova Scotia Scots* (Toronto, 1974).

Campbell H.F. 'Notes on the county of Sutherland in the eighteenth century', *Transactions of the Gaelic Society of Inverness* (*TGSI*), vol. XXVI (1904–7).

Campbell, J.L. *Songs Remembered in Exile* (Aberdeen, 1990).

————*The Book of Barra* (London, 1936).

————(ed.) *A Collection of Highland Rites and Customs, Copied by Edward Lluyd from the Manuscript of the Rev. James Kirkwood (1650–1709), and Annotated by him with the Aid of the Rev. John Beaton* (The Folklore Society, Cambridge, 1975).

————'Eviction at first hand. The clearing of Clanranald's Islands', *Scots Magazine* (January 1945).

Campbell, R.H. *Scotland since 1707* (Oxford, 1965).

————and J.B.A. Dow. *Source Book of Scottish Economic and Social History* (Oxford, 1968).

Cannadine, D. 'Aristocratic indebtedness in the 19th century: the case reopened', *Economic History Review*, vol. 30 (1977).

Carlyle, W.J. 'The changing distribution of breeds of sheep in Scotland, 1795–1956', *Agricultural History Review*, vol. 27 (1979).

Carpenter, S.D. MacD. 'Patterns of recruitment of the Highland Regiments of the British Army, 1756 to 1815', unpublished M.Litt. thesis, University of St Andrews, 1977.

Carr, H. 'Mexican agrarian response, 1910–1960', in E.L. Jones and S.J. Woolf (eds.), *Agrarian Change and Economic Development* (London, 1969).

Carrington, C.E. *The British Overseas* (Cambridge, 1950).

Carruthers, R. *The Highland Notebook* (Inverness, 1887).

Carter, I. 'The changing image of the Scottish peasantry, 1745–1980' in R. Samuel (ed.), *People's History and Socialist Theory* (London, 1981).

——'The Highlands of Scotland as an under-developed region' in E. de Kadt and C. Williams (eds.), *Sociology and Development* (London, 1974).

Cavendish, A.E.J. *An Reisimeid Chataich* (1928).

Chadwick, E. *Report on the Sanitary Condition of the Labouring Population of G. Britain* (Edinburgh, ed. 1965 [1842]).

Chambers, J.D. and Mingay, G.E. *The Agricultural Revolution, 1750–1880* (London, 1966).

Checkland, S.G. 'Scottish economic history', *Economica*, vol. 21 (1964).

——*Scottish Banking, A History, 1695–1973* (Glasgow, 1975).

Chisholm, C. 'The clearance of the Highland glens', *TGSI*, vol. 5 (1876–7).

Clapham, J.H. *Economic History of Modern Britain* (1926).

Clark, A. *An Enlightened Scott. Hugh Cleghorn (1752–1837)* (Duns, 1992).

Clark, G.K. *The Making of Victorian England* (London, 1962).

Clarke, J.B. *The Crofters' Act* (London, 1887).

Clark, S. *Social Origins of the Irish Land War* (Princeton, 1979).

Cloward, R.A. and F.F. Piven. 'Hidden protest: the channelling of female innovation and resistance', *Signs* 4 (Summer 1979), pp. 601–69.

Cobbett, W. *Rural Rides*, ed. G.D.H. and Margaret Cole (3 vols., London, 1930 edn.).

Cockburn, H. *Journal of Henry Cockburn, 1831–1854* (2 vols., Edinburgh, 1874).

——*Memorials of Henry Cockburn* (Edinburgh, 1856).

Collier, A. *The Crofting Problem* (Cambridge, 1953).

Collins, B. 'Proto-industrialization and pre-famine emigration', *Social History*, vol. 7 (1982).

Collins, E.J.T. 'The Economy of upland Britain, 1750–1850' in R.B. Tranter (ed.), *The Future of Upland Britain* (2 vols., Reading, 1978).

Connolly, S.J., Houston, R.A. and Morris, R.J. (eds.). *Conflict,*

Identity and Economic Development: Ireland and Scotland, 1600–1939. Carnegie Publishing (Preston, 1995).

Cookson, J.E. 'The Napoleonic Wars, military Scotland and Tory Highlandism in the early nineteenth century', *Scottish Historical Review* 78 (1999), pp. 60–75.

Cooper, D. *Hebridean Connection* (London, 1977).

——*Road to the Isles* (London, 1979).

——*Skye* (London, 1970).

——*The Road to Mingulay* (1985).

Cooper, P. *An Old Story Retold: The So-Called Evictions from the Macdonald Estates in the Island of North Uist, Outer Hebrides, 1849* (Aberdeen, 1881).

Coull, J.R. 'Fisheries in the north-east of Scotland before 1880', *Scottish Studies (SS)*, vol. 13 (1969).

Cowan, R. *Vital Statistics of Glasgow* (Edinburgh, 1838).

Cowie, R. *Shetland, Descriptive and Historical* (Aberdeen, 1879).

Cozens-Hardy, B. (ed.) *Diary of Sylas Neville, 1767–1788* (London, 1950).

Craig, D. *On the Crofter's Trail: In Search of the Clearance Highlanders* (London, 1997 [1990]).

Cramb, A. *Who Owns Scotland Now?* (Edinburgh, 1996).

Crawford, I. 'Contribution to the history of domestic settlement in North Uist', *SS*, vol. 9, (1965).

Cregeen, E.R. (ed.) *Argyll Estate Instructions* (Scottish History Society, Edinburgh, 1964).

——'The changing role of the House of Argyll in the Scottish Highlands' in N.T. Phillipson and Rosalind Mitchison (eds.), *Scotland in the Age of Improvement* (Edinburgh, 1970).

——'The House of Argyll and the Highlands' in I.M. Lewis (ed.), *History and Social Anthropology* (London, 1968).

——'Oral sources for the social history of the Scottish Highlands and Islands', *Oral History*, vol. 2 (1974).

——'Oral tradition and agrarian history in the West Highlands', *Oral History*, vol. 2 (1974).

——'The tacksmen and their successors', *SS*, vol. 13 (1969).

Crichton Smith, I. *Consider the Lilies*, 2nd edn. (Edinburgh: Canongate Classics, 1987 [1968]).

Crotty, R.D. *Irish Agricultural Production* (Cork, 1966).

Crouzet, F. 'Wars, blockade and economic change in Europe 1792–1815', *Journal of Economic History*, vol. 24 (1964).

Crowley, D.W. 'The Crofters' Party 1885–1892', *SHR*, XXXV (1956).

Cullen, L.M. *An Economic History of Ireland since 1660* (London, 1972).

———(ed.) *The Formation of the Irish Economy* (Cork, 1976).

Cumming, S.F.G. *In The Hebrides* (London, 1883).

Cummings, A.J.G. and Devine, T.M. *Industry, Business and Society in Scotland since 1700* (Edinburgh, 1994).

Daiches, D. (ed.) *New Companion to Scottish Culture* (Edinburgh, 1993).

Dalriad [Lord Cohn Campbell] *The Crofter in History* (Edinburgh, 1885).

Daly, M. 'Revisionism and Irish History: the Great Famine', in D.G. Boyce and A. O'Day (eds.) *The Making of Modern Irish History: Revisionism and the Revisionist Controversy* (London, 1996).

Darby, H.I. (ed.) *A New Historical Geography of England* (Cambridge, 1973).

Darling, F.F. *Island Years* (London, 1940).

——— *The Story of Scotland* (London, 1945).

——— *West Highland Survey* (Oxford, 1955).

Dawson, J.H. *The Abridged Statistical History of the Scottish Counties* (Edinburgh, 1862).

Day, J.P. *Public Administration in the Highlands and Islands of Scotland* (London, 1918).

de Crevecoeur, J.H. St J. *Letters from an American Farmer* (London, 1782; 1962 edition).

Deane, P. and Col, W.A. *British Economic Growth 1688–1959* (Cambridge, 1969).

Defoe, D. *A Tour Through The Whole Island Of Great Britain* (Penguin edn., 1971).

Dempster, G. *A Discourse on the Proceedings of the British Fisheries Society* (London, 1788).

——— *In Memoriam* (privately printed, 1889).

De Serville, P. *Port Phillip Gentlemen* (Melbourne, 1980).

Devine, T.M. 'Highland migration to Lowland Scotland, 1760–1860', *SHR*, vol. 62 (1983).

———'The rise and fall of illicit whisky-making in Northern Scotland c. 1780–1840', *Scottish Historical Review*, vol. 54 (1975).

———'Temporary Migration and the Scottish Highlands in the nineteenth century', *Economic History Review (EHR)*, vol. 32 (1979).

———*Clanship to Crofter's War* (Manchester, 1994).

———*Exploring the Scottish Past* (Edinburgh, 1985).

———*Lairds and Improvement in the Scotland of the Enlightenment* (Dundee, 1979).

———*The Transformation of Rural Scotland* (Edinburgh, 1994).

———*Conflict and Stability in Scottish Society, 1700–1850* (Edinburgh, 1990).

Devine, T.M. and Mitchison, R. (eds.). *People and Society in Scotland vol. I: 1760–1830* (Edinburgh, 1988).

Devine, T.M and Orr, W.J. *The Great Highland Famine* (Edinburgh, 1988).

de Vries, J. *The Dutch Rural Economy in the Golden Age, 1500–1700* (London, 1974).

Dewey, Clive. 'Celtic agrarian legislation and the Celtic revival: historicist implications of Gladstone's Irish and Scottish Lands Acts 1870–1886', *Past and Present*, no. 64 (1974).

———'The rehabilitation of the peasant proprietor in nineteenth century economic thought', *History of Political Economy*, vol. 6 (1974).

De Wolfe, B. (ed.) *Discoveries of America* (New York, 1997).

Dodd, A.H. *The Industrial Revolution in North Wales* (Cardiff, 1933; 1951 edition).

Dodgshon, R.A. *From Chiefs to Landlords* (Edinburgh, 1998).

———*Land and Society in Early Scotland* (Oxford, 1981).

———'Livestock production in the Scottish Highlands before and after the Clearances', *Rural History* 9 (1998).

———'West Highland and Hebridean settlement prior to crofting and the Clearances: a study in stability or change?', *Proceedings of the Society of Antiquaries of Scotland*, 123 (1993) 419–38.

———'Agricultural change and its social consequences in the southern uplands, 1600–1780' in T.M. Devine and David Dickson (eds.), *Ireland and Scotland 1600–1850* (Edinburgh, 1983).

———'The economics of sheep farming in the southern uplands during the Age of Improvement, 1750–1833' *EHR*, vol. XXIX (1976).

———'The removal of runrig in Roxburghshire and Berwickshire, 1680–1766' *SS*, vol. 16 (1974).

Donaldson, G. *The Scots Overseas* (London, 1966).

Donaldson, J. *General View Of The Agriculture Of The County Of Banff* (Edinburgh, 1794).

Donaldson, J.E. *Caithness In The Eighteenth Century* (Edinburgh, 1938).

Donnachie, I. and Macleod, I. *Old Galloway* (Newton Abbott, 1974).

Donnelly, J.S. *The Land and People of Nineteenth Century Cork* (London, 1975).

Douglas, T. (Earl of Selkirk), *Observations on the Present State of The Highlands of Scotland* (London, 1805).

Dovring, J.F. 'The transformation of European agriculture', in *Cambridge Economic History of Europe*. (Cambridge, 1965), vol. VI.

Dugdale, B.E. *Arthur James Balfour* (2 vols. London, 1939).

Dunbabin, J.P.D. *Rural Discontent in Nineteenth Century Britain* (London, 1974).

Dunderdale, G. *The Book of the Bush* (London, 1898).

Dunlop, J. *The British Fisheries Society 1786–1893* (Edinburgh, 1978).

———'The British Fisheries Society: 1787 Questionnaire', *Northern Scotland*, vol. 2, no. 1 (1974–5).

Edmondston, A. *A View of the Ancient and Present State of the Zetland Islands* (2 vols., Edinburgh, 1809).

Edwards, M.M. *The Growth of the British Cotton Trade, 1780–1815* (Manchester, 1967).

Egremont, M. *Balfour* (London, 1980).

Ellice, E. *A Letter to Sir George Grey on the Administration of the Poor Law in The Highlands* (London, 1855).

Elliot, R. *Special Report on Sutherland and the West Highlands* (pamphlet, 1848).

Engels, F. *The Condition of the Working Class in England in 1844* (London, 1952 edition).

Erickson, C. *Emigration from Europe, 1815–1914* (London, 1976).

——*Invisible Immigrants* (London, 1972).

Extracts from Letters of the Rev. Dr McLeod, Glasgow, Regarding the Famine and Destitution in the Highlands (Glasgow, 1847).

Fairhurst, H. 'Rosal: a Deserted Township in Strath Naver, Sutherland', *Proceedings of the Society of Antiquities of Scotland*, vol. 100 (1967–8).

——'The surveys for the Sutherland Clearances 1813–1820', *SS*, vol. 8 (1964).

——and G.I. Petrie. 'Scottish Clachans II: Lix and Rossal', *Scottish Geographical Magazine*, vol. 80 (1964).

Fairhurst, J. 'The rural settlement pattern of Scotland with special reference to the West and North', in R.W. Steel and R. Lawton (eds.) *Liverpool Essays in Geography* (London, 1967).

Falk, B. *The Bridgewater Millions* (1942).

Fea, J. *The Present State of the Orkney Islands* (Edinburgh, 1775).

Ferguson, W. *Scotland 1689 to the Present* (Edinburgh, 1968).

Fergusson, J. (ed.) *Letters of George Dempster to Sir Adam Fergusson, 1756–1813* (London, 1934).

Fernstein, C.H. 'Pessimism perpetuated: real wages and the standard of living in Britain during and after the Industrial Revolution?' *Journal of Economic History,* 58, (1998).

Findlater, E.J. *Highland Clearances: the Real Cause of Highland Famines* (Edinburgh, 1855).

Fischer, W. 'Rural industrialization and population change', *Comparative Studies in Society and History*, vol. 15 (1973).

Fleming, R. (ed.) *The Lochaber Emigrants to Glengarry* (Toronto, 1994).

Flinn, M.W. 'Malthus, emigration and potatoes in the Scottish north-west, 1770–1870' in L.M. Cullen and T.C. Smout (eds.), *Comparative Aspects of Scottish and Irish Economic and Social History 1600–1900* (Edinburgh, 1977).

————*et al. Scottish Population History* (Cambridge, 1977).

————'The stabilisation of mortality in pre-industrial Western Europe', *Journal of European Economic History*, vol. 3 (1974).

Floud, Roderick and McCloskey, Donald (eds.), *The Economic History of Britain since 1700. I. 1770–1860* (Cambridge, 1981).

Forbes, D. *The Sutherland Clearances, 1806–1820* (Ayr, 1976).

Forsyth, R. *The Beauties of Scotland* (5 vols., Edinburgh, 1808).

Foster, S. and Smout, T.C. *The History of Soils and Field Systems* (Aberdeen, 1994).

Fraser, Sir W. (ed.). *The Sutherland Book* (3 vols., Edinburgh, 1892).

Fraser, W.H. and Morris R.J. (eds.) *People and Society in Scotland vol. II: 1830–1914*.

Fraser-Mackintosh, C. *Letters of Two Centuries* (Inverness, 1890).

————*Antiquarian Notes* (Sitrling, 1913).

————'The Depopulation of Aberarder in Badenoch', *Celtic Magazine*, vol. 11 (1877).

Freeman, T.W. *Pre-Famine Ireland* (Manchester, 1957).

Fry, M. *The Dundas Despotism* (Edinburgh, 1992).

Fullarton, Allan and C.R. Baird. *Remarks on the Evils at Present Affecting the Highlands and Islands of Scotland* (Glasgow, 1838).

Fussell, G.E. and Goodman, C. 'Eighteenth century traffic in livestock', *Economic History*, vol. III (1936).

Gaffney, V. *The Lordship Of Strathavon* (Aberdeen, 1960).

Gaffney, V. 'Summer Shealings', *SHR*, vol. 38 (1959).

Gailey, R.A. 'Agrarian improvement and the development of enclosure in the South West Highlands of Scotland', *SHR*, vol. 42 (1963).

————'Mobility of tenants on a Highland estate in the early nineteenth century', *SHR*, vol. 40 (1961).

————'The role of subletting in the crofting community', *SS*, vol. V (1961).

Garnett, T. *Observations on a Tour through the Highlands and Part of the Western Isles of Scotland* (2 vols., London, 1811).

Gaskell, P. *Morvern Transformed* (Cambridge, 1968; 1980 edition).

Gauldie, E. *Cruel Habitations* (London, 1974).

Gayer, A. *et al. The Growth and Fluctuation of the British Economy 1790–1850* (2 vols., Oxford, 1953).

Geikie, A. *Scottish Reminiscences* (Glasgow, 1904).

George, H. *Scotland and Scotsmen* (Glasgow, 1884).

Gibbon, E. *Decline And Fall Of The Roman Empire*, abridged edn., D.M. Low (ed.), (London, 1963).

Gibbon, J.M. *Scots in Canada* (London, 1911).

Gibson, R. *Toppling the Duke – Outrage at Ben Bragghie* (Evanton, 1996).

Gill, C. (ed.) *Dartmoor. A New Study* (Newton Abbott, 1970).

Gillespie, J. 'The cattle industry in Scotland', *Transactions of the Royal Highland and Agricultural Society of Scotland*, 5th series, vol. 10 (1898).

Gonner, E.C.K. *Common Land and Enclosure* (2nd edn., London, 1966).

Goodman, D. and M. Reddift. *From Peasant to Proletarian* (Oxford, 1981).

Gower, Ronald (Lord). *My Reminiscences* (4th edn. London, 1885).

Graham, I.C.C. *Colonists from Scotland: Emigration to North America 1707–1783* (Ithaca, 1954).

Grant, A. *Letters from the Mountains* (3 vols., London, 1807).

Grant, I.F. 'The Highland open field system', *Geographical Teacher*, Autumn (1926).

———*The Economic History of Scotland* (London, 1934).

———*Everyday Life on an Old Highland Farm, 1769–1782* (London, 1924).

———*Highland Folk Ways* (London, 1961).

———*The Macleods, The History Of A Clan* (London, 1959).

———'The social effects of the agricultural reforms and enclosure movement in Aberdeenshire', *Economic History*, vol. 1 (1926).

Grant, M.W. 'Why always Sutherland?' typescript (n.d.).

———*Golspie's Story* (Golspie, 1991 ed.).

Gray, A. *The Development of Economic Doctrine* (London, 1931).

Gray, J.M. *Lord Selkirk of Red River* (London, 1963).

Gray, M. 'The abolition of runrig in the Highlands of Scotland', *EHR*, vol. V (1952).

———'Some accounts of individual Highland sporting estates', *Economic History*, no. 3 (January 1928).

———'Settlement in the Highlands, 1750–1850', *SS*, vol. VI (1962).

———'The Consolidation of the Crofting System', *Agricultural History Review*, vol. 5 (1957).

———'Economic welfare and money income in the Highlands, 1750–1850', *Scottish Journal of Political Economy*, vol. 2 (1955).

———*The Fishing Industries of Scotland 1790–1914* (Aberdeen, 1978).

———*The Highland Economy 1750–1850* (Edinburgh, 1957).

———'The Highland potato famine of the 1840s', *EHR*, vol. 7 (1954–5).

———'The kelp industry in the Highlands and Islands of Scotland', *Economic History Review*, vol. 4 (1951).

———'Migration in the rural Lowlands of Scotland, 1750–1850' in T.M. Devine and David Dickson (eds.), *Ireland and Scotland 1600–1850* (Edinbugh, 1983).

———'Scottish emigration: the social impact of agrarian change in the rural Lowlands, 1775–1875', *Perspectives in American History*, vol. 7 (1973).

Greg, W.R. 'Highland destitution and Irish emigration', *Quarterly Review*, vol. 90 (1851).

Grierson, T. *Autumnal Rambles among the Scottish Mountains* (Edinburgh, 1850).

Grimble, I. *Chief of Mackay* (London, 1965).

———'Emigration in the time of Rob Donn, 1714–1778', *SS*, vol. 7 (1963).

———'Gael and Saxon in Scotland', *Yale Review*, vol. 52 (1962).

———'John Mackay of Strathan Melness, Patron of Rob Donn', *Scottish Gaelic Studies*, vol. 10 (1964).

———'Patrick Sellar' in Gordon Menzies (ed.), *History is my Witness* (London, 1977).

———'The Rev. Alexander Pope's Letter to James Hogg, 1774', *Scottish Gaelic Studies*, vol. 11 (1966).

———*The Trial of Patrick Sellar* (London, 1962).

———'Unsceptred Isle' in D.C. Thomson and I. Grimble (eds.), *The Future of the Highlands* (London, 1968).

———*The World of Rob Donn* (Edinburgh, 1979).

Guillet, E.C. *Early Life in Upper Canada* (Toronto, 1933).

———*The Great Migration* (Toronto, 1933).

Gunn, D. *History of Manitoba* (Ottawa, 1880).

Gunn, N.M. 'The tragedy of the Highland Clearances', *Radio Times*, 10 December 1954.

Guttsman, W.L. *The English Ruling Class* (London, 1969).

Haber, L.F. *The Chemical Industry during the Nineteenth Century* (Oxford, 1958).

Haldane, A.R.B. *The Drove Roads Of Scotland* (Edinburgh, 1968).

——*New Ways Through The Glens* (Edinburgh, 1962).

Hall, J. *Travels in Scotland by an Unusual Route* (2 vols., London, 1807).

Hall, R. *The Highland Sportsman and Tourist* (London, 1885).

Hallett, G.P. Randall and E.G. West. *Regional Policy for Ever?* (London, 1973).

Hamilton, H. *An Economic History of Scotland in the Eighteenth Century* (Oxford, 1963).

——*The Industrial Revolution in Scotland* (Oxford, 1932).

Handley, J.E. *The Navvy in Scotland* (Cork, 1970).

——*Scottish Farming in the Eighteenth Century* (London, 1953).

Hanham, H.J. 'Mid-century Scottish nationalism' in R. Robson (ed.), *Ideas and Institutions in Victorian Britain* (London, 1967).

——'The problem of Highland discontent, 1880–1885', *Transactions of the Royal Historical Society*, vol. 19 (1969).

Hansen, M.L. *The Atlantic Migration* (New York, 1961).

Harris, B. 'Patriotic commerce and national revival: the Free British Fishery Society and British politics, c. 1749–58' *English Historical Review* 114, 285–313, (1999).

Hart, J. 'Sir Charles Trevelyan at the Treasury', *English Historical Review*, vol. 75, no. 294 (1960).

Hartwell, R.M. 'A revolution in the character and destiny of British wool' in N.B. Harte and K.G. Ponting (eds.), *Textile History and Economic History* (Manchester, 1973).

Hawkins, A. *Reshaping Rural England: A Social History* (London, 1991).

Hechter, M. *Internal Colonialism: the Celtic Fringe in British National Development, 1536–1966* (London, 1975).

Henderson, J. *General View of the Agriculture of the County of Sutherland* (London, 1812).

———*Caithness Family History* (Edinburgh, 1884).

Heney, H.M.E. *In a Dark Glass* (Sydney, 1961).

Heron, R. *General View Of The Hebrides* (Edinburgh, 1794).

Heywood, C. 'The role of the peasantry in French Industrialisation, 1815–80', *Economic History Review*, vol. 34 (1981).

Highland Emigration Society. Report of the Highland Emigration Society from its Formation in April 1852 until April 1853 (London, 1853).

Hildebrandt, R.N. 'Migration and economic change in the Northern Highlands during the nineteenth century, with particular reference to the period 1851–91', unpublished Ph.D. thesis, University of Glasgow, 1980.

Himmelfarb, G. *Victorian Minds* (London, 1968).

Hirschman, A.O. *Essays in Trespassing* (Cambridge, 1981).

———*The Strategy of Economic Development* (New Haven, 1965).

'Historical pamphlets of Inverness-shire', vol. 1, 'Emigrants from Skye to Australia', Inverness Public Library.

Hobsbawm, E.J. *The Age Of Capital* (London, 1975).

———*The Age Of Revolution*, 1789–1848 (New York, 1964).

———*Industry and Empire* (Penguin edn., 1969).

———'Capitalism and agriculture; the Scottish Reformers in the eighteenth century', *Annales*, vol. 33 (1978).

———'Scottish reformers of the eighteenth century and capitalist agriculture' in E.J. Hobsbawm (ed.), *Peasants in History* (Calcutta, 1980).

Hobson, P.M. 'Congestion and depopulation, a study in rural contrasts between West Lewis and West Sutherland', unpublished Ph.D. thesis, University of St Andrews, 1952.

Hogg, J. *A Tour In The Highlands In 1803* (Paisley, 1888).

Holland, S. *Capital versus the Regions* (London, 1976).

———*The Regional Problem* (London, 1976).

Hollander, S. *The Economics of Adam Smith* (London, 1973).

Homer, P.B. *Observations on a Short Tour Made in the Summer of 1803 to the Western Highlands of Scotland* (London, 1804).

Horner, F. *The Economic Writings of Francis Homer in the Edinburgh Review 1802–6*, ed. F.W. Fetter (London, 1957).

Houston, G. 'Farm Wages in Central Scotland from 1814 to 1870', *Journal of the Royal Statistical Society*, series A, vol. 118 (1955).

Houston, R.A. 'Scottish education and literacy, 1600–1800: an international perspective' in T.M. Devine (ed.) *Improvement and Enlightenment* (Edinburgh, 1989).

Houston, R.R. 'The impact of economic change in Sutherland 1755–1851', unpublished PhD thesis, University of Edinburgh, 1980.

Howison, J. *Sketches of Upper Canada* (Edinburgh, 1825).

Howitt, W. *The Rural Life Of England* (Shannon, 1971 edn.).

Hufton, O. 'Women in revolution, 1789–1796', *Past and Present*, no. 83 (1971).

Hughes, E. 'The eighteenth century estate agent' in H. A. Cronne, T.W. Moody and D.B. Quinn (eds.), *Essays in British and Irish History* (London, 1949).

Hunt, E.H. *Regional Wage Variations in Britain 1850–1914* (Oxford, 1973).

Hunter, J. 'The emergence of the crofting community: the religious contribution, 1798–1843', *Scottish Studies*, vol. 18 (1974).

—————*The Making of the Crofting Community* (Edinburgh, 1976).

—————'The politics of land reform 1873–1895', *Scottish Historical Review*, vol. 53 (1974).

—————'Sheep and deer: highland sheep farming, 1850–1900', *Northern Scotland*, vol. 1 (1973).

—————*A Dance Called America* (Edinburgh, 1994).

—————*The Claim of Crofting* (Edinburgh, 1991).

Hunter, J. (ed.) *For the People's Cause: From the Writings of John Murdoch* (Edinburgh, 1986).

Hunter, J. *The Essex Landscape* (Chelmsford, 1999).

Hyde, E.D. 'The British Fisheries Society: its settlement and the Scottish Fisheries, 1750–1850', unpublished Ph.D. thesis, University of Strathclyde, 1973.

Hymer, S. and Resnick, S. 'A model of an agrarian economy with non-agricultural activities', *American Economic Review*, vol. 59 (1969).

Innes, C. *Lectures on Scottish Legal Antiquities* (Edinburgh, 1872).

—————*Sketches of Early Scotch History and Social Progress* (Edinburgh, 1861).

Innes, S.A. ' "They must worship industry or starve": Scottish resistance to British imperialism in Gunn's *The Silver Darlings*', *Studies in Scottish Literature* (1993), pp. 28 133–149.

Irvine, A. *An Inquiry into the Causes and Effects of Emigration from the Highlands and Western Isles of Scotland* (Edinburgh, 1802).

James, J.A.J. and Mark, T. (eds.) *Capitalism in Context* (Chicago, 1994).

Johnson, S. *Johnson's Journey to the Western Islands of Scotland and Boswell's Journal of a Tour to the Hebrides with Samuel Johnson LL.D*, edited by R.W. Chapman (Oxford, 1924).

Johnston, H.J.M. *British Emigration Policy 1815–30* (Ox ford, 1972).

Johnston, J.F.W. 'On the state and prospects of British Agriculture', *Edinburgh Review*, vol. 84 (1846).

Johnston, J.G. *The Truth, Consisting of Letters Just Received from Emigrants to the Australian Colonies* (Edinburgh, 1839).

Johnston, S.C. *A History of Emigration from the United Kingdom to North America 1763–1912* (London, 1966 edn.).

Johnston, T. *The History of the Working Classes in Scotland* (Glasgow, 1922).

——— *Our Scots Noble Families* (Glasgow, 1926).

Jones, D. *Before Rebecca. Popular Protest in Wales 1793–1835* (London, 1973).

Katz, M. *The People of Hamilton, Canada West* (Cambridge, MA., 1975).

Kellas, J.G. 'The Crofters' War 1882–1888', *History Today*, vol. 12 (1962).

Kellas, J.O. 'The Liberal Party and the Scottish Church Disestablishment Crisis', *English Historical Review*, LXXIX (1964).

Kellas, J.G. 'The Liberal Party in Scotland 1876–1895', *SHR*, XLIV (1964).

Kennedy, J. *The Days of the Fathers in Ross-shire* (3rd edn,. Edinburgh, 1861).

Kennedy, L. and T.B. Grainger. *The Present State of the Tenancy of Land in the Highland and Grazing Districts in Great Britain* (London, 1829).

Ker, A. *Report to Sir John Sinclair on the State of Sheep Farming* (Edinburgh, 1791).

Kincaid, B. 'Scottish immigration to Cape Breton, 1758–1838', unpublished MA thesis, University of Dalhousie, 1964.

Knox, J.A. *A View of the British Empire, More Especially Scotland* (3rd edn.,, London, 1785; London, 1978).

Ladurie, E.L. 'A Reply to Professor Brenner', *Past and Present*, no. 79 (1978).

Lamont, W. (ed.) *Historical Controversies and Historians* (London, 1998).

Lang, P.L. *The Langs of Selkirk, updated 1910–1992* (Warrnambool, n.d.c. 1993).

Larkin, J.A. *The Pampangans* (University of California Press, 1972).

Lawrence, E.P. *Henry George in the British Isles* (East Lansing, 1957).

Lawson, W.R. 'The poetry and the prose of the crofter question', *National Review*, vol. 4 (1884–5).

Lawton, R. 'Regional population trends in England and Wales, 1750–1971', in John Hobcraft and Phillip Rees (eds.), *Regional Demographic Development* (London, 1979).

Leavitt, I. and Smout, T.C. *The State of the Scottish Working Class in 1843* (Edinburgh, 1979).

Lebow, R.N. *J.S. Mill and the Irish Land Question* (Philadelphia, 1979).

Lee, J. 'The Ribbonmen' in T.D. Williams (ed.), *Secret Societies in Ireland* (Dublin, 1973).

Lees, J.C. *A History of the County of Inverness* (Edinburgh, 1897).

Leibenstein, H. *Economic Backwardness and Economic Growth* (New York, 1963).

Leigh, M.M. 'The Crofting Problem 1790–1883', *Scottish Journal of Agriculture*, vol. 11–12 (1928–9).

Leighton, R. (ed.) *Correspondence of Charlotte Grenville, Lady Williams Wynn* (London, 1920).

Leneman, L. *Living in Atholl, 1685–1785* (Edinburgh, 1986).

Leneman, L. (ed.) *Perspectives on Scottish Social History* (Aberdeen, 1988).

Lenman, B. *An Economic History Of Modern Scotland 1660–1976* (London, 1977).

Leopold, J. 'The Levellers' revolt in Galloway in 1724', *Scottish Labour History Journal*, vol. 14 (1980).

Lesingham-Smith, C. *Excursions through the Highlands and Islands of Scotland in 1835 and 1836* (London, 1837).

Leslie, W. *General View of the Agriculture of the Counties of Nairn and Moray* (1813).

Leveson Gower, F. (ed.) *Letters of Harriet Countess Granville, 1810–1845*, 2 vols. (1894).

Letters to the Rev. Dr Norman Macleod Regarding the Famine in the Highlands (Glasgow, 1847).

Lettice, J. *Letters on a Tour through Various Parts of Scotland in the Year 1792* (London, 1794).

Levi, L. *On the Economic Condition of The Highlands of Scotland* (London, 1857).

Levitt, I. and Smout, C. *The State of the Scottish Working Class in 1843* (Edinburgh, 1979).

Leyden, J. *Journal of a Tour in the Highlands and Western Islands of Scotland in 1800* (Edinburgh, 1903).

Lindner, S.B. *Trade and Trade Policy for Development* (New York, 1967).

Little, J.I. *Crofters and Habitants* (Montreal, 1991).

Lobban, R.D. 'The migration of Highlanders into Lowland Scotland (c. 1750–1890) with particular reference to Greenock', unpublished Ph.D. thesis, University of Edinburgh, 1969.

Loch, J.C.S. 'Poor relief in Scotland: its statistics and development 1791 to 1891', *Journal Of The Royal Statistical Society*, vol. LXI (1892).

Loch, J. *An Account of the Improvements on the Estates of the Marquess of Stafford* (London, 1815; enlarged edn., London, 1820).

———*Facts as to the Past and Present State of the Estate of Sutherland* (published anonymously, 1845).

Lockhart, D.G. 'Patterns of migration and movement of Labour to the planned villages of North East Scotland', *Scottish Geographical Magazine*, (1983).

Lockhart, J.G. *Memoirs Of The Life Of Sir Walter Scott* (7 vols., Edinburgh, 1837).

Logue, K.J. *Popular Disturbances in Scotland*, 1780–1815 (Edinburgh, 1977).

Low, D. *On Landed Property and the Economy of Estates* (London, 1844).

Lyons, F.S.L. *Ireland since the Famine* (London, 1971).

McArthur, M.M. *Survey of Lochtayside 1769* (Scottish History Society Publications, 3rd series, XXVII, Edinburgh, 1936).

McConnell, P. 'Experiences of a Scotsman on the Essex clays', *Journal of the Royal Agricultural Society of England*. 3rd series, vol. 2, 311–25 (1891).

MacCormick, D. *Hebridean Folksongs* (Oxford, 1969).

MacCulloch, J. *A Description of the Western Islands of Scotland* (3 vols., London, 1819).

——— *The Highlands and Western Isles of Scotland* (4 vols., London, 1824).

McCulloch, J.R. *A Descriptive and Statistical Account of the British Empire* (2 vols., London, 1854).

——— *A Dictionary of Commerce* (London, 1834).

MacDermid, G.E. 'The religious and ecclesiastical life of the North West Highlands 1750–1843', unpublished Ph.D. thesis, University of Aberdeen, 1967.

MacDonagh, O. *Ireland* (Englewood Cliffs, 1968).

——— *A Pattern of Government Growth 1800–1860* (London, 1961).

Macdonald, C. 'Transition in the Highlands of Scotland', *Scottish Review* (July 1888).

Macdonald, C.S. 'Early Highland emigration to Nova Scotia and Prince Edward Island, 1770–1853', *Nova Scotia Historical Society Collections*, vol. 23 (1941).

Macdonald, D. *Lewis, a History of the Island* (Edinburgh, 1978).

Macdonald, D.G.F. *Cattle, Sheep and Deer* (London, 1872).

McDonald, Forrest, and E.S. McDonald. 'The ethnic origins of the American People, 1790', *William and Mary Quarterly*, vol. 37 (April 1980).

MacDonald J.R. *Cultural retention and adaptation among the Highland Scots of North Carolina*, D. Phil. thesis (Edinburgh, 1991).

Macdonald, J. *Travels (1745–1779). Memoirs of an Eighteenth Century Footman* (London, 1927).

——*General View of the Agriculture of the Hebrides* (London, 1811).

MacDonald, R.C. *Sketches of the Highlanders: with an Account of their Early Arrival in North America* (St John, New Brunswick, 1843).

Macdonald, R.H. *The Emigration of Highland Crofters* (Edinburgh, 1885).

Macdonald, S. 'The role of the individual in agricultural change: the example of George Culley of Fenton, Northumberland', in H.S.A. Fox and R.A. Butlin (eds.), *Change in the Countryside: Essays on Rural England, 1500–1900* (London, 1973).

Macfarlane, A. *The Origins of English Individualism* (Oxford, 1978).

MacGill, W. *Old Ross-shire and Scotland as Seen in the Tain and Balnagowan Documents* (Inverness, 1909).

McGrath, J. *The Cheviot, the Stag and the Black Black Oil* (Kyleakin, 1974).

Macinnes, A. 'Crofters' Holdings Act of 1886: a hundred-year sentence?' *Radical Scotland*, no. 25 (1987).

——'Social mobility in medieval and early modern Scottish Gaeldom: the controvertible evidence', *Transactions of the Gaelic Society of Inverness*, LVIII (1993–4).

Macinnes, J. *The Evangelical Movements in the Highlands of Scotland 1699–1800* (Aberdeen, 1951).

Macintyre, L.M. 'Sir Walter Scott and the Highlands', unpublished Ph.D. thesis, University of Glasgow, 1976).

Mackay, A. *Sketches of Sutherland Characters* (Edinburgh, 1889).

——*The Book of Mackay* (Edinburgh, 1906).

Mackay, D.I. and N.K. Buxton. 'The North of Scotland – a case for redevelopment?' *Scottish Journal of Political Economy*, vol. 12 (1965).

Mackay, G.G. *On the Management of Highland Property* (Edinburgh, 1858).

Mackay, H.M. *Notes on the Successive Buildings used for Country, Municipal and Judicial Purposes of the County of Sutherland and*

Burgh of Dornoch (privately published, Edinburgh, 1896).

Mackay, I.R. 'Glenalladale's settlement, Prince Edward Island', *Scottish Gaelic Studies*, vol. 10 (1963).

McKay, M. 'Nineteenth century Tiree emigrant communities in Ontario', *Oral History*, vol. 9 (1981).

———(ed.) *The Rev. Dr John Walker's Report on the Hebrides in 1764 and 1771* (Edinburgh, 1980).

———'A Highland Minister's Diary', *Cornhill Magazine*, vol. 152 (1935).

Mackay, W. 'Industrial life in the Highlands in the older time', in [Highland Village Association Ltd.], *Home Life of the Highlanders 1400–1746* (Glasgow, 1911).

———*Sidelights on Highland History* (Inverness, 1925).

Mackelvie, P.H. *An Account of the Scottish Regiments with the Statistics of Each, From 1808 to March 1861* (Edinburgh, 1861).

Mackenzie, A. *An Analysis of the Report of the Crofter Royal Commission* (Inverness, n.d.).

———*The Highland Clearances – a Strange Return by the Highland Chiefs for the Fidelity of the Clans* (Inverness, 1881).

———*The History of the Highland Clearances* (Inverness, 1883).

———*A History of The Clan Mackenzie* (Inverness, 1889).

———*History of the Macdonalds* (Inverness, 1883).

———*The Isle of Skye in 1882–1883* (Inverness, 1883).

———(ed.) *The Trial of Patrick Sellar* (Inverness, 1883).

———*History of The Frasers of Lovat* (Inverness, 1896).

Mackenzie, C. 'On the settlement of crofters on estate of Kilcoy', *Transactions of the Royal Highland and Agricultural Society of Scotland*, series, vol. V (1937).

Mackenzie, G.S. *Letter to the Proprietors of Land in Ross-shire* (Edinburgh, 1803).

———*General View of the Agriculture of the Counties of Ross and Cromarty* (London, 1813).

Mackenzie, K.S. 'Changes in the ownership of land in Ross-shire, 1756–1853', *TGSI* (1897).

Mackenzie, O. *A Hundred Years in the Highlands* (London, 1972).

Mackenzie, W.C. *A Short History of the Scottish Highlands and Islands* (London, 1908).

————*The Highlands and Isles of Scotland* (London, 1949).

Mackenzie, W.M. *Hugh Miller. A Critical Study* (London, 1905).

MacKerral, A. *Kintyre In The Seventeenth Century* (Edinburgh, 1948).

————'The tacksman and his holdings in the south-west Highlands', *SHR*, vol. 26 (1947).

Mackinnon, N.J. 'Strath, Skye, in the Mid-Nineteenth Century', *TGSI*, vol. 51(1978–80).

Mackintosh, H.B. *Elgin, Past and Present* (Edinburgh, 1914).

Mackintosh, T.D. 'Factors in emigration from the Islands of Scotland to North America, 1772–1803', unpublished M.Litt. thesis, University of Aberdeen, 1979.

Maclaine, A. *Population of the Highlands of Scotland* (Edinburgh, 1857).

McLaren, M. *Shell Guide to Scotland* (London, 1972).

McLauchlan, T. *The Depopulation System in the Highlands* (Edinburgh, 1849).

Maclean, C. *Island on the Edge of the World: Utopian St Kilda and its Passing* (London, 1972).

Maclean, D. *The Effect of the 1745 Rising on the Social and Economic Conditions of the Highlands* (Edinburgh, n.d.).

Maclean, J.P. *An Historical Account of the Settlements of Scotch Highlanders in America Prior to the Peace of 1783* (Glasgow and Cleveland, 1900).

MacLean, M. *The People of Glengarry: Highlanders in Transition, 1745–1820* (Montreal, 1991).

————'Peopling Glengarry County: the Scottish origins of a Canadian Community' in D. Johnson and C. Lecelle (eds.), *Historical Papers* (Ottawa, 1982).

Maclean, S. 'The poetry of the Highland Clearances', *TGSI*, vol. 38 (1937–41).

Macleay, D. *Scotland Farewell: The People of the Hector* (Scarborough, Ontario, 1980).

MacLeod, D. *History of the Destitution in Sutherlandshire* (Edinburgh, 1841).

————*Gloomy Memories in the Highlands of Scotland* (1892 edition reprinted, Bettyhill, 1996).

Macleod, J.F.M. 'Notes on Waternish in the nineteenth century', *Transactions of the Gaelic Society of Inverness*, LIX (1994–6).

MacLeod, J.N. *Memorials of the Rev. Norman Macleod* (Edinburgh, 1898).

MacLeod, R. 'The Crofters: how to benefit them', *Blackwood's Magazine*, vol. 139 (1886).

Macleod, R.C. 'The Western Highlands in the Eighteenth Century', *SHR*, vol. 1 (1922).

McMaster, G. *Scott and Society* (Cambridge, 1981).

Macmillan, D.S. *Scotland and Australia, 1788–1850: Emigration, Commerce and Investment* (Oxford, 1967).

MacMillan, S. *The Emigration of Lochaber MacMillans to Canada in 1812* (Paisley, 1958).

MacMillan, S. *Bygone Lochaber* (Glasgow, 1971).

Macnab, P.A. *The Isle of Mull* (Newton Abbott, 1970).

MacPhail, I.M.M. 'The Skye military expedition 1884–85', *TGSI*, vol. XLVIII (1972–4).

———'Prelude to the Crofters' War, 1870–1880', *TGSI*, vol. 49 (1974–6).

———'The Skye Military Expedition of 1884–85', *TGSI*, vol. 48 (1972–4).

MacPhee, H. 'The Trail of the Emigrants', *TGSI*, vol. 46 (1969–70).

MacSween, M.D. 'Settlement in Trotternish, Isle of Skye, 1700–1858', unpublished B.Litt. thesis, University of Glasgow, 1962.

Maddison, A. *Economic Progress and Policy in Developing Countries* (London, 1970).

Magnusson, M. *The Clacken and the Slate: The Story of the Edinburgh Academy, 1824–1974* (1974).

Maguire, W. A. *The Downshire Estates in Ireland 1801–1845* (Oxford, 1972).

Malmesbury, Earl of (J.H. Hanris). *Memoirs of an Ex-Minister* (London, 1885).

Malthus, T.R. *An Essay on the Principle of Population* (London, 1972 edn.).

Manning, B. 'The Peasantry and the English Revolution', *Journal Of Peasant Studies*, vol. 2 (1975).

Mantoux, P. *The Industrial Revolution in the Eighteenth Century* (London, 1964).

Marryat, J. *Thoughts on the Abolition of the Slave Trade and Civilization of Africa* (1816).

Martell, J.S. *Immigration to and Emigration from Nova Scotia, 1815–1838* (Halifax, 1942).

Martin, M. *Description of the Western Isles of Scotland* (London, 1703).

Marx, C. [K.] 'Sutherland and Slavery, or The Duchess at Home', *The People's Paper*, 12 March 1853.

——— *The American Journalism of Marx and Engels* (New York, n.d.).

——— *Capital* (3 vols., Moscow, nd.).

——— *Collected Works* (Moscow, 1976).

——— *Ireland and the Irish Question. A Collection of Writings by Karl Marx and Frederick Engels* (New York, 1972).

——— *The Poverty of Philosophy* (New York, 1963 edn.).

Mason, J. 'Conditions in the Highlands after the '45', *SHR*, XXVI (1947).

Mason, J.W. 'The Duke of Argyll and the land question in late nineteenth century Britain', *Victorian Studies*, vol. 21 (1978).

Mason, R. and Macdougall, N. (eds.) *People and Power in Scotland* (Edinburgh, 1992).

Mather, A. 'The environmental impact of sheep farming in the Scottish Highlands', in T.C. Smout (ed.) *Scotland Since Pre-History* (1993).

Mather, F.C. *After the Canal Duke* (Oxford 1970).

Mathias, P. *The First Industrial National* (London, 1969).

Mathur, A. 'The anatomy of disguised unemployment', *Oxford Economic Papers*, vol. 16 (1964).

Mayhew, H. *London Labour and London Poor* (4 vols., London, 1861–2; reprinted 1967).

Mearns, A. 'The minister and the bailiff: a study of presbyterian clergy in the northern Highlands during the clearances', *Scottish Church History Society Records*, XXIV (1990).

Meek, D.E. 'Gaelic Poets of the Land Agitation', *TGSI*, vol. 48 (1972–4).

Meek, D. (ed.) *Tuath is tighearna. Tenants and Landlords* (Edinburgh, 1995).

Meikle, H.W. *Scotland and the French Revolution* (Edinburgh, 1912).

Mercer, J. *Hebridean Islands, Colonsay, Gigha, Jura* (London, 1974).

Merivale, H. *Lectures on Colonization and Colonies* (London, 1861 edn.).

Meyer, D. *The Highland Scots of North Carolina, 1732–1776* (Chapel Hill, 1961).

Michie, R.C. *Money, Mania and Markets* (Edinburgh, 1981).

Miller, H. *The Cruise of The Betsy* (Edinburgh, 1858).

———*Essays* (Edinburgh, 1875).

———*Leading Articles on Various Subjects* (Edinburgh, 1870).

———*My Schools and Schoolmasters* (Edinburgh, 1874 edn.).

———*Sutherland as it was, and is; or, How a Country may be Ruined* (Edinburgh, 1843).

Miller, R. 'Orkney: A land of increment', in R. Miller and J.W. Watson (eds.) *Geographical Essays In Memory of A.G. Ogilvie* (London, 1959).

Miller, R. *Orkney* (London, 1976).

Mills, D.R. *English Rural Communities. The Impact of a Specialised Economy* (London, 1973).

Milward, A.S. and Saul, S.B. *The Economic Development of Continental Europe 1780–1870* (London, 1973).

Mingay, O.E. *Enclosure and the small farmer in the age of the Industrial Revolution* (London, 1968).

Mingay, E.G. *The Gentry* (London, 1976).

Mitchell, J. *Reminiscences of my Life in the Highlands* (London, 1883).

Mitchison, R. 'The Government and the Highlands, 1707–1745', in N.T. Phillipson and Rosalind Mitchison (eds.), *Scotland in the age of Improvement* (Edinburgh, 1970).

———*Agricultural Sir John. The Life of Sir John Sinclair of Ulbster 1754–1835* (London, 1962).

———'The Highland Clearances', *Scottish Economic and Social History*, vol. 1 (1981).

———*A History of Scotland* (London, 1970).

———'The movement of Scottish corn prices in the seventeenth and eighteenth centuries', *Economic History Review*, vol. 18 (1965).

Moisley, H.A. 'The Deserted Hebrides?' *SS* 10, 44–68 (1966).

Mokyr, J. *Why Ireland Starved. A Quantitative and Analytical History of the Irish Economy, 1800–1850* (London, 1983).

Morgan, E.V. 'Regional problems and common currencies', *Lloyds Bank Review*, no. 110 (October 1973).

Morgan, V. 'Agricultural wage rates in late eighteenth-century Scotland', *Economic History Review*, vol. 24 (1971).

Morse, S.L. 'Immigration to Nova Scotia, 1839–1851', unpublished MA thesis, University of Dalhousie, 1946

Mowat, I.R.M. *Easter Ross 1750–1850* (Edinburgh, 1980).

Mulock, T. *The Western Highlands and Islands of Scotland Socially Considered, With Reference to Proprietors and People* (Edinburgh, 1850).

Murdoch, A. 'A Scottish document concerning emigration to North Carolina in 1772.' *The North Carolina Historical Review*, LXVII (1990).

———'Emigration from the Scottish Highlands to America in the eighteenth century', *British Journal of Eighteenth Century Studies*, 21 (1998).

Murray, N. *The Scottish Handloom Weavers 1790–1850* (Edinburgh, 1978).

Murray, T. *The Literary History of Galloway* (Edinburgh, 1822).

Murray, W.H. *Companion Guide to the West Highlands of Scotland* (London, 1968).

———*Islands of Western Scotland* (London, 1973).

Napier, Lord 'The Highland Crofters. A Vindication of the Report of the Crofters' Commission', *Nineteenth Century*, vol. XVII (1855).

Neale, K. *Essex: A History* (Chichester, 1997).

Neeson, J.M. *The Commoners: Common Right, Enclosure and Social Change in England, 1700–1820* (Cambridge, 1993).

———'Opposition to enclosure' in A. Charlesworth (ed.), *An Atlas of Rural Protest in Britain 1518–1900* (London, 1983).

Newsome, A.R. 'Records of emigrants from England and Scotland to North Carolina 1774–5', *North Carolina Historical Review* vol. 11 (1934).

New Statistical Account of Scotland (15 vols., Edinburgh, 1835–45).

Nicholson, C. (ed.) *Iain Crichton Smith. Critical Essays* (Edinburgh, 1992).

Nicolson, A. *History of Skye* (Glasgow, 1930).

Nicolson, J.R. *Shetland* (Newton Abbott, 1972).

Nicolson, N. *Lord of the Isles* (London, 1960).

Noble, J. *Miscellanea Invernessiana* (Stirling, 1902).

North, D.C. *The Economic Growth of the United States 1790–1860* (Englewood Cliffs, 1960).

O'Farrell, P. 'Emigrant attitudes and behaviour as a source for Irish History', *Historical Studies*, vol. 10 (1976).

O'Grada, C. 'Demographic adjustment and seasonal migration in nineteenth century Ireland' in L. M. Cullen and F. Furet (eds.), *Irlande et France* (Paris, 1980).

———'The investment behaviour of Irish Landlords, 1850–1875', *Agricultural History Review*, vol. 23 (1975).

———'Seasonal migration and post-famine adjustment in the West of Ireland', *Studia Hibernica*, vol. 13 (1973).

Okun, B. and Richardson, R.W. 'Regional income inequality and internal population migration', *Economic Development and Cultural Change*, vol. 9 (1961).

'An Old Highlander', 'Home Truths on the Crofter Agitation', *Blackwood's Edinburgh Magazine*, vol. 138 (1885).

Oldroyd, D.R. *The Highland Controversy: Constructing Geological Knowledge through Fieldwork in the Nineteenth Century Britain* (Chicago, 1990).

Omand, D. *The Caithness Book* (Inverness, 1972).

———(ed.) *The Sutherland Book* (Golspie, 1985).

Orr, Willie. *Deer Forests, Landlords and Crofters* (Edinburgh, 1982).

Otter, William (ed.) *The Life and Remains of the Rev. Edward Daniel Clarke LL.D.* (London, 1824).

Pacione, M. 'Rural problems and planning for real in Skye and Lochalsh', *Scottish Geographical Magazine* (1996) 112, 20–8.

Paget, J. *The New Examen* (Halifax, 1934).

Parker, A.W. *Scottish Highlanders in Colonial Georgia* (Athens, Georgia, 1997).

Parker, W.N. and E.L. Jones (eds.). *European Peasants and their Markets* (Princeton, 1976).

Paszkowski, L. *Sir Paul Edmund de Strzelecki* (Melbourne, 1997).

Paton, D.M. 'Brought to a wilderness: the Reverend D. MacKenzie of Farr and the Scottish Clearances' *Northern Scotland* 13, 75–101 (1993).

Patterson, George. *A History of the County of Pictou,* Nova Scotia (Montreal, 1877).

Pennant, T. *A Tour of Scotland and Voyage to the Hebrides* (London, 1774).

Pennell, J.P. and E.R. *Our Journey to the Hebrides* (London, 1890).

Perren, Richard. 'The effects of agricultural depression on the English estates of the Dukes of Sutherland, 1870–1900', unpublished Ph.D. thesis, University of Nottingham, 1968

———'The landlord and agricultural transformation, 1870–1900', *Agricultural History Review,* vol. 18 (1970).

Phillipson, N.T. and Mitchison, R. *Scotland in the Age of Improvement* (Edinburgh, 1970).

Picton, J.A. 'The Crofters' cry for more land', *Contemporary Review,* vol. 48 (1885).

Plant, M. 'The servant problem in eighteenth-century Scotland', *SHR,* vol. 29 (1950).

Ployen, C. *Reminiscences of a Voyage to Shetland, Orkney, and Scotland in the Summer of 1839* (Lerwick, 1894).

Plumb, J.H. *The First Four Georges* (London, 1966).

Pollard, S. 'Industrialisation and the European Economy', *EHR,* vol. 26 (1973).

———*The Genesis of Modern Management* (London, 1965).

———and D.W. Crossley. *The Wealth of Britain* (London, 1968).

Prattis, J.I. *Economic Structures in the Highlands of Scotland* (The Fraser of Allander Institute Speculative Papers, no. 7, Glasgow, 1977).

Prebble, J. *Culloden* (London, 1961).

———*Glencoe* (London, 1966).

———*The Highland Clearances* (London, 1963).

———*Mutiny* (London, 1975).

———*The King's Jaunt* (1988).

Pritchett, J.P. *The Red River Valley 1811–1849. A Regional Study* (Toronto, 1942).

Pryde, G.S. *Scotland from 1603 to the Present Day* (London, 1962).

Rae, J. 'The Crofter problem', *Contemporary Review*, vol. 47 (1885).

Ramsay, F. (ed.) *Day Book of David Campbell of Shawfield 1767* (Aberdeen, 1991).

Ramsay, J. *Scotland and Scotsmen of the Eighteenth Century* (2 vols., Edinburgh, 1888).

Razzell, P. *Essays in English Population History* (London, 1994).

Redford, A. *Labour Migration in England, 1800–1850* (Manchester, 1964).

Rendall, J. *The Origins of the Scottish Enlightenment* (1978).

Richards, D. *Masks of Difference* (Cambridge, 1994).

Richards, E. 'The decline of St Kilda: demography, economy and emigration,' *Scottish Economic and Social History* 14, 55–75 (1992).

——'Fate and culpability in the Highland Clearances', in the *Yearbook of the Scottish History Teachers Association*, 17–42 (1989).

——'Margins of the Industrial Revolution', in *The Industrial Revolution and British Society*, ed. P. O'Brien and R. Quinault (Cambridge, 1993).

——*Patrick Sellar and the Highland Clearances* (Edinburgh, 1999).

——'St Kilda and Australia: emigrants in peril, 1852–3', *SHR* 71, 129–55 (1993).

——'Agricultural change, modernization and the Clearances' in D. Omand (ed.), *The Ross and Cromarty Book* (Inverness, 1984).

——'An anatomy of the Sutherland fortune: income, consumption, investments and returns, 1780–1880', *Business History*, vol. 21 (1979).

——'Australia and the Scottish Connection, 1788–1914' in R.A. Cage (ed.), *The Scots Abroad* (London, 1984).

——'The Highland Scots of South Australia', *Journal of the Historical Society of South Australia*, no. 4 (1978).

——*A History of the Highland Clearances: Agrarian*

Transformation and the Evictions 1746–1886 (London, 1982).

——'How tame were the Highlanders during the clearances?' *SS*, vol. 17 (1973).

——'The Sutherland clearances: new evidence from Dunrobin', *Northern Scotland,* 2 (1976).

——'The Military Register and the Pursuit of Patrick Sellar', *Scottish Economic and Social History,* 16 (1996).

——*A History of the Highland Clearances: Vol 2, Emigration, Protest, Reasons,* (1985).

——'The Highland passage to colonial Australia', *Scotlands* (1995).

——'The Land Agent' in G.E. Mingay (ed.) *The Victorian Countryside* (2 vols., London, 1981).

——*The Last Scottish Food Riots* (London, 1982).

——*The Leviathan of Wealth* (London, 1973).

——'The mind of Patrick Sellar (1780–1851)', *SS*, vol. 15 (1971).

——'Patterns of Highland discontent, 1790–1860' in John Stevenson and Roland Quinault (eds.), *Popular Protest and Public Order* (London, 1976).

——'Problems on the Cromartie Estate, 1851–3', *SHR*, vol. 52 (1973).

——'The prospect of economic growth in Sutherland at the time of the clearances, 1809 to 1813', *SHR*, vol. 49 (1970).

——'Structural Change in a Regional Economy: Sutherland and the Industrial Revolution, 1780–1830', *EHR*, vol. 26 (1973).

——'Varieties of Scottish emigration in the nineteenth century', *Historical Studies* 21 (Melbourne, 1985), 473–94.

——and Clough, M. *Cromartie: Highland Life, 1650–1914* (Aberdeen, 1989).

Rinn, J.A. 'Scots in bondage. Forgotten contributors to colonial society', *History Today,* vol. 30 (1980).

Rixson, D. *Knoydart: A History* (Edinburgh, 1999)

Robertson, A. *Where are the Highlanders?* (Edinburgh, n.d.).

Robertson, J. *General View of the Agriculture of the Southern Districts of the County of Perth* (London, 1794).

Robertson, P. *Report of the Trial of Patrick Sellar, Esq. Factor of the*

Most Noble the Marquis and Marchioness of Stafford for the crimes of Culpable Homicide, Real Injury, and Oppression. Before the Circuit Court of Justiciary, held at Inverness, on Tuesday 23 April, 1816 (Edinburgh, 1816).

Robson, J. *General View of the Agriculture of Argyll and the Western part of Inverness-Shire* (London, 1794).

Ross, D. *The Glengarry Evictions* (Glasgow, 1853).

———— *The Russians of Ross-shire* (Glasgow, 1854).

————*Real Scottish Grievances* (Glasgow, 1854).

———— *The Scottish Highlanders: Their Present Sufferings and Future Prospects* (Glasgow, 1852).

Rostow, W.W. *Stages of Economic Growth. A Non-Communist Manifesto* (London, 1960).

Rudé, G. 'The Pre-Industrial Crowd', in G. Rudé, *Paris and London in the Eighteenth Century* (London, 1970).

———— *The Crowd in History* (New York, 1964).

Russel, A. 'The Highlands – Men, Sheep and Deer', *Edinburgh Review*, vol. 106 (1857).

Rymer, L. 'The kelp industry in North Knapdale', *SS*, vol. 18 (1974).

Sage, D. *Memorabilia Domestica, or Domestic Life in the North of Scotland* (Wick, 1889; 2nd edn., 1899).

St John, C. *A Tour in Sutherlandshire* (2 vols., London, 1849).

Saltmarsh, J. and Darby, H.C. 'The infield-outfield system on a Norfolk manor', *Economic History*, vol. III (1935).

Saville, J. *Rural Depopulation in England and Wales 1851–1951* (London, 1957).

Scarisbrick, J.J. *Henry VIII* (London, edn. 1976).

Schaw, J. *Journal of a Lady of Quality*, ed. E.W. Andrews (New Haven, 1939).

Scott, H. *Fasti Ecclesiae Scoticanae* (3 vols., Edinburgh, 1915–28).

Scott, J.C. *Weapons of the Weak. Everyday Forms of Peasant Resistance* (New Haven, 1985).

Scott, W., *Guy Mannering* (1957 edn).

———— *The Letters of Sir Walter Scott* ed. H.J.C. Grierson, 12 vols. (London, 1932–37).

Scrope, G.P. *Some Notes on a Tour in England, Scotland and Ireland* (London, 1849).

Selkirk, Earl of (Thomas Douglas). *Observations on the Present State of the Highlands of Scotland* (Edinburgh, 1805).

Selkirk, P.L. *The Langs of Selkirk* (Melbourne, 1910).

Sellar, E.M. *Recollections and Impressions* (Edinburgh, 1908).

Sellar, P. *Statement* (1825).

——*Farm Reports III, County of Sutherland. Strathnaver, Morvich and Culmaily Farms*, Library of Useful Knowledge (London, 1831).

Sellar, T. *The Sutherland Evictions of 1814* (London, 1883).

Senior, N.S. *Journals, Conversations and Essays Relating to Ireland* (2 vols., London, 1868).

Seton, G. *St Kilda, Past and Present* (Edinburgh, 1878).

Shairp, J.C. *Glen Desseray and other Poems* (London, 1888).

Shannon, C.B. Review of W.E. Vaughan, *Landlords and Tenants, in AHR* 102:5 (1997), pp. 1490–2

Sharpe, R. *Raasay: A Study In Island* History (London, 1977).

Shaw, C.B. *Pigeon-holes of Memory: The Life and Times of Dr John MacKenzie, 1803–1886* (Palo Alto, 1988).

Shaw, F.J. 'Landownership in the Western Isles in the seventeenth century', *SHR*, vol. 56 (1977).

Shaw, L. *History of the Province of Moray* (3 vols. Glasgow, 1882).

Shepperson, G. 'Harriet Beecher Stowe and Scotland, 1852–3', *SHR*, vol. 32 (1953).

Shepperson, W.S. *British Emigration to North America* (Minneapolis, 1957).

Simpson, D. 'Investment, employment and government expenditure in the Highlands, 1951–60', *Scottish Journal of Political Economy*, vol. 10 (1963).

Simpson, D.R.F. 'An economic analysis of crofting agriculture', unpublished Ph.D. thesis, Harvard University, 1962.

Sinclair, C. *Scotland and the Scotch* (Edinburgh, 1850).

Sinclair, D.M. 'Highland emigration to Nova Scotia', *Dalhousie Review*, vol. 23 (1943–4).

Sinclair, J. *Address to the Society for the Improvement of British Wool* (Edinburgh, 1791).

——*Analysis of the Statistical Account of Scotland* (2 vols., London, 1825).

————*General Report on the Agricultural State and Political Circumstances of Scotland* (Edinburgh, 1814).

————*General View of the Agriculture of the Northern Counties of Scotland* (London, 1795).

————*Memoirs of the Life and Works of the late Right Honourable Sir John Sinclair, Bart* (2 vols., Edinburgh, 1837).

————(ed.) *Statistical Account of Scotland* (21 vols, Edinburgh, 1791–9; reprinted, East Ardsley, 1975–).

Singer, W. 'On the introduction of sheepfarming into the Highlands', *THAS*, 1st series, vol. III (1807).

Skene, W. *Celtic Scotland* (Edinburgh, 1880).

Skinner, A. *A System of Social Science* (Oxford, 1979).

Skovgaard, K. 'Consolidation of agricultural land in Denmark', *International Journal Of Agrarian Affairs* vol. 1, no. 4 (1952).

Slaven, A. *The Development of the West of Scotland 1750–1960* (London, 1975).

Slaven, A. and Checkland, S. (eds.) *Dictionary of Scottish Business Biography 1860–1960* vol. 1 (Aberdeen, 1986).

Slicher van Bath, B.H. *The Agrarian History of Western Europe* (London, 1963).

Smith, A. *The Wealth of Nations* (Glasgow edn., 1976).

————*A Summer in Skye* (Edinburgh, 1912 edn).

Smith, A.M. 'Annexed estates in the eighteenth-century Highlands', *Northern Scotland*, vol. 3, no. 1, (1977–8).

————*Jacobite Estates of the Forty Five* (Edinburgh, 1982).

Smith, E. *The Irish Journals of Elizabeth Smith 1840–1850*, ed. David Thomson and Moyra McGusty (Oxford, 1980).

Smith, J. *General View of the Agriculture of Argyll* (Edinburgh, 1798).

Smout, T.C. 'Famine and famine relief in Scotland' in L. M. Cullen and T.C. Smout (eds.), *Comparative Aspects of Scottish and Irish Economic and Social History 1600–1900* (Edinburgh, 1977).

————*A History of the Scottish People, 1560–1830* (London, 1969).

————'The landowner and the planned village in Scotland, 1730–1830', in N.T. Phillipson and R. Mitchison (eds.) *Scotland in the Age of Improvement* (Edinburgh, 1970).

————'An ideological struggle: the Highland Clearances', *Scottish International*, vol. 5, no. 2 (February 1972).

————'Scotland and England: is dependency a symptom or a cause of under-development?' *Review*, vol. 3 (1980).

————'Scottish landowners and economic growth, 1650–1850', *Scottish Journal of Political Economy*, XVIII (1964).

————(ed.) *Scotland since Pre-History* (Aberdeen, 1993).

Society for the Support of Gaelic Schools. *Annual Reports* (Edinburgh, 1810–22).

Solow, B.L. *The Land Question and the Irish Economy, 1870–1903* (Cambridge, MA, 1971).

Somers, R. *Letters from the Highlands* (London, 1848).

Southey, R. *Journal of a tour in Scotland in 1819* (London, 1929).

Spencer, H. *An Autobiography*, 2, vols. (1904).

Spring, D. *English Landed Estates in the Nineteenth Century: their Administration* (Baltimore, 1963).

Stark, W. (ed.) *Jeremy Bentham's Economic Writings* (London, 1952).

Steel, T. *The Life and Death of St Kilda* (Edinburgh, 1965).

Stevenson, D. *Alasdair Maccolla and the Highland Problem in the Seventeenth Century* (Edinburgh, 1980).

Stewart, A.A. *Highland Parish or the History of Fortingall* (Glasgow, 1928).

Stewart, D. *Sketches of the Character, Manners, and Present State of the Highlanders of Scotland: with Details of the Military Service of the Highland Regiments (2 vols., Edinburgh, 1822; 2nd edition, 1825).*

Stoddart, A.M. *John Stuart Blackie: A Biography* (2 vols., London, 1895).

Stowe, H.B. *Sunny Memories of Foreign Lands* (London, 1854).

Survey of the Province of Moray (Aberdeen, 1790).

Strawhorn, J. *The History of Irvine* (Edinburgh, 1985).

Strzelecki, P.E. de, *Physical Description of New South Wales and Van Diemens Land* (2 vols., 1845).

Sutherland, A. *A Summer Ramble in the Northern Highlands* (London, 1825).

————*Victoria and its Metropolis* (Melbourne, 1888).

Sutherland, S.R. 'Ethics and economics in the Sutherland Clearances', *Northern Scotland*, vol. 2, no. 1 (1974–5).

Sutton, K. 'Population resettlement – traumatic upheavals and the Algerian experience', *Journal Of Modern African Studies*, vol. 15 (1977).

Symons, J.A. *Scottish Farming, Past and Present* (Edinburgh, 1959).

Tate, W.E. 'Opposition to parliamentary enclosure in eighteenth century England', *Agricultural History*, vol. 19 (1945).

———'Parliamentary counter-petitions during the enclosures of the eighteenth and nineteenth centuries', *English Historical Review*, vol. 59 (1944).

Tawney, R.H. *The Agrarian Problem in the Sixteenth Century* (London, 1912).

Taylor, A.J. *Laissez-faire and State Intervention in Nineteenth Century Britain* (1972).

Teignmouth, Lord (C.J. Shore). *Sketches of the Coasts and Islands of Scotland and of the Isle of Man* (2 vols., London, 1836).

The Journal of the Rev. John Wesley (4 vols. London, 1906).

The Trial of Patrick Sellar, new edition with introductory remarks by Alexander Mackenzie (Inverness, 1883).

Thirsk, J. *Tudor Enclosures* (London, 1959).

Thom, W. 'Journal of a tour in the North of Scotland' *New Agricultural and Commercial Magazine*, vol. I (1811).

Thomas, B. *The Welsh Economy* (Cardiff, 1962).

———*Migration and Economic Growth* (Cambridge, 1954).

Thomas, D. *Agriculture in Wales During the Napoleonic Wars* (Cardiff, 1963).

Thomas, P.D.G. *The House of Commons in the Eighteenth Century* (Oxford, 1971).

Thompson, E.P. 'English trade unionism and other labour movements before 1790', *Society for the Study of Labour History*, Bulletin no. 17 (1968).

———'History from below', *Times Literary Supplement*, 7 April 1968

———*The Making of the English Working Class* (New York, 1963).

Thompson, F. *The Highlands and Islands* (London, 1974).

Thomson, A. 'On the settlement of crofters at Banchory', *THAS*,

2nd series, vol. V (1837).

Thomson, D. *An Introduction to Gaelic Poetry* (London, 1974).

Thomson, D.C. and Grimble, I. (eds.) *The Future of the Highlands* (London, 1968).

Thomson, James. *The Value and Importance of the Scottish Fisheries* (London, 1849).

Thomson, W.P.L. *The Little General and the Rousay Crofters* (Edinburgh, 1981).

Thornber, I, 'Some Morvern songwriters of the nineteenth century', *Transactions of the Gaelic Society of Inverness*, vol. LIII (1982–4) pp. 1–90.

Tilly, C. 'Collective violence in European perspective' in H.D. Graham and T.P. Gurr (eds.), *Violence in America: Historical and Comparative Perspectives* (New York, 1969).

——'Did the cake of custom break?' in John M. Merriman (ed.), *Consciousness and Class Experience in Nineteenth Century Europe* (New York, 1979).

——'Proletarianization and rural collective action in East Anglia and elsewhere, 1500–1900', *Peasant Studies*, vol. 10 (1982).

Tivy, J. 'Easter Ross: A residual crofting area', *Scottish Studies*, vol. IX (1965).

Toomey, K. 'Emigration from the Scottish Catholic bounds, 1770–1810, and the role of the clergy'. D.Phil. thesis (Edinburgh, 1991).

The Topographical, Statistical and Historical Gazeteer of Scotland (Edinburgh, 1844).

Tranter, R.B. (ed.) *The Future of Upland Britain* (2 vols., Reading, 1978).

Trevor-Roper, H. 'The invention of tradition: the Highland tradition of Scotland', in Eric Hobsbawm and Terence Ranger (eds.), *The Invention of Tradition* (Cambridge, 1983).

Turnock, D. *Patterns Of Highland Development* (London, 1970).

——'Stages of agricultural improvement in the Uplands of Scotland's Grampian Region', *Journal of Historical Geography*, 3 (1977).

Ure, D. *General view of the Agriculture of the County of Dunbarton* (London, 1794).

Vaughan, W.E. *Landlords and Tenants in Ireland, 1848–1904* (Dublin, 1984).

———*Landlords and Tenants in Mid-Victorian Ireland* (Oxford, 1994).

———'An assessment of the economic performance of Irish landlords, 1851–1881' in F.S.L. Lyons and A.A.J. Hawkins (eds.), *Ireland under the Union* (Oxford, 1980).

———'Landlord and Tenant Relations in Ireland between the Famine and the Land War, 1850–1878' in L.M. Cullen and T.C. Smout (eds.), *Comparative Aspects of Scottish and Irish Economic and Social History 1600–1900* (Edinburgh, 1977).

Viner, J. 'Guide to John Rae's *Life of Adam Smith*' in John Rae, *Life of Adam Smith* (reprinted, 1965).

Walker, D.M. *The Oxford Companion to Law* (Oxford, 1980).

———*The Scottish Jurists* (Edinburgh, 1985).

Walker, J. *An Economical History of the Hebrides and Highlands of Scotland* (2 vols., Edinburgh, 1812).

———*Report on the Hebrides in 1764 and 1771*, ed. M.M. McKay (Edinburgh, 1980).

Wallace, A.R. *Land Nationalisation*.

Watson, A. and Allan, E. 'Depopulation by clearances and non-enforced emigration in the north-east Highlands', *Northern Scotland* 10 (1990).

Watson, D. *Caledonia Australis* (Sydney, 1984).

Watson, J.A.S. 'The Rise and development of the sheep industry in the Highlands', *THAS*, 5th series, vol. 44 (1982).

Watson, J. and W. *Morayshire Described* (Elgin, 1868).

White, J.T. *The Scottish Border and Northumberland* (London, 1973).

White, P. *Observations upon the Present State of the Scotch Fisheries* (Edinburgh, 1791).

White, P.C.T. *Lord Selkirk's Diary 1803–4* (Toronto, 1958).

Wicksteed, P. *The Common Sense of Political Economy* (2 vols., London, 1910).

Williams, T.D. (ed.). *Secret Societies in Ireland* (Dublin, 1973).

Wills, V, (ed.). *Reports on the Annexed Estates, 1755–1769* (Edinburgh, 1973).

———*Statistics of the Annexed Estates, 1755–1756* (Edinburgh, 1974).

Wilson, J. *A Voyage Round the Coasts of Scotland and the Isles* (Edinburgh, 1842).

Winberg, C. 'Population growth and proletarianization' in S. Akerman, H.C. Johansen and D. Graunt (eds.), *Chance and Change* (Odense, 1978).

Withers, C.W.J. 'Place, memory, monument: memorialising the past in contemporary Highland Scotland', *Ecumen* 1996, 3.

———'Destination and migration: labour mobility and relief from famine in Highland Scotland, 1836–1850', *Journal of Historical Geography* 14, 128–50 (1998).

———'Highland–Lowland migration and the making of the crofting community, 1755–1891', *Scottish Geographical Magazine*, 103 (1987).

———*Urban Highlanders* (Edinburgh, 1998).

Wood, G.H. 'Real wages and the standard of comfort since 1858', *Journal of the Royal Statistical Society*, vol. 62 (1909).

Wrigley, E.A. 'The process of modernisation and the Industrial Revolution in England', *Journal of Interdisciplinary History*, vol. 3 (1972).

———and R.S. Schofield. *The Population History of England, 1541–1871* (London, 1981).

Wylie, J. *Disruption Worthies of the Highlands. Another Memorial of 1843* (Edinburgh, 1877).

Wynn, C.W. *Correspondence of Charlotte Grenville, Lady Williams Wynn*, ed. R. Leighton (no place, 1920).

Yanaihara, T. *A Full and Detailed Catalogue of Books which Belonged to Adam Smith's Library* (Tokyo, 1951).

Young, D. *Scotland* (London, 1971).

Young, G.M. 'Scott and the Historians', *Sir Walter Scott Lectures*, 1940–1948 (University of Edinburgh, 1946).

Young, K. *Arthur James Balfour* (London, 1963).

Young, R. *Annals of the Parish and Burgh of Elgin* (Elgin, 1879).

———*The Parish of Spyniein the County of Elgin* (Elgin 1871).

———*Notes on Burghead, Ancient and Modern* (Elgin, 1868).

Youngson, A.J. *After the Forty Five* (Edinburgh, 1973).

———*Beyond The Highland Line* (London, 1974).

Zebel, S.H. *Balfour, A Political Biography* (London, 1973).

Index